富血小板血浆在肌骨疼痛中的应用

主编：伍少玲　马　超

编者：（以姓氏笔画为序）

马　超（中山大学孙逸仙纪念医院康复医学科）

马海云（中山大学孙逸仙纪念医院康复医学科）

王少玲（中山大学孙逸仙纪念医院康复医学科）

伍少玲（中山大学孙逸仙纪念医院康复医学科）

刘翠翠（中山大学孙逸仙纪念医院康复医学科）

许　珍（中山大学孙逸仙纪念医院康复医学科）

余少君（中山大学孙逸仙纪念医院康复医学科）

汪衍雪（中山大学孙逸仙纪念医院康复医学科）

郑耀超（中山大学孙逸仙纪念医院康复医学科）

袁　泽（中山大学孙逸仙纪念医院康复医学科）

栾　烁（中山大学孙逸仙纪念医院康复医学科）

翟羽佳（中山大学孙逸仙纪念医院康复医学科）

SPM 南方传媒　｜　广东科技出版社　全国优秀出版社

· 广 州 ·

图书在版编目（CIP）数据

富血小板血浆在肌骨疼痛中的应用/伍少玲，马超主编. —广州：广东科技出版社，2022.10

ISBN 978-7-5359-7878-3

Ⅰ.①富…　Ⅱ.①伍…②马…　Ⅲ.①血小板—血浆—临床应用—肌肉疾病—疼痛—研究②血小板—血浆—临床应用—骨疾病—疼痛—研究　Ⅳ.①R685②R681

中国版本图书馆CIP数据核字（2022）第100832号

富血小板血浆在肌骨疼痛中的应用
Fuxuexiaoban Xuejiang Zai Jigu Tengtong Zhong De Yingyong

出 版 人：严奉强

责任编辑：马霄行

封面设计：林少娟

责任校对：陈　静

责任印制：彭海波

出版发行：广东科技出版社

（广州市环市东路水荫路11号　邮政编码：510075）

销售热线：020-37607413

http://www.gdstp.com.cn

E-mail：gdkjbw@nfcb.com.cn

经　　销：广东新华发行集团股份有限公司

排　　版：创溢文化

印　　刷：广州市彩源印刷有限公司

（广州市黄埔区百合三路8号　邮政编码：510700）

规　　格：787 mm×1 092 mm　1/16　印张17.75　字数355千

版　　次：2022年10月第1版

　　　　　2022年10月第1次印刷

定　　价：90.00元

如发现因印装质量问题影响阅读，请与广东科技出版社印制室联系调换（电话：020-37607272）。

慢性肌筋膜和骨关节肌肉疼痛是临床常见病症，困扰着许多中老年患者，其治疗也是临床医生颇感棘手的问题。随着我国人口老龄化的加速和全民健身的开展，慢性骨骼肌肉退行性疾病和运动损伤的发生率逐年增高，使这一问题更为突出。

人体软骨、肌腱、韧带、骨组织等的自我修复能力弱，损伤后恢复困难，其重要原因是损伤局部缺乏足够的生长因子，或生长因子活性不佳等，无法启动和调控组织的修复过程。近年来，富血小板血浆（PRP）疗法为上述慢性病的治疗带来了新的希望。

PRP是通过离心法从全血中提取的血小板浓缩液，含有高浓度的血小板、白细胞和纤维蛋白等成分。血小板激活后可分泌多种生长因子，白细胞可预防感染，纤维蛋白能在局部组织构建修复所需的三维结构。这些浓缩的PRP成分可以为组织提供"充足的营养"，为组织修复搭建理想的微环境，促进软组织和骨骼的修复。

随着PRP基础研究的不断深入，其在临床上的应用也越来越广泛。PRP在康复医学、运动医学和美容整形等领域的应用尤其受到关注。中华医学会骨科分会关节外科学组在《膝骨关节炎阶梯治疗专家共识（2018年版）》中提出，PRP可作为修复手段改善关节透明软骨损伤。由于PRP来源于自体，其安全、有效的特性被越来越多的医生和患者所接受。

中山大学孙逸仙纪念医院康复医学科经过多年的临床应用和基础研究发现，PRP对膝骨关节炎、股骨头无菌性坏死、骨不连和慢性肌腱损伤等有良好的临床疗效。同时，该科室拥有的超声引导疼痛注射技术在国内处于领先地位，能确保PRP的精准注射。

一项新的技术总是需要在临床上经历应用、总结、推广、提高的过程。目前，PRP注射技术在康复医学中的临床应用正处于兴起阶段，其标准化制备流程、规范临床应用等问题需要大家共同努力解决。为此，伍少玲和马超教授组织编写了《富血小板血浆在肌骨疼痛中的应用》一书，为推进PRP技术的应用和发展抱薪出力。我希望更多的康复医生能从此书中受益，更熟练地掌握此项技术，以造福广大慢性骨关节肌肉疼痛和运动损伤患者。

中山大学教授
广东省医学会会长　姚志彬

富血小板血浆（platelet-rich plasma，PRP）是自体血经离心浓缩后获得的血小板浓缩液。由于PRP源于自体、无免疫原性反应、制作简单、对机体损伤小，因此安全有效。大量研究表明：PRP含有多种细胞因子和生长因子，可加速损伤愈合，促进组织修复，减轻疼痛。自20世纪70年代开始，PRP在口腔颌面外科、美容及整形外科、疼痛科和康复医学科得到广泛的临床应用。本书从PRP的概述、制备、在骨关节疼痛中的应用、在软组织修复中的应用、在神经修复中的应用、治疗技术的质量控制、研究展望及超声引导下的注射技术等方面详细介绍了PRP的作用原理、制作方法、相关基础研究情况及其在康复医学科常见疾患中的临床应用等，希望借此进一步推动国内PRP技术的应用与研究。

中山大学孙逸仙纪念医院康复医学科团队经过多年临床应用，证实PRP在康复医学领域有着广阔的应用前景，特别是在退行性骨关节痛、慢性肌肉韧带损伤、软组织损伤、外周神经痛和骨折骨不连方面有很好的疗效，并且于2017年率先在国内康复医学领域招收进修生，举办专题培训班推广"超声引导下富血小板血浆治疗技术"，累计培训学员上千人，备受同道关注。值得注意的是，PRP治疗技术虽然在临床上应用广泛，但也受到制备因素等的制约。因此，为提高其临床疗效，首先要把握好适应证，其次要掌握PRP制备技术，减少不利的影响因素，做到保证质量和精准治疗。近年来，我们在临床应用过程中逐渐发现，由于治疗的适应证把握不当、PRP中血小板浓度偏低等情况的出现，导致PRP临床治疗效果不佳。应广大学员和临床医生的要求，我们密切结合临床实际应用，组织团队整理近年来PRP相关的研究成果和临床经验编成此书。

本书也是中山大学孙逸仙纪念医院康复医学科研究团队阶段性PRP研究成果和临床应用经验的总结，仅为抛砖引玉之作。书中难免有不足之处，还请各位专家同道及时指正。

伍少玲 马 超

2022年5月

目 录

第一章

富血小板血浆概述

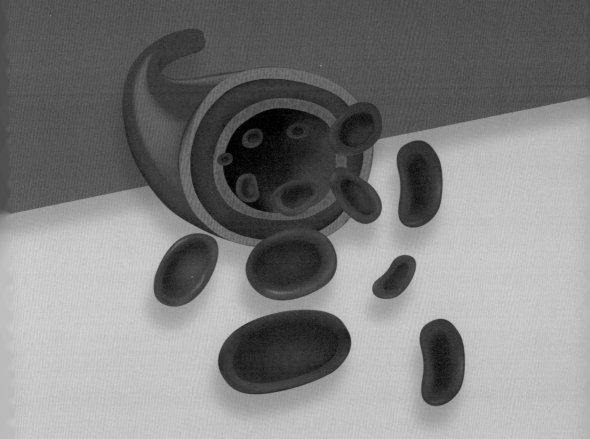

第一节 血小板生理学

富血小板血浆（platelet-rich plasma，PRP）是指通过高速离心的方法从自体血中抽提出来的血小板浓缩液（platelet concentrate）。由于PRP可以促进骨关节和软组织的修复，且无免疫排斥，制作简单，近年来逐渐被骨科、口腔颌面外科、心胸外科、神经外科和整形美容科等所接受。

富血小板血浆主要成分为血小板，血小板由骨髓造血组织中的巨核细胞产生。多功能造血干细胞在造血组织中经过定向分化形成原始的巨核细胞，又进一步发展成为成熟的巨核细胞。成熟巨核细胞膜表面有许多凹陷，伸入细胞质之中，相邻的凹陷细胞膜在凹陷深部相互融合，使巨核细胞部分细胞质与母体分开。最后这些被细胞膜包围的与巨核细胞细胞质分离开的成分脱离巨核细胞，通过骨髓造血组织中的血窦进入血液循环成为血小板。新生成的血小板先进入脾脏，约有1/3的血小板在此储存。储存的血小板可与进入血液循环的血小板自由交换，以维持血中血小板的正常含量。

血小板本身为细胞碎片，体积很小，形状不规则，常成群分布在红细胞之间。循环血中正常状态的血小板呈两面微凹的椭圆形或圆盘形，称为循环型血小板。血小板虽无细胞核，但具有细胞器，以及散在分布的颗粒成分。循环型血小板一旦与创伤处的非血管内膜表面接触，即会迅速扩展，其中的颗粒向中央集中，并伸出数个伪足，即成树突型血小板，并释放大部分颗粒，血小板互相融合就形成黏性变形血小板。树突型血小板如及时消除其刺激因素就能恢复成循环型血小板，黏性变形血小板则难以逆转。血小板膜是附着或镶嵌有蛋白质双分子层的脂膜，膜中含有多种糖蛋白,且膜外附有由血浆蛋白、凝血因子和纤维蛋白溶解系统相关分子组成的血浆层[1-2]。

生理上血小板参与了止血、凝血过程。当血管破损时,血小板因受到损伤部位激活因素刺激而出现聚集,形成血小板凝块,起初级止血作用;接着血小板通过释放凝血酶,使纤维蛋白原转变为纤维蛋白,纤维蛋白互相交织使血小板凝块与血细胞缠结成血凝块,即血栓形成。同时血小板的突起伸入纤维蛋白网内,随着血小板微丝(肌动蛋白)和肌球蛋白的收缩,血凝块出现收缩,血栓变得更坚实,能更有效地止血,起二级止血作用。伴随着血栓的形成,血小板释放血栓素A2、致密颗粒和α颗粒,通过与表面相连的管道系统释放腺苷二磷酸(ADP)、5-羟色胺、凝血酶敏感蛋白、细胞生长因子、凝血因子Ⅴ、凝血因子Ⅷ、凝血因子Ⅻ和血管通透因子等多种活性物质,通过激活周围血小板、促进血管收缩、促进纤维蛋白形成等多种方式产生正反馈,增强凝血效果,同时增强损伤部位的炎症和免疫反应。

血小板数量减少(血小板减少症)或功能减退(血小板功能不全)可引起血小板疾病,导致血栓形成不良和出血。严重的血小板疾病可引起典型的出血,如多发性瘀斑,最常见于小腿,或在受轻微外伤的部位出现小的散在性瘀斑,或黏膜出血(鼻出血,胃肠道、泌尿生殖道和阴道出血)和手术后大量出血。临床上常采用血小板计数、血块收缩试验(CRT)、全血凝固分析法(WBCA)、活化凝血时间测定法(ACT)、血小板计数比值(PCR)、快速血小板功能分析法(RPFA)等检测血小板凝血功能,并结合血小板黏附试验、血小板释放反应、血小板花生四烯酸(AA)代谢产物测定、血小板膜蛋白检测结果进行筛查诊断。

第二节　富血小板血浆的成分和作用机制

制备设备和技术不同，则PRP中血浆、红细胞、白细胞和血小板的含量也就不同，因此临床应用和基础研究所用的PRP并不都是相同的。当PRP被激活时，α颗粒通过脱颗粒引起生长因子的分泌，其中包括血小板源性生长因子（platelet derived growth factor，PDGF）、白细胞介素-1受体拮抗剂（interleukin-1 receptor antagonist，IL-1Ra）、可溶性肿瘤坏死因子受体（soluble tumor necrosis factor receptor，sTNFR）、转化生长因子（transforming growth factor，TGF）、血小板因子4（platelet factor 4，PF4）、血管内皮生长因子（vascular endothelial growth factor，VEGF）、血小板源表皮生长因子（platelet-derived epidermal growth factor，PDEGF）、胰岛素样生长因子（insulin-like growth factor，IGF）、骨钙素（osteocalcin，OCN）、骨粘连蛋白、纤维蛋白原、纤维连接蛋白和血小板应答蛋白-1（thrombospondin-1，TSP-1）等。这些因子通过调控细胞微环境、激活相关通路，进而对肌腱干细胞的增殖分化以及软骨的修复起促进作用[3]，详见表1。

表1　富血小板血浆主要成分的潜在效应

成分	潜在效应
PDGF	促进血管生成、巨噬细胞活化 促进成纤维细胞增殖、趋化及胶原合成 增强骨细胞的增殖
TGF	促进成纤维细胞增殖 促进Ⅰ型胶原和纤维连接蛋白的合成 诱导骨基质沉积，抑制骨吸收

续表

成分	潜在效应
PF4	刺激中性粒细胞 化学刺激成纤维细胞
VEGF	刺激血管内皮细胞形成血管
PDEGF	刺激表皮再生 通过角质形成细胞的增殖和皮肤成纤维细胞的刺激促进伤口愈合 提高其他增长因素的产量和影响
IGF	对成纤维细胞有趋化作用并刺激蛋白质合成 增强骨形成

第三节　富血小板血浆的分类及其衍生物

　　白细胞和血小板有相近的沉降系数，且含量都较少，在离心时很难将二者分开；为了更准确地描述PRP的临床应用，2006年Everts等学者提出了富白细胞PRP这一概念。Dohan等根据白细胞含量将PRP大致分为两种：贫白细胞PRP（LP-PRP）和富白细胞PRP（LR-PRP），二者的制备方法有所差异[4]。

　　贫白细胞PRP（LP-PRP）的制作方法是由Anitua在1999年发明的，其制备设备由西班牙的BTI公司生产。该方法通过一次转速较小的离心使加入抗凝剂的全血由上到下分为4层，最顶层的是不含血小板的上清液，中间悬液是富含血小板的PRP，PRP下面一层是白细胞层，红细胞位于最底层。该技术的特点是不收集白细胞层，但是因为白细胞层也会有大量的血小板，故用此方法制备的PRP中血小板浓度相比其他方法略低，因此该方法现在应用较少。

富白细胞PRP（LR-PRP）是目前应用最多的PRP产品，是通过二次离心制备出的含有高浓度白细胞的PRP，其代表设备是美国强生公司生产的血小板富集制备系统。其制备原理是根据血液中各组分的沉降系数不同，在第一次离心后将血液分成3层，最底层是沉降系数最大的红细胞，最上层是上清液，交界处有一薄层，即富血小板层。第一次离心后，弃去上清液或者弃去红细胞层，然后改变离心力再次离心，可使更多的血小板分离出来。由于白细胞和血小板有类似的沉降系数，故在二次离心后沉积在红细胞层上面的是含有高浓度白细胞的PRP。目前一般认为一次离心采用低速离心、二次离心采用高速离心有助于获得高浓度的PRP，但也有研究者对此并不认同，认为PRP产品质量可能与所用的设备和人为因素有关。LR-PRP可能有更好的抗炎作用，因为白细胞释放出的递质会诱导包括炎性细胞在内的多种细胞聚集和黏附，利于组织修复。因此现在大多数研究文献中所提到的PRP是指LR-PRP。与LR-PRP相对应的LP-PRP则含有很低浓度的白细胞或者不含有白细胞。

根据应用形式又可以将PRP分为未激活PRP和激活后的PRP，后者又包括了PRP凝胶和PRP释放物或提取物（又叫富含生长因子的PRP）。PRP凝胶是指血小板被激活后，在释放生长因子的同时，释放出纤维蛋白原聚合为纤维蛋白，纤维蛋白连接成网状而形成的肉眼可见的凝胶，该凝胶有一定黏附性和强度。PRP释放物通常用于描述血小板活化后释放入血浆或血清中的含有生长因子和活性蛋白的上清液。激活PRP的方法有添加氯化钙、添加凝血酶、添加氯化钙和凝血酶、采用物理方法（冻结和融化）等4种，至于哪一种激活方法激活得更充分，尚无定论。当PRP在体外应用或将PRP作为止血剂或组织包埋的媒介时，必须体外激活血小板。对于在体内应用是否需要体外激活是有争议的，因为体内有足够的内源性凝血酶原激酶。目前最常用的体外激活方法是添加氯化钙和凝血酶以启动凝血过程，从而得到PRP凝胶和释放物，再经过快速离心后就可得到生长因子。物理方法激活是通过低温（–80℃）冻结PRP后再常温（37℃）融化，以使血小板破裂，从而释放生长因子，离心去除细胞碎片后即可得到PRP释放物。另外，从理论上讲，当PRP接触到富含胶原蛋白的损伤的肌肉骨骼组织时也可以被激活，并且被激活后可能会维持更长的生长因子释放时间。

除此之外，"PRP"与"血小板浓缩物"曾经一度被很多学者认为是等同的，其实血小板浓缩物是不含有血浆的血小板固体物，不会再发生凝集，与PRP的特性不符。近年来出现了第二代血小板浓缩物，即PRF。PRF是由法国的Dohan等首先制备而成的，最初被用于口腔颌面部手术中。PRF与PRP都含有高浓度的血小板，但两者有根本的区别。首先，PRF是固态的，这与其制备步骤有关。其次，与PRP相比，PRF的制备要简单得多：将不加抗凝剂的血液样本放入离心管中，在约400g的离心力下离心10min后得到的位于血浆和红细胞之间的凝块就是PRF，PRF内含有大量的白细胞。另外，PRF与PRP凝胶之间的主要区别在于形成的方式不同。PRF是在离心过程中自然而缓慢形成的，使纤维蛋白原转变为纤维蛋白的凝血酶是生理存在的，这就保证了PRF的纤维蛋白之间有更紧密的连接和更好的弹性。而PRP凝胶是通过添加氯化钙或者凝血酶来启动凝血过程的最后几个步骤，使纤维蛋白突然聚合。这种快速的反应要求有较大量凝血酶的参与。这种聚合机制将会在很大程度上影响纤维蛋白网的机械和生物学特性。

除此之外，其他PRP常见衍生物如表2所示。与传统PRP相比较而言，这些衍生物一般是部分提取步骤的产物或组分比例不同的产物，但目前不同衍生物的特殊之处仍有待研究，本章节暂不赘述。

表2　PRP常见衍生物

名称缩写	全称	常用中文名称
A-PRF	advanced platelet-rich fibrin	富含血小板纤维蛋白
ACP	autologous conditioned plasma	自体条件血浆
AGF	autologous growth factors	自体生长因子
APG	autologous platelet gel	自体血小板凝胶
C-PRP	clinical platelet-rich plasma	临床用富含血小板血浆
i-PRF	injectable platelet-rich fibrin	可注射型富血小板纤维蛋白
PFC	platelet-derived factor concentrate	血小板源因子浓缩液
P-PRP	pure platelet-rich plasma	纯富血小板血浆
PFS	platelet fibrin sealant	血小板纤维蛋白胶
PLG	platelet-leukocyte gel	血小板-白细胞凝胶
PRF	platelet-rich fibrin	富血小板纤维蛋白
PRFM	platelet-rich fibrin matrix	富血小板纤维蛋白基质
PRGF	preparation rich in growth factors	富生长因子制剂

第四节　富血小板血浆的应用评价

　　富血小板血浆不仅可作为一种辅助治疗手段，而且已经逐渐成为一种独立的治疗手段，其相关制剂在各个医疗领域逐渐得到广泛应用。富血小板血浆产生治疗作用的基本科学原理是：在损伤部位注射的血小板通过释放许多生物活性因子（生长因子、细胞因子、溶酶体）和黏附蛋白来启动组织修复，这些生物活性因子和黏附蛋白负责启动止血级联反应、新结缔组织的合成和血运重建。此外，血浆蛋白（如纤维蛋白原、凝血酶原和纤维连接蛋白）存在于贫血小板血浆（PPP）组分中。富血小板血浆浓缩物可以刺激生长因子的超生理性释放，从而加速慢性损伤的愈合，加速急性损伤修复过程。在组织修复过程的各个阶段，各种各样的生长因子、细胞因子和局部作用的调节因子通过内分泌、旁分泌、自分泌等机制来促进最基本的细胞功能。

富血小板血浆的主要优点是安全、方便，更重要的是，富血小板血浆是一种自体产物，与常用的皮质类固醇相比，没有已知的不良反应。然而，目前对于可注射的富血小板血浆的成分和配方没有明确的规定，并且富血小板血浆成分在血小板和白细胞含量、红细胞污染程度及PDGF浓度方面差异很大。

最初，成功抽提富血小板血浆的唯一标准是血小板浓度高于全血值的标本。直到最近，富血小板血浆作为一种自体血衍生产品在市场上被商业化，较为标准的制备流程为医务人员提供了在特定的病理和疾病中使用自体血小板生长因子技术的能力。如今在不同适应证的情况下，首先需要有充分的证据和充分的临床研究来预先确定富血小板血浆的潜在治疗效果。

利用富血小板血浆的新兴自体细胞疗法有可能在各种再生医学治疗计划中发挥巨大作用，以满足肌肉骨骼系统（MSK）和脊柱疾病、骨关节炎（OA）、慢性复杂难治性疼痛的医学需求。

第五节　富血小板血浆的国内外研究现状

尽管再生治疗策略取得了不少进展，但肌肉骨骼系统疾病仍然是一项临床挑战。富血小板血浆的出现使一些治疗瓶颈得以突破，为康复科、骨科提供了新的治疗思路和方向。体外研究发现，富血小板血浆和胰岛素的存在可促进人脂肪干细胞向软骨细胞和成骨干细胞的分化。研究发现，在骨软骨损伤模型中，尽管国际软骨修复学会（ICRS）宏观评分在富血小板血浆组和生理盐水组无显著性差异，然而主观宏观评价表明，富血小板血浆治疗提供了一个更大的组织填充度与较少的裂缝，使关节形态逐渐恢复

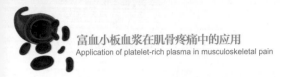
正常，组织中糖胺聚糖和Ⅱ型胶原的含量也较高[5-8]。

自2012年首次对富血小板血浆治疗骨关节炎（OA）进行随机对照试验以来，均主要是与关节内注射透明质酸（HA）疗法进行比较。总的来说，结果显示富血小板血浆注射是一种安全的治疗方法，至少在短期内（12个月）有缓解OA症状的作用，对病情较轻的年轻患者可能效果更显著[9-10]。由于方法学上的差异和研究间的显著异质性，关于富血小板血浆在OA中的作用还没有明确的结论，需要进一步的高质量研究来确定富血小板血浆的临床和成本效益、最有可能受益的患者以及最佳的治疗方案。一项荟萃分析[11]发现，在注射后6个月，富血小板血浆和HA在缓解疼痛和改善功能方面具有相似的效果。而与生理盐水相比，富血小板血浆在注射后6个月、12个月的疼痛缓解和功能改善方面更为有效，并且在6个月、12个月时疼痛和功能的评分——西安大略大学和麦克马斯特大学骨关节炎指数评分（WOMAC评分）均超过最小临床重要差异度（minimum clinically important difference，MCID）阈值。更重要的是，与HA和生理盐水相比，富血小板血浆不会增加不良事件的风险[12]。

富血小板血浆可以与常规治疗相结合作为辅助治疗。例如，在兔骨软骨病变中，与未使用富血小板血浆的镶嵌成形术相比，使用富血小板血浆进行镶嵌成形术可以产生更好的愈合反应和与相邻表面更好的整合，并在3周内获得更好的组织学评分[13]。同时，临床研究发现，富血小板血浆在平均16.3个月的随访中可以提高关节镜下治疗距骨骨软骨损伤的功能评分[14]。不少研究表明，富血小板血浆组具有较高的国际软骨修复学会评分和较好的移植物整合度。与单纯支架相比，富血小板血浆或骨髓抽吸浓缩物对组织填充的改善效果更好[14]。但也有研究指出，在骨软骨损伤绵羊模型中，富血小板血浆的使用降低了胶原羟基磷灰石支架内的骨软骨再生[15]。与有富血小板血浆的支架相比，无富血小板血浆的支架具有明显更好的骨再生和软骨表面重建状态。通过显微计算机断层扫描、组织学、组织形态计量学、荧光显微镜和宏观评估发现，将富血小板血浆加入同种异体脱钙骨基质中并不能促进距骨骨软骨损伤的愈合[16]。

另外，大量证据支持使用富血小板血浆进行骨关节系统病变引起的疼痛的治疗[17]。椎间盘内注射富血小板血浆也是一种安全且可能有效的治疗椎间盘源性腰痛的方法。一项对29名接受椎间盘内注射富血小板血浆治疗椎间盘源性下腰痛的患者进行的临床研究发现，经过两年的随访，患者的疼痛和功能在统计学与临床上均有显著改善[18]。

同时，也有研究发现，与注射安慰剂相比，单次注射富血小板血浆对慢性大转子疼痛综合征（GTPS）没有显著改善作用[19]。对富血小板血浆镇痛效果差异的最好解释是，在富血小板血浆的制备和应用过程中，未能考虑到可以增加或消除其镇痛能力的变量。如何使血小板中5-羟色胺的含量最小，最大化减少引起炎症和疼痛的血小板含量，同时保持其生物活性，最大化提升血小板在损伤部位聚集的能力，诱导其快速和同步释放活性因子，并优化富血小板血浆操作步骤，是未来的研究方向。

（郑耀超）

参考文献

[1] WU P I, DIAZ R, BORG-STEIN J. Platelet-rich plasma[J]. Phys Med Rehabil Clin N Am, 2016, 27（4）：825-853.

[2] MARTÍNEZ-MARTÍNEZ A, RUIZ-SANTIAGO F, GARCÍA-ESPINOSA J. Platelet-rich plasma：myth or reality？[J]. Radiologia, 2018, 60（6）：465-475.

[3] MUSSANO F, GENOVA T, MUNARON L, et al. Cytokine, chemokine, and growth factor profile of platelet-rich plasma[J]. Platelets, 2016, 27（5）：467-471.

[4] DOHAN E D M, RASMUSSON L, ALBREKTSSON T. Classification of platelet concentrates：from pure platelet-rich plasma（P-PRP）to leucocyte- and platelet-rich fibrin（L-PRF）[J]. Trends Biotechnol, 2009, 27（3）：158-167.

[5] 左秀芹，尹飒飒，谢惠敏，等. 富血小板血浆在肌骨修复领域应用的适用性与相关规范[J]. 中国组织工程研究，2021，25（20）：3239-3245.

[6] 张长青，程飚. 富血小板血浆技术在临床的应用[M]. 上海：上海交通大学出版社，2019.

[7] 刘金鑫，张益，高甲科，等. 踝关节镜联合富血小板血浆治疗距骨软骨损伤的效果[J]. 精准医学杂志，2020，35（3）：253-256.

[8] 贾岩波，李伟，任逸众，等. 关节镜下微骨折术与微骨折术联合富血小板血浆治疗距骨软骨损伤的疗效比较[J]. 中国骨与关节损伤杂志，2020，35（8）：867-869.

[9] 孙仁义，贾堂宏. 关节腔内注射透明质酸钠与富血小板血浆治疗膝关节骨性关节炎的比较[J]. 中国组织工程研究，2020，24（14）：2164-2169.

[10] 饶东. 富血小板血浆联合透明质酸钠治疗老年晚期膝骨关节炎的临床研究[J]. 实用手外科杂志，2020，34（2）：152-154.

[11] 王养发，刘军，潘建科，等. 富血小板血浆与透明质酸治疗膝骨关节炎疗效对比的Meta分析[J]. 中国组织工程研究，2020，24（27）：4421-4428.

[12] 谢磊，刘佳，王华军，等. 关节腔注射透明质酸及富血小板血浆对老年膝骨关节炎的治疗作用比较[J]. 中国老年学杂志，2018，38（5）：1129-1131.

[13] ALTAN E, AYDIN K, ERKOCAK O, et al. The effect of platelet-rich plasma on osteochondral defects treated with mosaicplasty[J]. Int Orthop, 2014, 38（6）：1321-1328.

[14] GUNEY A, AKAR M, KARAMAN I, et al. Clinical outcomes of platelet rich plasma（PRP）as an adjunct to microfracture surgery in osteochondral lesions of the talus[J]. Knee Surg Sports Traumatol Arthrosc, 2015, 23（8）：2384-2389.

[15] KON E, FILARDO G, DELCOGLIANO M, et al. Platelet autologous growth factors decrease the osteochondral regeneration capability of a collagen-hydroxyapatite scaffold in a sheep model[J]. BMC Musculoskelet Disord, 2010, 11：220.

[16] VAN BERGEN C J, KERKHOFFS G M, ÖZDEMIR M, et al. Demineralized bone matrix and platelet-rich plasma do not improve healing of osteochondral defects of the talus：an experimental goat study[J]. Osteoarthritis Cartilage, 2013, 21（11）：1746-1754.

[17] MOHAMMED S, YU J. Platelet-rich plasma injections：an emerging therapy for chronic discogenic low back pain[J]. J Spine Surg, 2018, 4（1）：115-122.

[18] MONFETT M, HARRISON J, BOACHIE-ADJEI K, et al. Intradiscal platelet-rich plasma（PRP）injections for discogenic low back pain：an update[J]. Int Orthop, 2016, 40（6）：1321-1328.

[19] ALI M, ODERUTH E, ATCHIA I, et al. The use of platelet-rich plasma in the treatment of greater trochanteric pain syndrome：a systematic literature review[J]. J Hip Preserv Surg, 2018, 5（3）：209-219.

第二章

富血小板血浆的制备

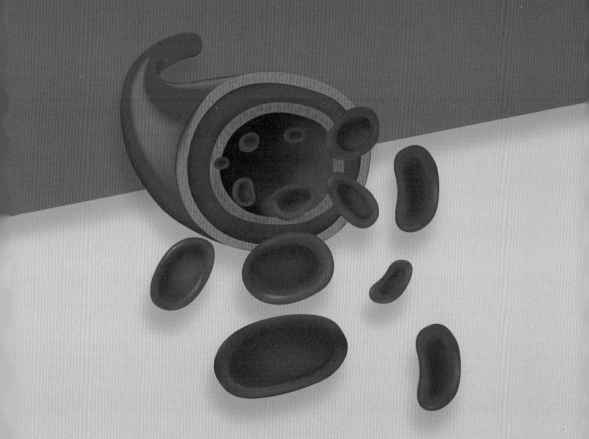

第一节　富血小板血浆的分离原理与技术

　　富血小板血浆（PRP）是通过离心的方法从自体血液中提取的血小板及血浆的浓聚物，即血小板浓度高于基础值的血浆，其血小板浓度一般为（0.15～0.45）×10^6/μL[1-2]。PRP制品中的核心物质是血小板，血小板内的α颗粒、致密颗粒、溶酶体等结构会在血小板被激活后释放生长因子、细胞因子、多种蛋白质、外泌体、血小板微颗粒等各种活性物质，从而促进组织的再生与修复[3-8]。研究表明，临床治疗用PRP的血小板浓度以（0.2～1）×10^6/μL为宜，更高浓度的血小板并不能带来更大的临床获益[9]。

　　目前PRP的制备方法标准化程度低，可变性大，制备出的PRP的纯度、含量和质量差异也较大。根据制备方法的不同，PRP可分为血小板富集血浆（PeRP）、血小板富集物（PRC）、血小板浓缩物、富白细胞PRP（LR-PRP）、富血小板纤维蛋白（PRF）、富生长因子制剂（PRGF）、富血小板纤维蛋白基质（PRFM）、自体条件血浆（ACP）、血小板凝胶、纯富血小板血浆（P-PRP）和血小板释放物等[10-14]。由于不同PRP产品含有不同浓度的血细胞（血小板、白细胞和红细胞）、血浆或纤维蛋白原，因此其血小板含量、纯度和生物特性不同，潜在疗效也不同。此外，一些临床试验是在没有明确定义或量化PRP生物学特性的情况下进行的，导致PRP的临床疗效不同。

　　2018年国际血栓与止血委员会总结了无菌PRP的制备技术，将其分为3类[15]：重力离心技术，标准的细胞分离技术，自体选择性细胞过滤技术（血小板过滤提取法）。然而，用于临床的PRP的制备技术尚无统一标准。现有PRP的主要分离制备方法也无统一的标准，主要有密度梯度离心法（一次离心法或二次离心法或三次离心法）和血浆分离置换法两种不同的方法。

（1）密度梯度离心法：该法是根据血液中各成分沉降系数的不同，经密度梯度离心后提取沉降系数最大的红细胞层和最上层的上清液交界处的血浆，即为高浓度的血小板血浆（PRP）。按离心次数的不同，密度梯度离心法可分为一次离心法、二次离心法及三次离心法。大量研究表明，二次离心法获得的PRP浓度和质量最好，所以目前二次离心法是较普遍、常用的分离制备方法。二次离心法制备PRP的简要步骤[16]如下：将外周静脉血抽入含抗凝剂的无菌试管中；经第一次离心后，血液分为三层，上层为贫血小板血浆层，下层为红细胞层，中间层为高度浓缩的血小板和白细胞层；吸取上层、中层以及邻近中层的部分红细胞，转移至另一无菌试管；进行第二次离心，血浆分为三层，下层为红细胞层，上层为贫血小板血浆层，两层之间为富血小板血浆层；弃去大部分的上清液，留取适量的血清用以悬浮浓缩的血小板，获得的即为PRP。若想获得PRP凝胶，可加入微量凝血酶及氯化钙，激活其中的血小板即可。二次离心法制备简单，设备要求也不高，但仍未被临床广泛使用，主要是由于其存在以下问题：①开放式的制备方法容易受到污染；②两次血小板的转移，致血小板被污染和激活的概率增加；③操作人员的操作习惯和衡量尺度对PRP中血小板的浓度影响较大；④血小板获取率低，各指标变异系数较大。

实验室传统的密度梯度离心法有Anitua法、Petrungarp法、Landesberg法和Aghaloo法。这4种制备方法的操作过程均以人工为主，血液基本上都需要经二次离心，并且操作过程中需多次移液，因此操作者个人习惯和衡量尺度的差异难免会产生各种误差。研究发现，Landesberg法制备的PRP中，血小板的体积分数和活化率最高，是目前较理想的制备方法[17]。

Landesberg法采用低速离心，第一次离心用200g的离心力离心10min，然后将上清液至交界面以下3mm的成分移至另一离心管中进行第二次离心，仍以200g的离心力离心10min，弃去大部分的上清液，留取适量的血清用以悬浮浓缩的血小板，获得的即为PRP，采用此制备方法，10mL的全血可制备约1mL的PRP[18]。宋扬等[19]和笔者所在团队改进了二次离心法，采用采血的注射器作为离心管，以使整个制备过程能在密闭环境中完成，避免了操作过程中血液反复转移造成的血小板污染或激活。该方法通过特殊设计的注射器来提高PRP中血小板/生长因子的富集系数和利用率，减少了人工操作因素对制备过程的影响。此外，朱业华等[20]还采用血袋制备PRP，密闭性好，操作步骤简单，大大降低了污染的发生率，避免了血小板和白细胞的损失以及血小板的激活，提高了获得的血小板、白细胞及生长因子的浓度。在我国，较多的PRP研究者和临床使用者采用密度梯度离心法。现已有采用密度梯度离心原理设计的商品化的富血小板血浆分离装置/分离器，但由于价格昂贵，尚未在临床上普遍使用。

（2）血浆分离置换法：该法是利用专业医用血成分分离设备把全血通过离心的方式转变成富血小板血浆和浓缩血小板等医用成分血，主要应用于血库对血小板的采集和临床成分输血。目前已有40多种不同生产厂家的PRP制备装置和试剂盒能从自体全血中制造PRP，但尚无标准化的PRP制备方法。

此外，PRP制备系统的差异对获得的PRP量、血小板浓度和成分等也有显著的影响。有研究发现，采用PCCS、Vivostat和Harvest制备系统所获得的PRP量及PRP在120h内释放的PDGF量基本相同，而采用Fibrinet制备系统所获得的PRP量及PRP在120h内释放的PDGF量最低[21]。Vivostat制备系统所获得的PRP，在6h后出现的血小板膜破裂可能是引起PDGF过早释放的原因。Mazzucco等还发现，Plateltex R PRP制备系统和PCCS R、Vivo-stat

R、Harvest R、Fibrinet R、PRP-Landesberg及Curasan R等制备系统的PRP制备效率相似，所制备的PRP中血小板的含量亦无显著性差异[22]。Appel等[23]将传统的实验室制备方法与Curasan制备系统及PCCS制备系统所获得的PRP进行对比后发现，PCCS制备系统所获得的PRP中血小板含量最高，Curasan制备系统所获得的PRP中血小板提取率最大。

需要说明的是，关于PRP的制备目前尚无统一标准，不管是在实验室中提取PRP，还是使用商业化设备提取PRP都需要两步操作：第一步全血离心，分离出红细胞；第二步从血浆中将PRP分离出来。虽然商品化的PRP制备系统能快速且稳定地获取PRP，且获得的PRP与人工密度梯度离心法获得的PRP差异小，但因其价格昂贵，所以尚未大范围推广应用。目前，国内大都使用传统的实验室制备方法制备PRP。

第二节　影响富血小板血浆质量的因素

PRP的最终血小板浓度和质量取决于采血的时间段、采血体位、血的体积、悬浮一定浓度血小板的血浆体积、白细胞和/或红细胞的相对浓度、保存方法与时间、制备系统、离心温度、离心力、离心速度、离心时间、离心轴长度、离心管的长度和直径、离心管材质、离心设备型号以及纯化技术等，其中任何一项参数的变化都会使制备的PRP发生变化，其中的血小板、白细胞、生长因子的浓度也就不尽相同。另外，患者个体因素如年龄、所服药物、并发症、外周静脉血的情况、循环血中生长因子和细胞的组分等也会影响PRP的血小板浓度和质量。

1. 采血

国内PRP临床制备一般是从肘静脉采血[24]，但采血量波动性较大，为4～500mL，最常见的采血量为30mL（约占14.9%）。采血量的不同也不可避免地导致了PRP制备量的差异（0.4～30mL）。推荐根据临床PRP的用量计算采血量，有报道认为采血量为最终PRP用量的10倍左右。采血量与抗凝剂的体积比为10：1或9：1[24]。笔者所在团队中山大学孙逸仙纪念医院康复医学科进行PRP制备时的采血量为最终PRP用量的4～5倍，采血量与抗凝剂的体积比为9：1。由于血小板容易被激活，所以制备PRP时采血针头不宜过细，采血速度不宜过快，血液与抗凝剂应缓和混匀，现采现制备。需要注意的是，采血时应该避开女性患者的月经期，因为此时女性血液中的血小板凝集功能下降，PRP激活后形成的血凝块中所含生长因子较少。

2. 抗凝剂

PRP的质量和生物学效应与抗凝剂的种类密切相关。尽管枸橼酸盐类抗凝剂普遍应用于输血[25]，但Anitua等[26]和Marx等[27]建议使用枸橼酸盐或A型枸橼酸葡萄糖作为制备PRP的抗凝剂。Harrison[15]认为，在PRP的制备中采用乙二胺四乙酸盐（EDTA）作为抗凝剂优于枸橼酸盐或A型枸橼酸葡萄糖。此外，近来有研究表明，EDTA作为制备PRP的抗凝剂可引起PRP中血小板的肿胀和活化，但产生的血小板数量最多，而采用肝素作为PRP的抗凝剂可使血小板聚集，干扰血细胞的整体计数[28]。国内有学者研究发现，枸橼酸葡萄糖和柠檬酸-茶碱-腺苷-双嘧达莫是PRP制备中最理想的抗凝剂，因为它们能维持血小板的高活性[29]。

3. 离心设备及参数

现有文献报道，PRP的制备主要采用非商品化的离心法，但未对离心设备的参数进行详细的描述。制备PRP的离心次数、离心力（离心的转速）以及离心的时间需要根据不同的离心机进行调整。国内制备PRP主要采用二次离心法（80.2%），一次离心法使用较少（18.8%）[24]，主要参考Landesberg法的制备流程[18]。文献报道中，个别商品化的PRP制备套装有描述离心设备参数。

二次离心法在离心过程中，一般第二次离心的离心力不小于第一次离心的离心力，国内两次离心采用同一离心力的约占37.9%，第二次离心力大于第一次离心力的约占62.1%[18]。由于相关参考文献中未标注离心机的离心半径、离心管的直径和深度，所以离心力以及离心的时间设置差异较大。第一次离心时，常见的离心力设置有200g、1500g、250g和313g，离心时间大多为10min，也有报道采用20min、15min和4min的；第二次离心时，常见的离心力设置有1500g、200g和250g，离心时间大多为10min，也有报道采用15min的。中山大学孙逸仙纪念医院康复医学科进行PRP制备时，第二次的离心力（700g）大于第一次的离心力（400g），两次离心时间均为10min。

一次离心法在离心过程中采用的离心力（或转速）和时间也差异较大，离心力设置一般为150～1500g，离心时间设置一般为2～40min，离心参数设置异质性较高[18]。

研究表明，提高离心力可增加PRP的富集倍数，离心转速过低、离心时间过短将导致血小板的浓度较低，难以满足临床治疗的需要，而离心力过大、离心时间过长以及离心次数过多则会导致血小板的活化率增加[30]。Dugrillon等[31]研究发现，为提高血小板的富集倍数而提高离心力会导致血小板被破坏，最大的离心力应控制在800g以内。保证最佳的离心力、离心时间和离心次数对于临床治疗用PRP的制备至关重要。

研究还发现，PRP制备过程中血小板的沉降和分布也与离心套装材料设计密切相关，例如离心管的直径、深度、底部形状等[32]。

4. 温度

温度也会影响PRP的质量，通常认为离心的最佳温度是（20±2）℃，

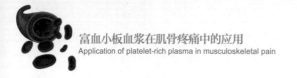
温度过高或过低都会使血小板活性降低或被激活[33]。

5. 保存

PRP制备后的储存时间和温度等也是影响PRP质量的重要因素[34-36]。有学者认为PRP制备好后，在抗凝状态下，室温下保存8h或更长时间，血小板的活性是稳定的。因PRP的制备操作过程简单，所以若所需PRP量较小，可现制现用。

需要注意的是，尽管PRP的制备过程并不复杂，但是在实验室制备的过程中必须保证无菌，且要保证血小板不被破坏或分解。目前，关于PRP临床应用的报道仍有些争议，这可能与使用的设备、使用条件、患者本身体质状况以及医生的操作熟练程度有关，因此需要进一步研究，制定PRP临床应用的统一标准。

第三节　富血小板血浆制备的标准化与检测方法

临床制备PRP的流程须标准化，以获得达到临床治疗标准的血小板浓度和活化率。这就需要采集全血的体积、采集全血的速度、离心速度、离心时间、提取量、纯化技术、离心温度、离心所用的耗材等均按统一的标准量化。以血小板浓度达到$1 \times 10^6/\mu L$作为制备PRP的标准，在相同制备条件下，制备出的血小板浓度可能有差异，如果血小板浓度过高，可以使用贫血小板血浆稀释调整血小板的浓度。

中山大学孙逸仙纪念医院康复医学科现有的标准化制备方法如下：

（1）采血部位及采血量：室温22℃，无菌条件下肘静脉缓慢采血20~40mL（3~6min），与抗凝剂枸橼酸钠充分混匀。忌抽血速度过快或与抗凝剂混匀的力度过大造成血小板机械性破坏或激活，忌血液与抗凝剂混匀不充分致血液凝固。

（2）采血时间：清晨抽血，原则是现采现制备，嘱患者晨起注意清淡饮食。

（3）离心力（离心转速）、离心次数、离心时间：第一次离心，离心力400g，离心时间10min；第二次离心，离心力700g，离心时间10min。

（4）PRP提取量：一般采集20～40mL血，获得PRP终体积约5mL。

目前PRP质量评价的关键指标之一就是血小板的浓度，文献中描述的PRP中血小板的浓度是全血的2～10倍，差别很大，这是造成当前PRP疗效不确定的关键因素。大多数学者认为血小板释放生长因子的最低浓度是$1 \times 10^6/\mu L$[37-39]。也有学者认为不同的组织和细胞所需要的血小板最低浓度不同，需要根据具体治疗目的选择不同的血小板浓度[40-42]。

此外，还有研究试图从离心力和离心时间、血小板富集率、生长因子释放量等多个指标评价PRP制品的质量[43-46]。但目前并未见到从血小板各项参数的角度来评价PRP质量的研究。

临床工作中，在判断所制备的PRP是否合格时，不需要也没必要去测定其中生长因子的浓度，可通过了解血小板浓度、血小板平均体积、血小板平均分布宽度以及血小板压积等参数来判断所制备PRP的质量[47]。在条件允许的情况下，可实时检测PRP中血小板的浓度。如果条件有限，则必须定期进行质控检测，以保证实验室制备方法的准确性。目前血小板浓度的检测方法主要有手工法、光学法及电阻抗法。临床上常用血细胞分析仪检测血小板浓度。

第四节　富血小板血浆制备中存在的问题

鉴于通过不同的制备方法和技术参数可获得不同组分、不同浓度的PRP，临床医生可根据不同患者的需要选择最适合的PRP产品。但时至今日，PRP的临床制备方法还没有统一的标准，不同的制备方法导致PRP的成分及其临床疗效不同，需要建立高效稳定的PRP制备方法，配备专门的经国家有关部门批准检验的无菌的套装包，为PRP的广泛应用提供质量保证。此外，不同方法制备的PRP中血小板的破坏程度、提取纯度不同，使得PRP中各种生长因子的浓度差异很大，各种因子的活性、生物学作用以及促进组织修复的机制等也难以完全阐明。遗憾的是，目前还没有足够的临床试验证据表明哪种制备方法是最理想的，这给临床医务工作者应用PRP造成了诸多困扰，但是了解获得和制备富血小板血浆的多种方法是必不可少的。

通过检索和分析已发表的有关PRP制备的文献可以发现，PRP的临床制备方法和流程尚无统一标准，包括采血量、血小板浓度、激活剂、离心设备、离心次数、离心力、离心时间和PRP制备量等均无统一标准。此外，如何评估患者的血小板功能、PRP中血小板的浓度和回收率，以及PRP中白细胞含有的大量炎性因子是否影响PRP疗效，如何将患者的损伤机制与PRP的个体化提取与治疗相结合等均无定论。PRP在临床应用前应坚持循证医学原则，建立更加可靠的、可重复的动物模型，进一步设计严格的、标准化的人群试验。目前虽然有部分高质量临床研究，但其研究结果存在不确定性，需要更高质量的研究或指南来规范和指导临床PRP的制备，需要大样本的多中心随机对照研究以明确该疗法的最佳临床应用路径。

（刘翠翠）

参考文献

[1] WEIBRICH G, KLEIS W K G, HAFNER G, et al. Growth factor levels in platelet-rich plasma and correlations with donor age, sex, and platelet count[J]. J Craniomaxillofacial Surg, 2002, 30（2）: 97-102.

[2] FOSTER T E, PUSKAS B L, MANDELBAUM B R, et al. Platelet-rich plasma: from basic science to clinical applications[J]. Am J Sports Med, 2009, 37（11）: 2259-2272.

[3] MASUKI H, OKUDERA T, WATANEBE T, et al. Growth factor and pro-inflammatory cytokine contents in platelet-rich plasma（PRP）, plasma rich in growth factors（PRGF）, advanced platelet-rich fibrin（A-PRF）, and concentrated growth factors（CGF）[J]. International Journal of Implant Dentistry, 2016, 2（1）: 19.

[4] ISOBE K, WATANEBE T, KAWABATA H, et al. Mechanical and degradation properties of advanced platelet-rich fibrin（A-PRF）, concentrated growth factors（CGF）, and platelet-poor plasma-derived fibrin（PPTF）[J]. International Journal of Implant Dentistry, 2017, 3（1）: 17.

[5] EREN G, GÜRKAN A, ATMACA H, et al. Effect of centrifugation time on growth factor and MMP release of an experimental platelet-rich fibrin-type product[J]. Platelets, 2016, 27（5）: 427-432.

[6] CHOUKROUN J, GHANAATI S. Reduction of relative centrifugation force within injectable platelet-rich-fibrin（PRF）concentrates advances patients'own inflammatory cells, platelets and growth factors: the first introduction to the low speed centrifugation concept[J]. European Journal of Trauma & Emergency Surgery, 2018, 44（1）: 1-9.

[7] GUO S C, TAO S C, YIN W J, et al. Exosomes derived from platelet-rich plasma promote the re-epithelization of chronic cutaneous wounds via activation of YAP in a diabetic rat model[J]. Theranostics, 2017, 7（1）: 81-96.

[8] PANAGIOTOU N, WAYNE D R, SELMAN C, et al. Microvesicles as vehicles for tissue regeneration: changing of the guards[J]. Current Pathobiology Reports, 2016, 4（4）: 181-187.

[9] MAZZOCCA A D, MCCARTHY M B R, CHOWANIEC D M, et al. Platelet-rich plasma differs according to preparation method and human variability[J]. J Bone Joint Surg Am, 2012, 94（4）: 308-316.

[10] DOHAN E D M, RASMUSSON L, ALBREKTSSON T. Classification of platelet concentrates: from pure platelet-rich plasma（P-PRP）to leucocyte- and platelet-rich

fibrin（L-PRF）[J]. Trends Biotechnol, 2009, 27（3）: 158-167.

[11] DOHAN E D M, BIELECKI T, MISHRA A, et al. In search of a consensus terminology in the field of platelet concentrates for surgical use: platelet-rich plasma （PRP）, platelet-rich fibrin（PRF）, fibrin gel polymerization and leukocytes[J]. Curr Pharm Biotechnol, 2012, 13（7）: 1131-1137.

[12] DOHAN E D M, ANDIA I, ZUMSTEIN M A, et al. Classification of platelet concentrates（platelet-rich plasma-PRP, platelet rich fibrin-PRF）for topical and infiltrative use in orthopedic and sports medicine: current consensus, clinical implications and perspectives[J]. Muscles Ligaments Tendons J, 2014, 4（1）: 3-9.

[13] MISHRA A, HARMON K, WOODALL J, et al. Sports medicine applications of platelet rich plasma[J]. Curr Pharm Biotechnol, 2012, 13（7）: 1185-1195.

[14] DE PASCALE M R, SOMMESE L, CASAMASSIMI A, et al. Platelet derivatives in regenerative medicine: an update[J]. Transfus Med Rev, 2015, 29（1）: 52-61.

[15] HARRISON P. The use of platelets in regenerative medicine and proposal for a new classification system: guidance from the SSC of the ISTH[J]. Journal of Thrombosis and Haemostasis, 2018, 16: 1895-1900.

[16] 吕敏, 裴国献, 刘勇, 等. 富血小板血浆的制备现状及研究进展[J]. 现代生物医学进展, 2013, 13（13）: 2574-2577, 2475.

[17] YUAN T, ZHANG C Q. Fabrication and principle of platelet-rich plasma in the repair of bone and soft tissues[J]. Chinese Journal of Clinical Rehabilitation, 2004, 8（35）: 7939-7941.

[18] LANDESBERG R, ROY M, GLICKMAN R S. Quantification of growth factor levels using a simplified method of platelet-rich plasma gel preparation[J]. J Oral Maxillofac Surg, 2000, 58（3）: 297-300.

[19] SONG Y, CHAO Y L, GONG P. Platelet-rich plasma made by a modified method promotes proliferation of rat osteoblast and human osteoblast in vitro[J]. Chinese J Reparative and Reconstructive Surgery, 2005, 9（3）: 178-182.

[20] ZHU Y H, MA C H, LUAN X J. The comparative study of effects between blood bag and in vitro on preparation of platelet-rich plasma[J]. Journal of Southern Medical University, 2012, 30（10）: 2399-2401.

[21] LEITNER G C, GRUBER R, NEUMÜLLER J, et al. Platelet content and growth factor release in platelet-rich plasma: a comparison of four different systems[J]. Vox Sang, 2006, 91（2）: 135-139.

[22] MAZZUCCO L, BALBO V, CATTANA E, et al. Platelet-rich plasma and platelet gel preparation using Plateltex[J]. Vox Sang, 2008, 94（3）: 202-208.

[23] APPEL T R, POTZSCH B, MÜLLER J, et al. Comparison of three different preparations of platelet concentrates for growth factor enrichment[J]. Clin Oral Implants

Res, 2002, 13（5）：522-528.

[24] 卫愉轩, 张昭远, 范峥莹, 等. 中国富血小板血浆临床制备方法的研究进展[J]. 中华关节外科杂志（电子版）, 2020, 14（2）：196-200.

[25] TATSUMI N. Universal anticoagulants for medical laboratory use[J]. J Jpn Soc Thromb Hemost, 2002, 13（2）：158-168.

[26] ANITUA E, PRADO R, TROYA M, et al. Implementation of a more physiological plasma rich in growth factor（PRGF）protocol：anticoagulant removal and reduction in activator concentration[J]. Platelets, 2016, 27（5）：459-466.

[27] MARX R E. Platelet-rich plasma（PRP）：what is PRP and what is not PRP?［J］. Implant Dent, 2001, 10（4）：225-228.

[28] AIZAWA H, KAWABATA H, SATO A, et al. A comparative study of the effects of anticoagulants on pure platelet-rich plasma quality and potency[J]. Biomedicines, 2020, 8（3）：42-56.

[29] LEI H, GUI L, LIU Z J. [The study of anticoagulants selection in platelet-rich plasma preparation]［J］. Zhonghua zheng xing wai ke za zhi. Chinese journal of plastic surgery, 2015, 31（4）：295-300.

[30] MAN D, PLOSKER H, WINLAND B J E. The use of autologous platetet-rich plasma（platelet gel）and autologous platelet-poor plasma（fibrin glue）in cosmetic surgmT[J]. Plast Reconstr Surg, 2001, 107（1）：229-237.

[31] DUGRILLON A, EICHLER H, KERN S, et al. Autologous concentrated platelet-rich plasma（cPRP）for local application in bone regeneration[J]. International Journal of Oral & Maxillofacial Surgery, 2002, 31（6）：615-619.

[32] PIAO L F, PARK H M, JO C H, et al. Theoretical prediction and validation of cell recovery rates in preparing platelet-rich plasma through a centrifugation[J]. Plos One, 2017, 12（11）：e0187509.

[33] WANG X, LI R G, DUAN X M. The research progress of platelet preservation methods on 22℃[J]. Chinese Medical Journal of Metallurgical Industry, 2004, 21（5）：396-398.

[34] DU L J, MIAO Y, LI X, et al. A novel and convenient method for the preparation and activation of PRP without any additives：temperature controlled PRP[J]. Biomed Research International, 2018：1761865.

[35] HOSNUTER M, ASLAN C, ISIK D, et al. Functional assessment of autologous platelet-rich plasma（PRP）after long-term storage at-20 degrees C without any preservation agent[J]. Journal of Plastic Surgery & Hand Surgery, 2017, 51（4）：235-239.

[36] HAUSCHILD G, GEBUREK F, GOSHEGER G, et al. Short term storage stability at room temperature of two different platelet-rich plasma preparations from equine donors and

potential impact on growth factor concentrations[J]. BMC Veterinary Research, 2016, 13（1）: 7-16.

[37] SUCHETHA A, LAKSHMI P, BHAT D, et al. Platelet concentration in platelet concentrates and periodontal regeneration-unscrambling the ambiguity[J]. Contemporary Clinical Dentistry, 2015, 6（4）: 510-516.

[38] PICCIN A, PIERRO A M D, CANZIAN L, et al. Platelet gel: A new therapeutic tool with great potential[J]. Blood Transfus, 2017, 15（4）: 1-8.

[39] ULUSAL G B. Platelet-rich plasma and hyaluronic acid: an efficient biostimulation method for face rejuvenation[J]. Journal of Cosmetic Dermatology, 2017, 16（1）: 112-119.

[40] JALOWIEC J M, D'ESTE M, BARA J J, et al. An in vitro investigation of platelet-rich plasma-gel as a cell and growth factor delivery vehicle for tissue engineering[J]. Tissue Engineering Part C Methods, 2016, 22（1）: 49-58.

[41] RUGHETTI A, GIUSTI I, D'ASCENZO S, et al. Platelet gel-released supernatant modulates the angiogenic capability of human endothelial cells[J]. Blood Transfusion, 2008, 6（1）: 12-17.

[42] GIUSTI I, RUGHETTI A, D'ASCENZO S, et al. Identification of an optimal concentration of platelet gel for promoting angiogenesis in human endothelial cells[J]. Transfusion, 2010, 49（4）: 771-778.

[43] ARORA S, DODA V, KOTWAL U, et al. Quantification of platelets and platelet derived growth factors from platelet-rich-plasma（PRP）prepared at different centrifugal force（g）and time[J]. Transfusion & Apheresis Science, 2016, 54（1）: 103-110.

[44] FRAUTSCHI R S, HASHEM A M, BRIANNA H, et al. Current evidence for clinical efficacy of platelet rich plasma in aesthetic surgery: a systematic review[J]. Aesthetic Surgery Journal, 2017, 37（3）: 353-362.

[45] GENTILE P, SCIOLI M G, BIELLI A, et al. Concise review: the use of adipose-derived stromal vascular fraction cells and platelet rich plasma in regenerative plastic surgery[J]. Stem Cells, 2017, 35（1）: 117-134.

[46] QIAO J, AN N, OUYANG X Y, et al. Quantification of growth factors in different platelet concentrates[J]. Platelets, 2017, 28（8）: 774-778.

[47] 宣力, 田举, 宣敏, 等. 二次离心法制备富血小板血浆中血小板相关参数的分析[J]. 华南国防医学杂志, 2017, 31（8）: 514-517, 530.

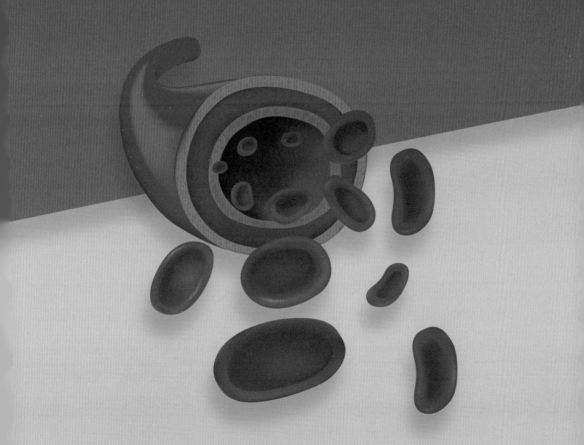

第三章

富血小板血浆在骨关节疼痛中的应用

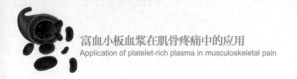
第一节　富血小板血浆在肩关节疼痛中的应用

肩关节疼痛是目前最常见的肌肉骨骼疼痛之一[1]。肩关节疼痛最常见的原因是机械性因素导致的肩袖肌腱、韧带和三角肌下滑囊周围相关结构的损伤。若无及时有效的治疗或进行了不适当的运动可能引起损伤进一步发展，疼痛明显加重，最终可导致关节功能障碍甚至残疾。PRP是自体全血经离心分离产生的高浓度血小板混悬物，能释放多种生长因子，促进细胞增殖和血管生成，目前已逐渐成为骨关节相关疾病的常用治疗手段，本节主要介绍PRP在肩部疼痛疾病中的应用。

一、肩袖损伤

肩袖损伤是覆盖于肩关节的肩胛下肌、冈上肌、冈下肌、小圆肌等肌腱组织损伤的总称。

1. 概述

肩袖损伤是引起肩关节疼痛和活动障碍的最主要原因，严重影响患者的日常生活质量，在中老年人群中更为常见。随着社会人口的老龄化，肩袖损伤的发病率呈现明显的上升趋势。肩袖肌腱和韧带缺乏血供，损伤后难以自愈，以往的治疗方法局限性大，使肩袖损伤成为肩肘外科和运动医学领域研究的热点、难点。目前比较常用的治疗指南是美国骨科医师学会（American Academy of Orthopaedic Surgeons，AAOS）循证临床实践指南（clinical practice guideline，CPG）工作组提出的，于2010年首次颁布。该指南提出了适用于全球的肩袖疾病的诊断、评估、预防和治疗的临床实践指导，但由于缺乏AAOS循证标准的资料，所以2010年版指南中缺乏"强烈推荐"的治疗方案。

　　2019年CPG工作组正式发布了新一版指南，对2010年版指南推荐中尚不明确的条目进行了重新评估和更新。其中关于肩袖撕裂的治疗，高级别证据支持物理治疗和手术治疗均可以显著改善症状性的中小型全层肩袖撕裂患者报告结局（PRO评分），但物理治疗的患者肩袖撕裂尺寸、肌肉萎缩和脂肪浸润程度可能会在5~10年内持续进展。中等证据支持肩袖修复术后肩袖完整愈合的患者PRO评分和功能优于物理治疗或术后发生再撕裂的患者。简而言之，2019年版指南进一步明确：对于中小型的肩袖撕裂尤其是无症状的患者，保守治疗可作为首选；对于症状性患者，可以结合患者的手术预期、功能需求以及治疗意愿等，先行保守治疗，在后续随访中根据患者病情变化调整治疗方案。关于关节腔注射治疗，中等证据支持使用单次皮质类固醇（corticosteroid，CS）联合局部麻醉药注射，可短期改善患者的肩关节疼痛和功能受限。有限的证据支持应用关节腔透明质酸（hyaluronic acid，HA）注射治疗没有撕裂的肩袖病变。多项体内外研究提示，PRP释放的生长因子在人肌腱细胞增殖和机制代谢中有积极作用，但目前尚缺乏充足证据支持PRP用于肩袖疾病的治疗，有限证据支持应用PRP可降低术后肩袖再撕裂率，但是否推荐在肩袖手术中常规使用PRP则尚无定论[2]。

　　2. PRP治疗肩袖损伤的临床研究进展

　　已有多项基础研究表明PRP对肌腱修复有积极作用，但现有临床证据并不完全支持这个结论。为了验证PRP是否能够改善关节镜下肩袖修复术的再撕裂率和功能结果，Zhao等和Hurley等[3-4]分别于2015年和2019年就目前国内外关于PRP在关节镜下肩袖修复术中的应用的高质量随机对照试验（RCT）进行了荟萃分析。Zhao等的研究纳入了8项RCT，相关病例数

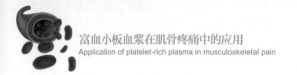

464例，临床证据1～2级，分析后发现，单纯手术组和手术联合PRP组在再撕裂率上无显著性差异。Hurley等增加了研究数量和患者数量，共纳入18项RCT，病例数1147例，研究结果显示，PRP能显著提高中小型完全撕裂肌腱的愈合率，对疼痛程度和临床功能也有明显的改善作用。

2016年，Zhang等[5]的一项RCT评估了PRP在关节镜下肩袖修复术中的作用，60例肩袖全层撕裂患者被随机分为试验组和对照组，对照组行关节镜双排肩袖修复术，试验组在手术后注射PRP，术后12个月时评估臂肩手障碍（DASH）评分、Constant Murley评分、视觉模拟评分法（VAS）、肩关节活动度等的改善情况，并采用MRI评估修复的完整性。结果发现，两组术后疼痛和功能状况均有显著改善，组间的改善程度未呈现显著性差异。但与对照组相比，试验组肌腱愈合率高，复发率显著降低，提示局部注射PRP对提高关节镜下双排肩袖修复术的效果有积极作用，证据等级为1级。

2019年，Cai等[6]报道了一项关于PRP和HA注射对肩袖撕裂疗效的RCT，重点分析了PRP注射作为保守治疗方法的作用。该研究纳入184例经MRI检查确诊为肩袖撕裂的患者，随机分为4组，分别进行生理盐水注射、HA注射、PRP注射、PRP联合HA注射。每位患者接受4次注射，时间间隔为1周。在治疗前及治疗后1个月、3个月、6个月和12个月评估Constant评分、ASES评分和VAS评分，1年后再次行MRI检查以评估肩袖撕裂的愈合情况。结果发现，治疗后PRP组和HA联合PRP组的各项评分明显提高，MRI检查结果显示PRP组和PRP联合HA组的肩袖撕裂面积均明显缩小。该研究为PRP注射在轻中度肩袖撕裂治疗中的有效性提供了有力的证据。

在2020年，Schwitzguebel等[7]的一项RCT结果不支持PRP在肩袖损伤的治疗中具有积极作用。在该研究中，80例经MRI确诊的症状性冈上肌撕裂患者被随机分为两组，分别接受超声引导下冈上肌内PRP或生理盐水注射（注射2次，时间间隔为1个月），治疗后7个月的疗效评估结果显示，两组在疼痛、关节功能、病灶减小等方面的改善均无显著性差异，且PRP组表现出更高的不良反应（如注射后疼痛、肩关节粘连、病灶扩大）发生率。该研究再次对PRP注射作为肩袖损伤保守治疗方法的安全性和有效性提出了质疑。

3. PRP治疗肩袖损伤的基础研究进展

目前多数基础实验和动物研究结果都表明，PRP能促进肌腱干细胞增殖并诱导血管内皮细胞生长因子的产生，促进受损肌腱周围新生血管形成，促进瘢痕愈合。早在2003年，Molloy等[8]对生长因子在肌腱修复中的作用的相关研究进行了系统综述，揭示了胰岛素样生长因子-Ⅰ（IGF-Ⅰ）、转化生长因子-β（TGF-β）、血管内皮生长因子（VEGF）、血小板源性生长因子（PDGF）和成纤维细胞生长因子（bFGF）等对肌腱修复的积极作用。研究者提出，尽管不同损伤区域肌腱细胞的修复过程不尽相同，但对于大多数类型的肌腱损伤，体内外研究都证实了生长因子的生物效应，提示生长因子及其衍生物（PRP）在提高肌腱愈合的效率和有效性方面具有一定的前景。

Marieke等[9]曾提出一个猜想：PRP可以促进细胞增殖和胶原蛋白的产生，从而诱导人肌腱细胞产生基质蛋白酶和内源性生长因子。他们将人肌腱细胞分别置于含有不同浓度PRP激活物（PRCR）和贫血小板血浆释放物（PPCR）的胎牛血清培养基中培养，分别在第4天、第7天和第14天检测细胞数量、总胶原量，Ⅰ型胶原和Ⅲ型胶原的基因表达情况，基质金属蛋白酶（MMP-1、MMP-3、MMP-13）、VEGF、TGF等因子的产生情况。结果表明，上述猜想得到了验证，PRCR和PPCR两组的细胞数量和总胶原量均有所增加，但相比于PPCR组，PRCR组的MMP-1和MMP-3表达明显

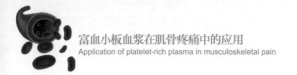
上调，VEGF的表达也显著增加，提示PRP可刺激细胞增殖和胶原蛋白的产生，增加基质金属蛋白酶和内源性生长因子的表达。该研究表明PRP可能会在一定程度上加速损伤肌腱周围基质的分解代谢，促进血管生成和纤维血管细胞形成。

2019年，Gabrielle等[10]评估了冻干壳聚糖（CS）和PRP组成的植入物是否能促进兔肩袖损伤模型的肌腱修复。其研究结果表明，CS-PRP植入物能通过加速大结节处的骨重塑，改善冈上肌腱与肱骨头的附着，抑制冈上肌腱的异位骨化。同时，CS-PRP植入物未引起明显不良反应。该研究证明，CS-PRP植入物可有效改善动物模型肩袖止点处腱-骨界面组织的愈合。

二、粘连性肩关节囊炎

粘连性肩关节囊炎（adhesive capsulitis，AC）即肩周炎，是指由多种原因导致的肩盂肱关节囊炎性粘连、僵硬，临床表现为肩关节周围疼痛、各方向主动和被动活动受限，以外旋受限为主，影像学检查可发现关节腔变狭窄及轻度骨质疏松。

1. 概述

已有研究证实，关节囊及周围韧带组织的慢性炎症和纤维化是AC的主要病理改变，纤维化导致的软组织弹性降低及盂肱关节有效容积减小，是肩关节活动受限的直接原因，但其基本病理生理过程仍不明确。临床上AC治疗的目标是减轻疼痛和改善活动范围，最终恢复肩关节功能。目前暂无治疗AC的金标准[11]，临床上仍以保守治疗为主，包括改变日常活动和运动方式、药物治疗、关节腔注射和物理治疗等。关节腔内CS注射成本低，减轻疼痛效果明显，是治疗AC最常用的方法。然而，有研究表明，CS注射与血糖升高、关节软骨损伤、肌腱断裂、局部皮肤脱色和皮下组织萎缩等多种不良反应密切相关。PRP有减轻疼痛、抗炎和促进再生作用，能促进慢性损伤组织的愈合，减轻关节的疼痛和僵硬，且关节腔注射安全有效，为AC的治疗提供了新的思路。

2. PRP治疗AC的临床研究进展

2016年，Aslani等[12]发表的一项病例报道初步展示了PRP在AC治疗中的有效性。同年，Kothari等[13]发表了一项临床研究，将195例肩周炎患者随机分成3组，分别进行PRP关节腔单次注射（2mL）、CS关节腔单次注射（甲基强的松龙80mg）和超声波治疗（两周内7次，1.5W/cm^2，1MHz，连续模式），在患者治疗前及治疗后3周、6周、12周进行评估。结果显示，与CS组和超声波组比较，PRP组患者在关节活动度（ROM）、VAS评分和快速DASH评分等方面均有显著改善，这表明PRP注射治疗肩周炎是有效的。

2019年，Apurba等[14]在一项前瞻性队列研究中比较了肩关节腔内行PRP注射和CS注射治疗AC的效果，研究中共纳入60例AC患者（病程不少于6个月），对照组（30例）接受CS注射（4mL），试验组（30例）接受PRP注射（4mL），随访时间为12周，随访期间暂停使用非甾体类药物。分别在注射后3周、6周、12周评估VAS评分、肩痛与残疾指数（SPADI）、肩部主动和被动活动度（ROM）等指标的改善情况，并记录患者满意度。结果显示，12周时PRP组VAS评分和SPADI评分分别下降58.4和55.1，而CS组分别下降48.7和45.8；在ROM方面，与CS组相比，PRP组在被动外展（−50.4 vs −39.4）、内旋（−36.8 vs −25.8）和外旋（−35.4 vs −25.9）等方面均有显著改善，两组观察期内均未发生明显不良反应，初步证实单次PRP注射在改善肩周炎患者的疼痛、功能障碍和关节活动度等方面优于CS注射，且具有较高的治疗满意度。

2020年，Thu等[15]报道了一项比较超声引导下肩关节腔内PRP注射和常规理疗对AC临床疗效的RCT，研究中共纳入64例患者，随机分组后分别实施PRP注射和物理治疗，随访时间为6周。结果显示，治疗后两组患者在VAS评分、DASH评分和ROM方面均有改善，两组间比较无显著性差异。但与常规理疗组比较，PRP组治疗后对乙酰氨基酚的用药量较少。

研究者提出，PRP注射治疗AC是安全有效的，尤其对于依从性差或有CS禁忌证的患者，PRP是比较有效的治疗手段。值得注意的是，上述研究均未对PRP的制备、血小板浓度、注射次数等进行标准化，且随访时间较短，因此，仍需更多高质量RCT来证明PRP在AC治疗中的积极作用。

3. PRP治疗粘连性肩关节囊炎的基础研究进展

迄今为止，AC的发病机制尚未完全明确，大多数学者认为AC的病理过程与关节囊及周围韧带组织的慢性炎症及纤维化有关。目前关于PRP治疗AC的基础研究相对较少。

2020年，Feusi等[16]发表了第一篇分析PRP对AC的治疗作用的标准化实验研究。研究者在20只SD大鼠中建立了肩周炎模型，随后将模型大鼠进行随机分组，对照组仅接受手术治疗，实验组在术后注射1次PRP。术后观察至第8周，取模型肩部组织进行切片，观察盂肱关节后部和下部组织炎症反应及滑膜重构的严重程度，采用半定量分级评估。结果显示，PRP组大鼠肩关节后部滑膜结构改变明显低于对照组，说明PRP注射可以改善AC模型大鼠肩关节的病变严重程度，且没有副作用。研究者提出，可将PRP关节腔注射作为早期肩周炎治疗的选择。

三、盂肱关节骨性关节炎

盂肱关节（glenohumeral，GH）骨性关节炎是指盂肱关节软骨的进行性丢失，可导致骨侵蚀、疼痛和功能下降。

1. 概述

盂肱关节骨性关节炎是常见的骨骼肌肉系统疾病之一，发病率仅次于膝关节和髋关节的骨性关节炎，65岁以上老年人患病率高达16.1%[17]。GH骨性关节炎多见于女性，大多数患者无外伤史或手术史，临床表现为疼痛、关节活动范围减小和关节功能进行性降低，病理特征为关节软骨损伤、软骨下骨硬化、骨赘形成、关节盂骨侵蚀、关节间隙狭窄和肱骨头半脱位。GH骨性关节炎的发病机制十分复杂。

目前的治疗手段包括保守治疗和手术治疗，一般的保守治疗包括日常活动方式调整、物理因子治疗、药物治疗和皮质类固醇注射等，但大多数保守治疗长期效果不明确[18]。最新一版的临床实践指南在2020年3月发布，该指南明确提出关节腔注射HA对GH骨性关节炎没有治疗作用，但关于PRP、骨髓间充质干细胞在GH骨性关节炎中的应用，证据级别仍是"不确定"，需要更多高质量的研究来证实其安全性、成本效益和临床疗效[19]。

2. PRP治疗GH骨性关节炎的临床研究进展

国内外关于PRP注射治疗GH骨性关节炎的临床研究很少。2016年，Lo等[20]发表了一项病例报道，评估同种异体真皮基质人工关节盂生物表面置换半关节置换术对GH骨性关节炎的疗效。该研究纳入55例接受人工关节盂半关节置换术的患者，平均随访时间为60个月。为优化手术方案、提高治疗效果，研究者在室温下解冻同种异体移植物，将其浸泡于PRP中备用。随访得到了满意的中期结果和较低的翻修率。研究者初步阐述了PRP的积极作用，但由于缺乏对照组，该研究最终无法说明PRP的生物效应。

2017年，Noh等[21]在一项临床研究中验证了氧化应激反应介质影响肩关节炎和肩袖撕裂（RCT）的假说。研究者提出，调节生长因子和氧化应激反应介质可能是预防退行性RCT的潜在治疗选择。该研究招募了12例RCT患者（无合并肩关节炎）作为对照组，又根据RCT和GH骨性关节炎的严重程度将另外24例患者分为RCT P1和RCT P2两组，其中，RCT P1组为轻度关节炎症合并RCT（撕裂≤2cm），RCT P2组为中度或重度关节炎症合并RCT（撕裂＞2cm）。所有患者根据病情接受盂唇修复术或肩袖修复术，并提取PRP 5mL做血清学检测。采用酶联免疫吸附法、免疫印迹法和胶原酶谱法分析滑膜液、血液、PRP和肌腱组织中的细胞因子、生长因子、血管生成物标志物。结果显示，RCT P组滑膜液中IL-8、TNF-α和IL-1β的诱导水平显著升高，滑膜液和血清中的IGF-Ⅰ和TGF-β1明显增多，在活性氧暴露的RCT P组滑膜液中，血管生成素Ang-1和Ang-2、Tie-2和低氧诱导因子1α均显著上调。RCT P组滑膜液中MMP-1的产生显著增加，而Ⅰ型胶原表达随着结缔组织生长因子表达的减少而减少，PRP中TGF-β1、Ang-1、Ang-2以及PDGF-AB高于对照组，但TNF-α和IL-1β在RCT P组中的浓度最低。由此推测，应用PRP可促进术后肌腱-骨的愈合和恢复，PRP可以促进组织再生和干细胞分化。此外，PRP中存在大量的血管生成素，有助于促进肌腱组织的血管生成。研究者强调，TGF-β1、Ang-1和Ang-2可能是修复RCT和影响肩关节炎的主要成分，该研究为PRP在肩关节炎和肩袖撕裂中的临床应用提供了初步证据，但需要进一步的临床研究加以证实。

结语：近年来，再生医学领域快速发展，PRP局部应用逐渐成为骨关节领域的常用治疗方法。PRP由自体全血制备而成，富含多种生长因子，在细胞增殖、分化和血管生成中发挥着关键作用，可促进肌腱愈合和组织修复。但目前PRP在肩关节相关疾病中的应用尚存在争议，国内外PRP相关研究仍未解决标准化制备、激活及储存等问题，临床上对注射次数、注射量及注射时间间隔等的意见尚未统一，未来需要更多高质量临床研究为PRP的临床应用提供有力证据。

（王少玲）

参考文献

[1] COOK T, LEWIS J. Rotator cuff-related shoulder pain：to inject or not to inject？[J]. J Orthop Sports Phys Ther，2019，49（5）：289-293.

[2] 张凯博，唐新，李箭，等. 2019年美国骨科医师学会（AAOS）肩袖损伤临床实践指南解读[J]. 中国运动医学杂志，2020，39（5）：403-412.

[3] ZHAO J G, ZHAO L, JIANG Y X, et al. Platelet-rich plasma in arthroscopic rotator cuff repair：a meta-analysis of randomized controlled trials[J]. Arthroscopy，2015，31（1）：125-135.

[4] HURLEY E T, LIM F D, MORAN C J, et al. The efficacy of platelet-rich plasma and platelet-rich fibrin in arthroscopic rotator cuff repair：a meta-analysis of randomized controlled trials[J]. Am J Sports Med，2019，47（3）：753-761.

[5] ZHANG Z X, WANG Y, SUN J Y. The effect of platelet-rich plasma on arthroscopic double-row rotator cuff repair：a clinical study with 12-month follow-up[J]. Acta Orthop Traumatol Turc，2016，50（2）：191-197.

[6] CAI Y, SUN Z X, LIAO B K, et al. Sodium hyaluronate and platelet-rich plasma for partial-thickness rotator cuff tears[J]. Med Sci Sports Exerc，2019，51（2）：227-233.

[7] SCHWITZGUEBEL A J, KOLO F C, TIREFORT J, et al. Efficacy of platelet-rich plasma for the treatment of interstitial supraspinatus tears：a double-blinded, randomized controlled trial[J]. Am J Sports Med，2019，47（8）：1885-1892.

[8] MOLLOY T, WANG Y, MURRELL G. The roles of growth factors in tendon and ligament healing[J]. Sports Med，2003，33（5）：381-394.

[9] DE MOS M, VAN DER WINDT A E, JAHR H, et al. Can platelet-rich plasma enhance tendon repair？ A cell culture study[J]. Am J Sports Med，2008，36（6）：1171-1178.

[10] DEPRES-TREMBLAY G, CHEVRIER A, SNOW M, et al. Freeze-dried chitosan-platelet-rich plasma implants improve supraspinatus tendon attachment in a transosseous rotator cuff repair model in the rabbit[J]. J Biomater Appl，2019，33（6）：792-807.

[11] RANGAN A, GOODCHILD L, GIBSON J, et al. Frozen shoulder[J]. Shoulder Elbow，2015，7（4）：299-307.

[12] ASLANI H, NOURBAKHSH S T, ZAFARANI Z, et al. Platelet-rich plasma for frozen

shoulder: a case report[J]. Arch Bone Jt Surg, 2016, 4（1）: 90–93.

[13] KOTHARI S Y, SRIKUMAR V, SINGH N. Comparative efficacy of platelet rich plasma injection, corticosteroid injection and ultrasonic therapy in the treatment of periarthritis shoulder[J]. J Clin Diagn Res, 2017, 11（5）: RC15–RC18.

[14] BARMAN A, MUKHERJEE S, SAHOO J, et al. Single intra–articular platelet–rich plasma versus corticosteroid injections in the treatment of adhesive capsulitis of the shoulder: a cohort study[J]. Am J Phys Med Rehabil, 2019, 98（7）: 549–557.

[15] THU A C, KWAK S G, SHEIN W N, et al. Comparison of ultrasound–guided platelet–rich plasma injection and conventional physical therapy for management of adhesive capsulitis: a randomized trial[J]. Journal of International Medical Research, 2020, 48（12）: 1–11.

[16] FEUSI O, KAROL A, FLEISCHMANN T, et al. Platelet–rich plasma as a potential prophylactic measure against frozen shoulder in an in vivo shoulder contracture model[J]. Arch Orthop Trauma Surg, 2020, 142（12）: 363–372.

[17] MACÍAS–HERNÁNDEZ S I, MORONES–ALBA J D, MIRANDA–DUARTE A, et al. Glenohumeral osteoarthritis: overview, therapy, and rehabilitation[J]. Disability and Rehabilitation, 2017, 39（16）: 1674–1682.

[18] ROSSI L A, PIUZZI N S, SHAPIRO S A. Glenohumeral osteoarthritis: the role for orthobiologic therapies: platelet–rich plasma and cell therapies[J]. JBJS Rev, 2020, 8（2）: e0075.

[19] KHAZZAM M, GEE A O, PEARL M. Management of glenohumeral joint osteoarthritis[J]. J Am Acad Orthop Surg, 2020, 28（19）: 781–789.

[20] LO E Y, FLANAGIN B A, BURKHEAD W Z. Biologic resurfacing arthroplasty with acellular human dermal allograft and platelet–rich plasma（PRP）in young patients with glenohumeral arthritis—average of 60 months of at mid–term follow–up[J]. Journal of Shoulder and Elbow Surgery, 2016, 25（7）: e199–e207.

[21] NOH K C, PARK S H, YANG C J, et al. Involvement of synovial matrix degradation and angiogenesis in oxidative stress–exposed degenerative rotator cuff tears with osteoarthritis[J]. Journal of Shoulder and Elbow Surgery, 2018, 27（1）: 141–150.

第二节　富血小板血浆在肘关节疼痛中的应用

富血小板血浆（PRP）在肘关节疼痛中的应用主要涉及肱骨外上髁炎、尺侧副韧带断裂和肘关节骨缺损等，其中对肱骨外上髁炎的治疗效果较为肯定且备受关注。

一、肱骨外上髁炎

肱骨外上髁炎（lateral epicondylitis，LE），又称网球肘，是伸肌总腱起点处的慢性损伤性炎症。

1. 概述

LE是引起肘部疼痛最常见的疲劳性损伤疾病，任何对肘部伸肌腱施加高应力的因素都是LE的危险因素。其发病机制为前臂伸肌过度收缩造成肌肉紧张，肌肉附着点肌腱退化甚至撕裂，以肱骨外上髁部位反复疼痛和活动受限为特点，疼痛可沿上肢向近端或远端放射，临床表现为局部压痛和活动痛。

治疗LE的方法主要包括应用非甾体抗炎药、物理因子治疗、冲击波治疗、局部糖皮质激素注射及手术等。PRP含有多种生长因子，可调控软骨、骨的生长修复，促使软骨细胞增殖分化、生长、黏附，修复关节退行性病变。因此，多数研究将PRP治疗LE作为一种新的有潜力的疗法。

2. PRP治疗LE的临床研究

2006年，Mishra等开展了首个应用PRP治疗慢性严重肘部肌腱病的随机对照研究[1]。共招募了20例经标准化理疗方案和保守治疗后仍有持

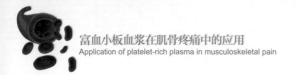

续性疼痛的LE患者，随机分为PRP注射组（15例）和布比卡因注射组（5例），采用VAS评分和改良的Mayo肘关节功能评分进行治疗效果评估，结果表明PRP治疗可以显著减轻疼痛。

Lim等研究探讨了PRP治疗LE患者细胞因子水平与临床疗效的关系，将156例LE患者随机分为单次PRP注射组和对照组（仅进行物理治疗），采用VAS评分、改良的Mayo肘关节功能评分和MRI进行评估，并检测治疗前后的全血和注射用PRP中细胞因子水平，与临床评分进行相关分析，结果发现注射后24周，PRP注射组患者疼痛和功能指标均有明显改善，PRP中血小板源性生长因子-AB（PDGF-AB）、血小板源性生长因子-BB（PDGF-BB）、转化生长因子-β（TGF-β）较全血明显升高，其中TGF-β与Mayo肘关节功能评分和MRI分级改善显著相关，提示PRP中TGF-β可能在肌腱愈合过程中起关键作用[2]。

Hastie等的一项回顾性研究收集了2012—2015年的LE病例，并比较开展PRP注射前后每年需要手术的病例数，结果发现开展PRP注射之前（2008—2011年），平均每年有12.75例患者接受手术，而在开展PRP之后（2012—2015年）该数据降低到4.25例，64例接受PRP治疗的患者中有56例（87.5%）的症状得到有效缓解，说明PRP是一种安全有效并能减轻症状的疗法，且开展PRP注射后需要手术的病例数减少[3]。

近年来，有关比较PRP和其他疗法治疗LE的随机对照临床研究受到关注。Thanasas等的一项PRP与自体血治疗慢性肘外上髁炎的随机对照临床试验中，28例患者被随机分成2组：PRP注射组和自体血注射组。在注射后6周、3个月和6个月分别采用VAS评分和Liverpool肘关节评分进行评估，发现PRP注射在6个月内缓解疼痛的效果优于自体血[4]。Alessio-Mazzola等比较了63例患者进行体外冲击波治疗与PRP治疗的效果，随访2年发现，PRP组治疗后患者症状缓解所用的平均时间明显缩短[5]。Gosens等将100

例慢性肘外上髁炎患者随机分为2组，分别接受皮质类固醇和PRP注射治疗，2年随访期间采用VAS评分和DASH评分进行评估，结果显示PRP组的治疗成功率明显高于皮质类固醇组[6]。董佩龙等将60例患者随机分为PRP组（30例）和糖皮质激素组（30例）进行注射治疗，在注射后1个月、3个月、12个月随访并采用注射部位炎性反应程度、VAS评分、Mayo肘关节功能评分及DASH评分进行评估，结果显示自体PRP及糖皮质激素局部注射治疗LE均能缓解疼痛、恢复肘关节功能，但糖皮质激素早期起效快、后期治疗效果缓和，而自体PRP治疗效果逐渐提高，且不增加治疗后的并发症[7]。

Farkash等首次采用新型可注射重组人胶原支架联合自体PRP治疗LE，该研究纳入40例患者，评估治疗后6个月的握力、功能残疾和超声肌腱外观的变化，结果发现患者的握力有不同程度的提高，68%的患者超声肌腱外观明显改善[8]。

2020年，Xu等荟萃分析了7个随机临床对照试验，涉及515例患者，结果显示在6个月的随访中，局部注射PRP在减轻疼痛和改善肘关节功能方面优于局部皮质类固醇治疗[9]。另一篇荟萃分析主要聚焦于PRP与肾上腺皮质激素在短期（1～3个月）和长期（≥6个月）内的疗效，作者经分析后认为PRP对长期疼痛的改善在统计学和临床上均优于肾上腺皮质激素[10]。

2018年，Le等综合了多篇PRP相关的临床文献，比较了富白细胞PRP（LR-PRP）和贫白细胞PRP（LP-PRP）治疗LE的疗效，得出循证医学建议。他们指出，PRP注射是一种有效的治疗LE的新方法，已有高质量的临床随机试验证实其具有短期和长期疗效，且有级别极高的证据证明LR-PRP是治疗LE的首选[11]。

然而，也有几项研究提出不同观点。Krogh等在一项PRP、糖皮质激素和生理盐水治疗LE的随机、双盲、安慰剂对照研究中提出，对LE患者注射PRP和糖皮质激素3个月后，疼痛缓解均不优于生理盐水注射[12]。Montalvan等将25例患者随机分为PRP组和生理盐水组，观察超声引导下肌腱内注射PRP或生理盐水注射（2次）在新近进展的LE患者中的疗效，在1个月、3个月、6个月和12个月后的随访中发现，两组患者VAS评分无明显差异[13]。欧洲肌肉骨骼放射学会在一篇基于德尔菲法的共识中提到，超声引导下PRP注射治疗慢性肘外上髁炎疗效良好，但与其他治疗方法（包括自体血、生理盐水、利多卡因注射或冲击波疗法）相比没有明显优势[14]。Linnanmaki等在2020年发表的一项随机对照研究也支持这一结论[15]。不同研究中使用的PRP制备方法、注射方案或联合康复治疗方案等的差异可能是导致研究结果不一致的原因。

近几年也有研究者将重心放在PRP联合微创手术治疗LE上。Carlier等采用超声经皮肌腱切断术联合PRP注射治疗261例顽固性LE患者，并采用VAS评分、快速DASH评分、网球肘功能评分、Mayo肘关节功能评分、肘关节自评评分、握力和返回工作岗位情况等进行疗效评估，治疗3个月后的评估结果显示该方法缓解疼痛、恢复握力快，患者满意度高，早期复工率高[16]。

3. PRP治疗LE的基础研究

关于PRP治疗LE的基础研究较少。2015年，有研究者分别采用LR-PRP和LP-PRP体外培养兔肌腱干细胞（tendon stem/progenitor cells，TSCs），应用免疫染色、实时定量聚合酶链反应、免疫印迹（Western blot）等方法检测细胞增殖，干细胞标志物的表达、合成和分解等，结果发现LR-PRP和LP-PRP均以剂量依赖性方式诱导细胞增殖，LR-PRP主要诱导肌腱细胞的分解代谢和炎性改变，而LP-PRP主要诱导合成代谢改变，提示虽然LR-PRP和LP-PRP在诱导TSCs分化为活跃的肌腱细胞时似乎都是"安全的"，但LR-PRP诱导的分解代谢和炎症反应可能并不利于受伤肌腱的愈合，而LP-PRP很强的诱导细胞合成代谢的潜能可能会导致过多的瘢痕组织形成[17]。

二、尺侧副韧带损伤

尺侧副韧带（ulnar collateral ligament，UCL）损伤是指当内侧肘关节所受力长期超过尺侧副韧带的抗拉强度时尺侧副韧带发生的慢性损伤[18]。

1. 概述

UCL损伤常发生在棒球运动员等需要做大量重复投掷动作的运动员中，可导致肘关节内侧疼痛和外翻不稳定[19]，极大地影响运动员的职业生涯。

一般来说，对于UCL完全撕裂的患者考虑手术干预，而对于青少年和不完全撕裂的患者则推荐非手术治疗，即早期康复并辅以生物治疗[20]。PRP富含多种生长因子，有助于招募细胞刺激血管生成和内皮细胞生长以增加血流量，从而启动加速愈合的级联反应[21]。

2. PRP在UCL损伤治疗中的临床研究

2013年，Podesta等首次将PRP应用于UCL撕裂，他们选取了34名MRI诊断为UCL部分撕裂且经至少2个月的非手术治疗而疗效不佳的运动员，在超声引导下对UCL进行单次LR-PRP（1A型）注射，并在注射后启动物理治疗。分别在注射前和返回赛场后每4周完成一次Kerlan-Jobe骨科（KJOC）评分、DASH评分和肱尺关节间隙的动态肌肉骨骼超声测量，直至患者恢复到受伤前的水平，平均随访70周。结果显示，30名患者在10～15周后恢复到受伤前的水平，与基线相比，运动员们的KJOC评分和

DASH评分提高，注射PRP前和末次随访时的外翻应力作用下的肱尺关节间隙平均测量值、应力性与非应力性肱尺关节间隙差都有下降，说明单次注射LR-PRP对肘关节部分性UCL撕裂有效[22]。Deal等在Podesta的基础上做了改进，对25例2级UCL损伤患者间隔2周进行2次LR-PRP（1B型）注射并给以肘部支架，治疗4周后每6周进行一次MRI随访，结果发现23例原发性损伤患者中，22名患者（96%）能够恢复比赛，并在MRI上显示UCL重建，而LR-PRP治疗失败的3名患者中有2名曾接受过UCL重建手术，说明2次LR-PRP注射对UCL部分性撕裂安全有效，但对于既往进行过UCL修复或重建手术的患者疗效似乎较差[23]。

Dines等回顾性研究了44例接受PRP注射治疗的部分性UCL撕裂的棒球运动员，研究者根据Conway量表修订版对最终随访时的体格检查结果进行分类，发现有15例（34%）预后极好，有17例（39%）预后良好，6名职业球员中有4名（67%）重返职业比赛，提示PRP治疗UCL功能不全的预后要好于既往的保守治疗[24]，且PRP注射对于韧带急性损伤的年轻运动员以及不愿意或无法进行韧带手术重建后长期康复的运动员尤其有益[24-25]。

上述研究证明PRP治疗UCL部分性撕裂有一定疗效，Kato等进而推测PRP治疗也可促进完全性UCL撕裂的愈合。他们招募了34例MRI诊断为部分性或完全性UCL撕裂的棒球运动员，在超声引导下采用18号针进行UCL钻孔后注射LP-PRP，在术前及术后6个月完成患者的VAS评分、DASH评分和外翻应力下的肱尺关节间隙超声测量，结果34例患者中有30例（88%）避免了UCL重建手术，这30例中有26例在术后6个月内恢复到伤前水平，平均时间为12.4周[26]。

然而，2019年Chauhan等进行了一项大型的队列研究，对PRP治疗UCL损伤的效果提出了质疑。他们将2011—2015年的544名UCL损伤的职业棒球运动员分为接受过PRP注射组（133名）和未接受PRP注射组（411名，仅接受康复治疗），对两组间患者结局和Kaplan-Meier生存分析进行比较，发现重返赛场的成功率为54%，其中接受PRP注射治疗的球员的成功率（46%）明显低于仅接受康复治疗的球员（57%）。与匹配的非PRP注射队列进行比较时发现，接受PRP注射治疗的球员恢复投掷和重返赛场所需的时间更长，这可能是因为给药时间延迟或PRP有潜在的帮助愈合的生物效应[27]。

结语：经过近20年的不断探索，已有证据表明PRP总体上可缓解肱骨外上髁炎的疼痛症状，相比于皮质类固醇注射的短期疗效，PRP有更好的长期疗效，但尚需进行更多的研究来探讨PRP产生疗效的具体机制。目前，有关PRP研究较大的制约因素是缺乏标准，制备方法、注射剂量、注射次数和不同治疗注射的组合等可能是决定PRP效果的重要影响因素，仍需要高质量的客观评估和更长的随访时间来确定PRP治疗肘关节疼痛的最佳注射方案。

（翟羽佳）

参考文献

[1] MISHRA A, PAVELKO T. Treatment of chronic elbow tendinosis with buffered platelet-rich plasma[J]. Am J Sports Med, 2006, 34（11）: 1774-1778.

[2] LIM W, PARK S H, KIM B, et al. Relationship of cytokine levels and clinical effect on platelet-rich plasma-treated lateral epicondylitis[J]. J Orthop Res, 2018, 36（3）: 913-920.

[3] HASTIE G, SOUFI M, WILSON J, et al. Platelet rich plasma injections for lateral epicondylitis of the elbow reduce the need for surgical intervention[J]. J Orthop, 2018, 15（1）: 239-241.

[4] THANASAS C, PAPADIMITRIOU G, CHARALAMBIDIS C, et al. Platelet-rich plasma versus autologous whole blood for the treatment of chronic lateral elbow epicondylitis: a randomized controlled clinical trial[J]. Am J Sports Med, 2011, 39（10）: 2130-2134.

[5] ALESSIO-MAZZOLA M, REPETTO I, BITI B, et al. Autologous US-guided PRP injection versus US-guided focal extracorporeal shock wave therapy for chronic lateral

epicondylitis: a minimum of 2-year follow-up retrospective comparative study[J]. J Orthop Surg（Hong Kong）, 2018, 26（1）: 1-8.

[6] GOSENS T, PEERBOOMS J C, VAN LAAR W, et al. Ongoing positive effect of platelet-rich plasma versus corticosteroid injection in lateral epicondylitis: a double-blind randomized controlled trial with 2-year follow-up[J]. Am J Sports Med, 2011, 39（6）: 1200-1208.

[7] 董佩龙, 唐晓波, 王健, 等. 富血小板血浆局部注射治疗肱骨外上髁炎的疗效[J]. 中华关节外科杂志, 2018, 12（5）: 608-613.

[8] FARKASH U, AVISAR E, VOLK I, et al. First clinical experience with a new injectable recombinant human collagen scaffold combined with autologous platelet-rich plasma for the treatment of lateral epicondylar tendinopathy（tennis elbow）[J]. J Shoulder Elbow Surg, 2019, 28（3）: 503-509.

[9] XU Q L, CHEN J Y, CHENG L. Comparison of platelet rich plasma and corticosteroids in the management of lateral epicondylitis: a meta-analysis of randomized controlled trials[J]. International Journal of Surgery, 2019, 67（9）: 37-46.

[10] HUANG K, GIDDINS G, WU L D. Platelet-rich plasma versus corticosteroid injections in the management of elbow epicondylitis and plantar fasciitis: an updated systematic review and meta-analysis[J]. Am J Sports Med, 2020, 48（10）: 2572-2585.

[11] LE A D K, ENWEZE L, DEBAUN M R, et al. Current clinical recommendations for use of platelet-rich plasma[J]. Curr Rev Musculoskelet Med, 2018, 11（4）: 624-634.

[12] KROGH T P, FREDBERG U, STENGAARD-PEDERSEN K, et al. Treatment of lateral epicondylitis with platelet-rich plasma, glucocorticoid, or saline: a randomized, double-blind, placebo-controlled trial[J]. Am J Sports Med, 2013, 41（3）: 625-635.

[13] MONTALVAN B, LE GOUX P, KLOUCHE S, et al. Inefficacy of ultrasound-guided local injections of autologous conditioned plasma for recent epicondylitis: results of a double-blind placebo-controlled randomized clinical trial with one-year follow-up[J]. Rheumatology（Oxford）, 2016, 55（2）: 279-285.

[14] SCONFIENZA L M, ADRIAENSEN M, ALBANO D, et al. Clinical indications for image-guided interventional procedures in the musculoskeletal system: a Delphi-based consensus paper from the European Society of Musculoskeletal Radiology（ESSR）-Part Ⅱ, elbow and wrist[J]. Eur Radiol, 2020, 30（4）: 2220-2230.

[15] LINNANMAKI L, KANTO K, KARJALAINEN T, et al. Platelet-rich plasma or autologous blood do not reduce pain or improve function in patients with lateral epicondylitis: a randomized controlled trial[J]. Clin Orthop Relat Res, 2020, 478（8）: 1892-1900.

[16] CARLIER Y, BONICHON F, PEUCHANT A. Recalcitrant lateral epicondylitis：early results with a new technique combining ultrasonographic percutaneous tenotomy with platelet-rich plasma injection[J]. Orthop Traumatol Surg Res, 2021, 107（2）：185-191.

[17] ZHOU Y Q, ZHANG J Y, WU H S, et al. The differential effects of leukocyte-containing and pure platelet-rich plasma（PRP）on tendon stem/progenitor cells-implications of PRP application for the clinical treatment of tendon injuries[J]. Stem Cell Res Ther, 2015, 6（1）：173.

[18] CAIN E L J, DUGAS J R, WOLF R S, et al. Elbow injuries in throwing athletes：a current concepts review[J]. Am J Sports Med, 2003, 31（4）：621-635.

[19] FREEHILL M T, SAFRAN M R. Diagnosis and management of ulnar collateral ligament injuries in throwers[J]. Curr Sports Med Rep, 2011, 10（5）：271-278.

[20] CLARK N J, DESAI V S, DINES J D, et al. Nonreconstruction options for treating medial ulnar collateral ligament injuries of the elbow in overhead athletes[J]. Curr Rev Musculoskelet Med, 2018, 11（1）：48-54.

[21] LOPEZ-VIDRIERO E, GOULDING K A, SIMON D A, et al. The use of platelet-rich plasma in arthroscopy and sports medicine：optimizing the healing environment[J]. Arthroscopy, 2010, 26（2）：269-278.

[22] PODESTA L, CROW S A, VOLKMER D, et al. Treatment of partial ulnar collateral ligament tears in the elbow with platelet-rich plasma[J]. Am J Sports Med, 2013, 41（7）：1689-1694.

[23] DEAL J B, SMITH E, HEARD W, et al. Platelet-rich plasma for primary treatment of partial ulnar collateral ligament tears：MRI correlation with results[J]. Orthop J Sports Med, 2017, 5（11）：1-6.

[24] DINES J S, WILLIAMS P N, ELATTRACHE N, et al. Platelet-rich plasma can be used to successfully treat elbow ulnar collateral ligament insufficiency in high-level throwers[J]. Am J Orthop（Belle Mead NJ）, 2016, 45（5）：296-300.

[25] GORDON A H, DE LUIGI A J. Adolescent pitcher recovery from partial ulnar collateral ligament tear after platelet-rich plasma[J]. Curr Sports Med Rep, 2018, 17（12）：407-409.

[26] KATO Y, YAMADA S, CHAVEZ J. Can platelet-rich plasma therapy save patients with ulnar collateral ligament tears from surgery? [J]. Regen Ther, 2019, 10（1）：123-126.

[27] CHAUHAN A, MCQUEEN P, CHALMERS P N, et al. Nonoperative treatment of elbow ulnar collateral ligament injuries with and without platelet-rich plasma in professional baseball players：a comparative and matched cohort analysis[J]. Am J Sports Med, 2019, 47（13）：3107-3119.

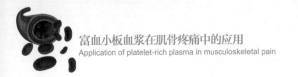
第三节　富血小板血浆在腕部和手部疼痛中的应用

富血小板血浆在腕部和手部疼痛中主要应用于腕部关节炎、狭窄性腱鞘炎和腕部骨折（桡骨远端、舟骨等的骨折）。

一、腕部关节炎

腕部关节炎包括第一腕掌关节炎（大多角掌骨关节炎/拇指基底部关节炎）、桡腕关节炎等疾病，是一种表现为腕掌部或拇指基底部疼痛的退行性疾病，常伴有掌骨关节半脱位或腕掌韧带松弛，严重时可影响手部功能及生活质量[1]。

1. 概述

腕掌关节炎是腕部和手部关节炎的常见类型，好发于第一腕掌关节，是一种渐进性致残疾病。影像学证据表明，第一腕掌关节炎的发病率高达25%～36%，其中1/3的患者存在临床症状。该病主要是由于腕掌关节半脱位导致掌骨内收，腕掌韧带松弛，掌指关节代偿性过伸，引起拇指"Z"字形外观改变[2]。

该病早期表现为第一腕掌关节肿胀、疼痛，随着疾病的发展，可出现骨关节膨大、活动受限、活动时伴有摩擦音，晚期可进展为持续性疼痛、关节畸形、活动严重受限。X线片的特征性改变为关节间隙变窄、关节边缘骨赘形成、软骨下骨硬化和囊性变[3]。临床上治疗腕掌关节炎的方法包括支具固定、药物治疗、物理治疗、局部注射及手术等。近年来随着技术的发展，PRP逐渐应用于骨关节炎疾病的治疗，并且获得了可靠的治疗效果。由于腕部骨骼的不规则性以及人们对腕部功能的高要求，手术及支具固定容易引起肌肉的萎缩、腕部功能的下降，因此探索可靠的临床治疗方法至关重要。

2. PRP在腕掌关节炎治疗中的临床研究

近年来关于PRP治疗腕掌关节炎的小样本研究在国内外逐渐开展，Medina-porqueres等[4]对1例腕掌关节炎进行了报道，该病例由于职业原因右手拇指根部慢性疼痛伴加重2年，伴随握力下降，被诊断为Ⅱ级腕掌关节炎。查体发现右手腕掌关节轻度积液，腕掌内侧压痛，内收活动范围受限，研磨试验及杠杆试验阳性。给予超声波、手法治疗、支具固定等保守治疗均未见明显好转。自体血浆制备后，将3mL PRP注射于腕掌关节内，一共注射3次，每次间隔1周。采用VAS评分、握力检测、Kapandji评分以及DASH评分客观评估治疗效果。结果显示该例患者未发生不良反应，治疗后6周报告疼痛明显减轻，日常活动相关的痛感消失。治疗后12个月患者恢复良好，拇指运动正常且无痛，握力恢复正常。Mayoly等[5]对3例桡腕关节炎患者进行微脂-PRP注射治疗，注射剂量为2.7~4mL。3例患者均未发生不良反应，注射3个月后3例患者的疼痛均减少一半以上，并且疼痛缓解的状况维持了1年左右。注射3个月后腕关节评分较治疗前明显改善，握力及关节活动度则未见明显变化。Markus等[6]对10例第一腕掌关节炎患者进行LP-PRP注射治疗，剂量为1~2mL，共注射2次，间隔4周。在治疗前及注射后3个月、6个月分别进行VAS评分、DASH评分、Mayo腕关节评分、握力及捏力测量。结果显示，注射后3个月、6个月与治疗前相比疼痛程度均明显下降，腕力均有改善，注射后6个月与治疗前相比握力明显增加。Malahias等[7]对33例第一腕掌关节炎患者进行前瞻性随机对照临床研究，试验组在超声引导下行PRP注射2次，对照组在超声引导下行皮质类固醇联合利多卡因注射2次，每次注射间隔2周。采用VAS评分

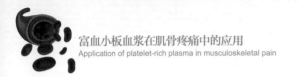

及DASH评分评估治疗效果，结果随访12个月后试验组VAS评分及DASH评分均优于对照组。

综合相关临床研究，PRP在腕掌关节炎的治疗上可获得持久疗效。但PRP在腕掌关节炎中的应用仍缺乏大样本、多中心的随机对照相关研究来进一步证实其治疗效果。

二、狭窄性腱鞘炎

狭窄性腱鞘炎（stenosing tenosynovitis，ST）是指因肌腱与腱鞘之间反复摩擦导致腱鞘肥厚狭窄引起的疾病[8]。

1. 概述

手部狭窄性腱鞘炎是常见的骨科疾病，根据发病位置可分为桡骨茎突腱鞘炎、指屈肌腱狭窄性腱鞘炎（扳机指）及尺侧腕伸肌腱狭窄性腱鞘炎。狭窄性腱鞘炎好发于女性及手工操作者，其中桡骨茎突腱鞘炎在女性中的发病率为1.3%，在男性中的发病率为0.5%[9]。该病是由于拇长展肌和拇短伸肌的肌腱反复持续拉伸，导致肌腱纤维化，其表面的伸肌支持带增厚，肌腱滑动时受阻，表现为在抓握、拇指外展时桡骨茎突疼痛发作[10]。扳机指的发病率为3%[11]，该病是屈肌腱与腱鞘的摩擦及两者之间的不平衡导致的慢性无菌性炎症。其临床表现为早期可触及手指根部结节，关节僵硬，随着病情进展可出现疼痛、手指屈伸活动受限、关节弹响[12]。目前狭窄性腱鞘炎在临床上常用的治疗方式为局部激素注射、夹板固定、小针刀松解术和手术。

2. PRP在狭窄性腱鞘炎治疗中的临床研究

Peck等[10]针对1例保守治疗、局部激素注射无效的桡骨茎突腱鞘炎患者，先进行开窗治疗，然后将3mL的PRP在超声引导下注射于拇长展肌与拇短伸肌之间。患者在治疗后3个月疼痛程度较治疗前减轻了74%，治疗后6个月疼痛程度减轻了36%。该文献报道表明，对保守治疗无效的腱鞘炎患者行超声引导下开窗联合PRP治疗，可有效缓解疼痛至少6个月。国内也有研究者报道，针对1例指屈肌腱腱鞘炎患者进行了PRP治疗[13]。该患者为47岁女性，长期从事家务劳动，因右手中指疼痛伴活动受限1个月就诊。查体发现右手中指掌指关节屈曲15°，主动屈曲障碍，屈曲后弹回困难，诊断为指屈肌腱腱鞘炎。患者入院后给予掌指关节间PRP注射，治疗后1周随访，患者疼痛明显减轻，但关节活动度无明显改善。治疗后10天疼痛基本消失，活动受限轻度改善，治疗后3个月手指无疼痛，活动自如。以上研究仅为单个病例报道，缺乏PRP治疗对腱鞘炎的随机对照临床试验研究。最近，Samuli Aspinen等[14]发表了一篇临床研究方案，对扳机指患者进行前瞻性、三盲、随机对照临床试验，未来该研究的结果可能会为PRP治疗扳机指的临床疗效提供一定的临床证据。为了增加PRP治疗狭窄性腱鞘炎的临床证据等级，需要更多的临床研究及基础研究进一步探讨PRP对该病的治疗效果及相关副作用。

三、腕部骨折

腕部骨折在临床上较为常见，多继发于手腕部外力撞击，包括桡骨远端骨折、舟骨骨折等。

1. 概述

由于腕部的位置特殊、骨折后易发生移位且稳定性差，因此腕部骨折愈合的时间较长。骨折不愈合或延迟愈合是腕部骨折的常见并发症，常见于桡骨远端骨折和舟骨骨折。桡骨远端骨折发生率占外科骨折的16%。舟骨位于腕部外侧，为形状不规则骨，腕部受到冲击后最先受累，舟骨骨折

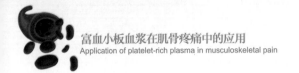
治疗后不愈合的发生率达10%[15]。骨折不愈合或延迟愈合可导致腕关节持续性疼痛、活动障碍及手功能下降。目前临床上常用的治疗方式为夹板、支具外固定及手术。

2. PRP在腕部骨折治疗中的临床研究

腕部骨折后长期固定会导致手部肌肉萎缩、关节僵硬及手功能下降。早期使用促进骨折愈合的保守治疗方式可在一定程度上避免出现长期固定的并发症。PRP中富含生长因子，已被证明可促进肌腱的愈合。近年来，PRP也被应用到促进骨折愈合的研究当中。Namazi[16]将30例桡骨远端骨折患者随机分为两组，对照组进行手术内固定治疗，试验组将自体3～5mL PRP注入腕关节内。两组在治疗后均进行6周的石膏固定。评估患者治疗前后的腕部评分（PRWE）、腕关节活动度、疼痛评分及日常活动能力，试验组注射PRP后3个月和6个月，腕部疼痛及日常活动能力均明显优于对照组，但关节活动度在3个月后只在腕关节屈伸方面有一定程度的改善，其余关节活动度两组之间无显著性差异。除桡骨远端骨折外，该研究者也对舟骨骨折进行了PRP的临床研究。其将14名骨折发生时间少于7天的急性腕舟骨骨折患者随机分为两组，试验组采用自体PRP制品1.5mL进行腕关节注射，对照组采用1.5mL生理盐水进行腕关节注射。注射后石膏固定2个月。通过X线、CT、腕部评估问卷及VAS评分评估患者的骨折愈合情况。分别在治疗后3个月、6个月进行随访。该研究的整个过程无局部或全身并发症的发生。研究发现，与对照组相比，试验组的疼痛程度和腕部功能评分显著改善，治疗后6个月腕关节尺骨偏斜显著改善，而其他腕关节运动（包括桡骨和尺骨的屈曲与伸展）未发现显著性差异。该研究表明PRP治疗可以更快地促进腕舟骨的愈合[17]。

虽然PRP在股骨骨折等相关研究中证明可通过促进新骨形成、改善生物力学作用而促进骨折愈合[18-19]，但PRP在腕部骨折方面的应用需要更多的临床及基础研究来探讨疗效及相关副作用。

（马海云）

参考文献

[1] LIAO J C, CHONG A K, TAN D M. Causes and assessment of subacute and chronic wrist pain[J]. Singapore Med J, 2013, 54（10）: 592-597.

[2] 田文，杨勇. 第一腕掌关节骨关节炎的治疗策略[J]. 中国骨与关节杂志，2020，9（11）: 803-805.

[3] 王晓南，韩宝平，李津，等. 拇指腕掌关节炎治疗进展[J]. 中国矫形外科杂志，2014，22（8）: 727-729.

[4] MEDINA-PORQUERES I, MARTIN-GARCIA P, SANZ-DE DIEGO S, et al. Platelet-rich plasma for thumb carpometacarpal joint osteoarthritis in a professional pianist: case-based review[J]. Rheumatol Int, 2019, 39（12）: 2167-2175.

[5] MAYOLY A, INIESTA A, CURVALE C, et al. Development of autologous platelet-rich plasma mixed-microfat as an advanced therapy medicinal product for intra-articular injection of radio-carpal osteoarthritis: from validation data to preliminary clinical results[J]. Int J Mol Sci, 2019, 20（5）: 1-13.

[6] LOIBL M, LANG S, DENDL L M, et al. Leukocyte-reduced platelet-rich plasma treatment of basal: a pilot study[J]. BioMed Research International, 2016（4）: 1-6.

[7] MALAHIAS M A, ROUMELIOTIS L, NIKOLAOU V S, et al. Platelet-rich plasma versus corticosteroid intra-articular injections for the treatment of trapeziometacarpal arthritis: a prospective randomized controlled clinical trial[J]. Cartilage, 2021, 12（1）: 51-61.

[8] DAY C S, WU W K, SMITH C C. Examination of the hand and wrist[J]. The New England journal of medicine, 2019, 380（12）: e15.

[9] ALLBROOK V. 'The side of my wrist hurts': De Quervain's tenosynovitis[J]. Australian journal of general practice, 2019, 48（11）: 753-756.

[10] PECK E, ELY E. Successful treatment of de Quervain tenosynovitis with ultrasound-guided percutaneous needle tenotomy and platelet-rich plasma injection: a case presentation[J]. PM & R: the journal of injury, function, and rehabilitation, 2013, 5（5）: 438-441.

[11] FIORINI H J, TAMAOKI M J, LENZA M, et al. Surgery for trigger finger[J/OL]. The Cochrane database of systematic reviews, 2018, 2（2）: CD009860. https://doi. org/10. 1002/14651858. CD009860. pub2.

[12] DAVID M, RANGARAJU M, RAINE A. Acquired triggering of the fingers and thumb in adults[J/OL]. BMJ（Clinical research ed）, 2017, 359: j5285. https://doi. org/10. 1136/bmj. j5285.

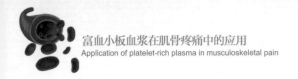
[13] 邱陈梅. 1例右手中指屈肌腱鞘炎患者采用PRP疗法效果观察[J]. 健康必读，2018
（23）：214.

[14] ASPINEN S, NORDBACK P H, ANTTILA T, et al. Platelet-rich plasma versus
corticosteroid injection for treatment of trigger finger：study protocol for a prospective
randomized triple-blind placebo-controlled trial[J]. Trials, 2020, 21（1）：984.

[15] PINDER R M, BRKLJAC M, RIX L, et al. Treatment of scaphoid nonunion：a
systematic review of the existing evidence[J]. The Journal of hand surgery, 2015, 40
（9）：1797-1805, e3.

[16] NAMAZI H, MEHBUDI A. Investigating the effect of intra-articular PRP injection on
pain and function improvement in patients with distal radius fracture[J]. Orthopaedics &
Traumatology：Surgery & Research, 2016, 102（1）：47-52.

[17] NAMAZI H, KAYEDI T. Investigating the effect of intra-articular platelet-rich plasma
injection on union：pain and function improvement in patients with scaphoid fracture[J].
J Hand Microsurg, 2016, 8（3）：140-144.

[18] GUZEL Y, KARALEZLI N, BILGE O, et al. The biomechanical and histological
effects of platelet-rich plasma on fracture healing[J]. Knee Surg Sports Traumatol
Arthrosc, 2015, 23（5）：1378-1383.

[19] SIMMAN R, HOFFMANN A, BOHINC R J, et al. Role of platelet-rich plasma in
acceleration of bone fracture healing[J]. Ann Plast Surg, 2008, 61（3）：337-344.

第四节　富血小板血浆在髋部疾病中的应用

富血小板血浆在髋部疾病中主要应用于髋骨性关节炎和股骨头无菌性
坏死。

一、髋骨性关节炎

髋骨性关节炎是指由于多种因素（肥胖、既往创伤、感染、先天畸形
等）导致的，以慢性、进行性髋部软骨变性和软骨下及关节周围新骨赘形
成为主要特点的退行性疾病[1]。

1. 概述

髋骨性关节炎起病隐袭，进展通常缓慢，表现为髋关节疼痛、僵硬、功能障碍逐渐加重，多见于中老年人群。主要症状包括活动或承重时步态异常和髋部疼痛，体格检查可见患髋屈曲、外旋和内收等畸形，患髋关节前方压痛伴活动受限、跛行步态，患肢可有短缩[2]。X线检查通常表现为关节间隙变窄、骨质增生等。目前髋骨性关节炎的主要治疗策略为减轻疼痛、改善关节功能，治疗方法包括非手术治疗和手术治疗，前者包括药物治疗、物理治疗和关节腔注射治疗（皮质类固醇、透明质酸）等，后者包括髋关节镜治疗、半髋关节/全髋关节置换术等[3-4]。

PRP关节腔注射治疗作为一种生物治疗方法，具有安全、简便、患者耐受性较好且无免疫排斥等优势，有助于促进软骨细胞增殖及细胞外基质合成，为关节修复提供较理想的微环境[5-7]。考虑到髋关节的解剖结构及患者的耐受程度，既往研究认为，9mL是单侧髋关节腔注射的上限推荐剂量[8]。近年来，国内外学者对PRP治疗髋骨性关节炎的疗效及安全性进行了初步探索。

2. PRP治疗髋骨性关节炎的临床研究进展

目前，PRP关节腔注射疗法的临床应用在下肢主要集中于膝骨关节炎。相比较而言，PRP在髋骨性关节炎治疗方面的循证医学依据尚显不足，尤其是高质量、大样本的随机对照试验研究较少[9-10]。2016年，Dallari等比较了超声引导下关节腔注射自体PRP（$n=44$）、透明质酸（hyaluronic acid，HA）（$n=36$）及PRP与HA联合注射（$n=31$）对髋骨性关节炎的临床疗效。患者纳入标准为基线VAS>2分（以10分为标准），患者年龄范围为18～65岁，并排除了大范围手术、过度关节畸形患者，以及合并风湿性疾病、感染性疾病、心血管或免疫系统疾病患者。各组注射方案统一为超声引导下每周注射1次，连续注射3周。主要观察指标包括治疗后2个月、6个月和12个月的VAS评分，次要指标包括Harris髋关节评分、WOMAC评分、PRP中生长因子浓度及其与临床预后的相关性。研究结果发现，随访期间PRP组患者VAS评分最低，随访至6个月时3组VAS评分分别为PRP组21分、HA组44分、联合注射组35分，且PRP中白细胞介素-10（interleukin-10，IL-10）含量与VAS评分变化呈中度相关性（$r=0.392$，$P=0.04$）。本研究证实了超声引导下PRP注射治疗髋骨性关节炎的有效性和安全性，且PRP与HA联合注射并无改善疼痛症状的额外获益[10]。

Sanchez等在更早期的非对照、前瞻性临床研究中纳入了40例髋骨性关节炎患者，随访至治疗后7周及治疗后6个月，VAS评分、WOMAC和Harris疼痛分量表评分均显著改善（$P<0.05$）[11]。2018年，Ali等对超声引导下PRP注射治疗髋骨性关节炎的临床研究现状进行了系统综述，共纳入3项高质量RCT研究、累计254例患者，结论认为PRP注射作为一种安全、高效的治疗方法，在较长期随访中（12个月）有效改善了患者的髋关节疼痛和功能障碍，不良反应较少见[12]。

3. PRP治疗髋骨性关节炎的基础研究进展

PRP治疗髋骨性关节炎相关动物模型的基础研究鲜见报道，既往研究更多集中于探讨PRP对体外培养的软骨细胞和组织在增殖、凋亡及细胞外基质分泌等方面的影响，与膝骨关节炎的基础研究存在共性。一般认为，白细胞浓度较高的富白细胞PRP（LR-PRP）通过多种细胞因子相关的分解代谢途径，可能诱发更多的不良反应；而白细胞浓度较低的贫白细胞PRP（LP-PRP）有助于调节炎症因子，从而更好地发挥刺激软骨细胞增殖和促进合成代谢的作用[13]。在关节炎疾病模型中，PRP不仅影响局部细胞和浸润细胞（主要成分为滑膜细胞和巨噬细胞），还作用于内皮细胞、免疫细胞及通路下游的软骨细胞和骨细胞[14]。值得注意的是，临床上关节炎组织的微环境因患者自身特点和疾病分期而异，且PRP疗效差异与关节内的特殊微环境密切相关，因此动物及体外细胞实验结论的推广仍需谨慎。

二、股骨头缺血性坏死

股骨头缺血性坏死又称股骨头坏死（osteonecrosis of the femoral head，ONFH），是股骨头静脉瘀滞、动脉血供受损或中断造成骨细胞及骨髓成分部分死亡，引起骨组织坏死并随后发生修复，导致股骨头结构改变及塌陷引起的髋关节疼痛及功能障碍[15]。

1. 概述

ONFH可分为创伤性和非创伤性两大类。在我国非创伤性ONFH的主要病因为应用皮质类固醇类药物、长期过量饮酒、自身免疫病等。ONFH的临床表现以髋部、臀部或腹股沟区疼痛为主，偶尔伴有膝关节疼痛，髋关节活动度受限（以内旋为主），MRI检查对ONFH的诊断具有较高敏感性。目前临床上对ONFH的治疗包括保护性负重、药物治疗（针对特定病因，建议选用抗凝剂，增加纤溶、扩张血管与降脂药物）、物理治疗（体外冲击波、高压氧等）及手术等[15-16]。

由于PRP成分多样、各组分间相互作用复杂，因此目前其治疗ONFH的作用机制尚在探索阶段，既往研究在促进组织修复、促进细胞增殖、诱导血管新生、调节细胞凋亡、缓解炎症反应等方面已有部分进展，但详细机制仍需进一步阐明[17]。

2. PRP治疗股骨头坏死的临床研究进展

目前，国内外有关PRP注射治疗ONFH的临床研究仍处于探索阶段，且多以个案或小样本形式报道。Jaewoo等报道了运用脂肪来源干细胞和PRP等联合治疗早期ONFH的个案：在超声引导下将含脂肪来源干细胞、

PRP、透明质酸的混合物注入发生病变的髋部，注射方案为每周1次，连续4周，在治疗后3个月、18个月、21个月分别进行连续MRI扫描、Harris髋关节评分、关节活动度（ROM）评估。结果显示患髋在治疗后3个月的疼痛评分、ROM和MRI表现均明显改善，且治疗后18个月和21个月的影像学随访结果示髋关节坏死完全治愈[18]。本病例虽然是早期ONFH治愈的个案，但对PRP治疗ONFH的临床应用具有重要意义。

Guadilla、Ibrahim等报道，经关节镜或超声引导下髋关节腔内PRP注射治疗后（个案），患髋疼痛缓解，运动功能及步行能力均有不同程度的改善，注射前后MRI评估证实坏死局部存在骨皮质增厚及股骨头重构等表现，随访1年疗效满意[19-20]。

2020年，中山大学孙逸仙纪念医院康复医学科团队报道了超声引导下髋关节腔PRP注射改善青少年ONFH国际骨微循环研究协会（ARCO）分期Ⅳ期的临床个案：患者16岁，女性，基线评估示VAS评分为7分/10分，双髋ROM明显受限，Harris髋关节评分为29分，WOMAC评分为59分，不能耐受长时间坐、站立及步行，MRI示双侧股骨头塌陷并有双侧髋关节间隙狭窄、关节腔大量积液。经PRP注射（每侧4.5mL，每周治疗1次，连续治疗5次）并配合常规康复治疗9个月后随访，患者VAS评分为3分，双髋ROM改善，Harris髋关节评分为64分，WOMAC评分为15分，且能耐受长时间坐、站立及短距离步行，复查MRI结果示双侧塌陷较前改善，积液明显减少，骨坏死体积减小，双侧关节间隙较前增大[21]。

2021年年初，中山大学孙逸仙纪念医院康复医学科团队回顾分析了2019年6月至2020年6月接受超声引导下髋关节腔PRP注射的29例股骨头坏死患者的临床特征和疗效，患者均接受4次注射，每次注射间隔1周。分别在治疗前和治疗后1个月、3个月、6个月时进行VAS评分、WOMAC评分、Harris髋关节评分等疗效评估和不良反应记录。结果显示，各指标在治疗后均有显著改善，且随访期间无不良反应报告。该研究初步证实超声引导下髋关节腔PRP注射能安全有效地缓解股骨头坏死患者的疼痛程度，改善髋关节功能，且效果持续至少6个月[22]。

2022年，笔者团队设计并发表了一项临床随机对照试验，证实每周1次、连续4周的体外冲击波治疗（ESWT）和超声引导下PRP治疗均能有效改善非创伤性ARCO Ⅰ～Ⅲ期ONFH患者的疼痛和功能障碍。试验结果显示，自治疗后3个月起，VAS评分、压力疼痛阈值（pressure pain threshold，PPT）、WOMAC评分、Harris评分随时间变化的组别效应有统计学差异（$P<0.05$，12个月随访PPT除外）。与ESWT组相比，随访至治疗后12个月即研究终点时PRP组患者的各项指标改善更显著，具体结果为：VAS评分平均差值=−0.82，95%CI [−1.39，−0.25]，$P=0.005$；WOMAC评分平均差值=−4.19，95%CI [−7.00，−1.37]，$P=0.004$；Harris评分平均差值=5.28，95%CI [1.94，8.62]，$P=0.002$。两组受试者在治疗及随访期间均未报告相关不良反应。由此得出结论，ESWT治疗和PRP治疗均有助于改善ONFH患者症状，超声引导下PRP注射在缓解疼痛和改善关节功能方面优于传统的保守物理疗法ESWT[23]。

PRP治疗ONFH的临床研究目前虽积累了部分证据，但针对不同分期ONFH患者疗效差异的观察研究尚且不足，尤其缺乏设计严谨、高质量的循证医学证据。此外，目前PRP制备、激活和储存方法尚未统一，LP-PRP与LR-PRP对ONFH的疗效比较研究尚未见报道，且未有公认疗效最佳的治疗浓度和剂量推荐，因此仍需要大样本RCT研究进一步验证。

3. PRP治疗股骨头坏死的基础研究进展

Tong等通过研究基于糖皮质激素诱导的小鼠ONFH模型发现，PRP有助于改善模型的组织学和关节炎评分，PRP处理后ONFH小鼠组织中IL-17a、IL-1β、肿瘤坏死因子-α、κB受体激活因子、IL-6、干扰素-γ表达下

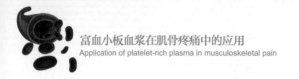

调；此外，PRP治疗后肝细胞生长因子、细胞间黏附分子-1、骨桥蛋白、血小板来源内皮细胞生长因子、血管内皮生长因子、血小板来源生长因子、胰岛素样生长因子-I和转化生长因子-β表达水平均升高[24]。

2017年，张长青团队报道ONFH模型大鼠通过尾静脉注射人PRP来源外泌体（PRP-Exos）可有效减轻骨坏死组织学及影像学表现，研究发现PRP-Exos在糖皮质激素诱导的内质网应激情况下，通过Akt/Bad/Bcl-2信号通路促进Bcl-2表达，具有预防ONFH模型大鼠细胞凋亡的潜能，从而可有效促进组织修复[25]。胡钟旭等在PRP联合骨髓间充质干细胞（bone marrow stem cells，BMSCs）治疗兔ONFH的研究中发现，PRP可促进BMSCs增殖，其机制可能与促进血管内皮生长因子及转化生长因子等关键生长因子的分泌有关[26]。中山大学孙逸仙纪念医院康复医学科团队在前期基础细胞实验中发现，PRP可以使大剂量地塞米松诱导的骨髓间充质干细胞的成骨分化、迁移、增殖能力改善，并且可以抑制其凋亡。进一步的动物实验发现，关节腔注射PRP联合人脐带间充质干细胞能在一定程度上延缓激素性股骨头坏死模型大鼠骨坏死的出现，其机制可能与促进血管内皮生长因子及Runt相关转录因子等与骨生成和血管生成相关因子表达上调、改善股骨头细胞凋亡情况有关。

目前PRP治疗ONFH在动物实验研究方面取得了初步进展，证实PRP可通过旁分泌、表观遗传学修饰等多种方式修复受损组织，且与磷酸三钙（TCP）、BMSCs等联合运用的协同作用研究也取得了阶段性进展。但因为动物模型限制等因素，几乎没有涉及较远期疗效的基础研究，动物实验的潜在临床转化价值仍有待进一步探讨。

结语：综上所述，髋骨性关节炎和ONFH都是制约患者运动功能、影响生活质量的重要因素，而目前常用的非手术、手术治疗手段均存在一定局限性，难以达到满意效果。如何进一步改善髋关节疾患的临床疗效是临床医生面临的重大挑战。现有研究证实，PRP关节腔注射有望改善患者疼痛症状，最大限度保留髋关节运动功能，而更远期疗效及相关机制日后仍需要更多前瞻性、大样本的高质量临床研究进一步完善、证实。

（余少君　栾烁　汪衍雪）

参考文献

[1] LEECH R D, EYLES J, BATT M E, et al. Lower extremity osteoarthritis: optimising musculoskeletal health is a growing global concern: a narrative review[J]. Br J Sports Med, 2019, 53（13）: 806-811.

[2] PRIETO-ALHAMBRA D, JUDGE A, JAVAID M K, et al. Incidence and risk factors for clinically diagnosed knee, hip and hand osteoarthritis: influences of age, gender and osteoarthritis affecting other joints[J]. Ann Rheum Dis, 2014, 73（9）: 1659-1664.

[3] QUINN R H, MURRAY J, PEZOLD R. Management of osteoarthritis of the hip[J]. J Am Acad Orthop Surg, 2018, 26（20）: e434-e436.

[4] REES H W, BARBA M. AAOS clinical practice guideline: management of osteoarthritis of the hip[J]. J Am Acad Orthop Surg, 2020, 28（7）: e292-e294.

[5] CHAHLA J, LAPRADE R F, MARDONES R, et al. Biological therapies for cartilage lesions in the hip: a new horizon[J]. Orthopedics, 2016, 39（4）: e715-e723.

[6] EVERTS P, ONISHI K, JAYARAM P, et al. Platelet-rich plasma: new performance understandings and therapeutic considerations in 2020[J]. Int J Mol Sci, 2020, 21（7794）: 1-36.

[7] BENNELL K L, HUNTER D J, PATERSON K L. Platelet-rich plasma for the management of hip and knee osteoarthritis[J]. Curr Rheumatol Rep, 2017, 19（5/6）: 24-34.

[8] YOUNG R, HARDING J, KINGSLY A, et al. Therapeutic hip injections: is the injection volume important?[J]. Clin Radiol, 2012, 67（1）: 55-60.

[9] BATTAGLIA M, GUARALDI F, VANNINI F, et al. Platelet-rich plasma（PRP）intra-articular ultrasound-guided injections as a possible treatment for hip osteoarthritis: a pilot study[J]. Clin Exp Rheumatol, 2011, 29（4）: 754.

[10] DALLARI D, STAGNI C, RANI N, et al. Ultrasound-guided injection of platelet-rich plasma and hyaluronic acid, separately and in combination, for hip osteoarthritis: a randomized controlled study[J]. Am J Sports Med, 2016, 44（3）: 664-671.

[11] SANCHEZ M, GUADILLA J, FIZ N, et al. Ultrasound-guided platelet-rich plasma injections for the treatment of osteoarthritis of the hip[J]. Rheumatology（Oxford）, 2012, 51（1）: 144-150.

[12] ALI M, MOHAMED A, AHMED H E, et al. The use of ultrasound-guided platelet-rich plasma injections in the treatment of hip osteoarthritis: a systematic review of the literature[J]. J Ultrason, 2018, 18（75）: 332-337.

[13] CAVALLO C, FILARDO G, MARIANI E, et al. Comparison of platelet-rich plasma formulations for cartilage healing: an in vitro study[J]. J Bone Joint Surg Am, 2014, 96（5）: 423-429.

[14] ANDIA I, MAFFULLI N. Platelet-rich plasma for managing pain and inflammation in osteoarthritis[J]. Nat Rev Rheumatol, 2013, 9（12）: 721-730.

[15] 中国医师协会骨科医师分会骨循环与骨坏死专业委员会, 中华医学会骨科分会骨显微修复学组, 国际骨循环学会中国区. 中国成人股骨头坏死临床诊疗指南（2020）[J]. 中华骨科杂志, 2020, 40（20）: 1365-1376.

[16] 曾祥洪, 梁博伟. 股骨头坏死保髋治疗的新策略[J]. 中国组织工程研究, 2021, 25（3）: 431-437.

[17] 郭海, 刘予豪, 姜山, 等. 富血小板血浆应用于早期非创伤性股骨头坏死的研究进展[J]. 中华关节外科杂志（电子版）, 2017, 11（6）: 651-654.

[18] PAK J, LEE J H, JEON J H, et al. Complete resolution of avascular necrosis of the human femoral head treated with adipose tissue-derived stem cells and platelet-rich plasma[J]. J Int Med Res, 2014, 42（6）: 1353-1362.

[19] GUADILLA J, FIZ N, ANDIA I, et al. Arthroscopic management and platelet-rich plasma therapy for avascular necrosis of the hip[J]. Knee Surg Sports Traumatol Arthrosc, 2012, 20（2）: 393-398.

[20] IBRAHIM V, DOWLING H. Platelet-rich plasma as a nonsurgical treatment option for osteonecrosis[J]. PM & R, 2012, 4（12）: 1015-1019.

[21] LUAN S, LIU C C, LIN C N, et al. Platelet-rich plasma for the treatment of adolescent late-stage femoral head necrosis: a case report[J]. Regen Med, 2020, 15（9）: 2067-2073.

[22] 王少玲, 栾烁, 范胜诺, 等. 超声引导髋关节腔富血小板血浆注射对股骨头坏死的疗效分析[J]. 华西医学, 2021, 36（5）: 617-622.

[23] LUAN S, WANG S L, LIN C N, et al. Comparisons of ultrasound-guided platelet-rich plasma intra-articular injection and extracorporeal shock wave therapy in treating ARCO Ⅰ-Ⅲ symptomatic non-traumatic femoral head necrosis: a randomized controlled clinical trial[J]. J Pain Res, 2022, 15: 341-354.

[24] TONG S C, YIN J M, LIU J. Platelet-rich plasma has beneficial effects in mice with osteonecrosis of the femoral head by promoting angiogenesis[J]. Exp Ther Med, 2018, 15（2）: 1781-1788.

[25] TAO S C, YUAN T, RUI B Y, et al. Exosomes derived from human platelet-rich plasma prevent apoptosis induced by glucocorticoid-associated endoplasmic reticulum

stress in rat osteonecrosis of the femoral head via the Akt/Bad/Bcl-2 signal pathway[J]. Theranostics, 2017, 7（3）: 733-750.

[26] 胡钟旭, 李东卿, 李贵涛, 等. 富血小板血浆联合骨髓间充质干细胞治疗家兔股骨头缺血坏死的研究[J]. 中华损伤与修复杂志（电子版）, 2014, 9（1）: 22-26.

第五节　富血小板血浆在膝部疾病中的应用

富血小板血浆（PRP）在膝部疾病中的临床应用涉及膝骨关节炎（knee osteoarthritis, KOA）、髌腱病（patellar tendinopathy, PT）、半月板损伤、前交叉韧带损伤及内侧副韧带损伤等。尽管PRP促进软骨、骨、肌腱、韧带等不同组织修复和再生的途径各有不同，但损伤组织对血液供应和生长因子信号通路的需求趋向是基本一致的。

一、膝骨关节炎

1. 概述

膝骨关节炎（KOA）是一种好发于中老年人群的退行性病变。流行病学数据显示，我国症状性KOA患病率高达8.1%。KOA患者常见的临床表现包括膝关节疼痛、屈伸活动受限、肿胀畸形及肌肉萎缩等，这种渐进的软骨组织破坏和关节功能恶化与关节软骨的再生潜力下降密切相关[1-2]。近年来，PRP注射作为一种较新的促进组织修复和镇痛的治疗方法，已被证实能够刺激软骨细胞和骨间充质干细胞增殖，促进软骨细胞外基质分泌，降低促炎细胞因子的分解代谢[3]。肌肉骨骼超声引导作为一种可实时、动态成像的方法，具有精准、安全、经济等优势，现已成为KOA注射治疗的常用辅助手段[4]。

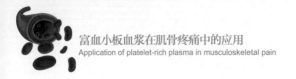

2. PRP治疗膝骨关节炎的临床研究进展

截至2016年的统计，全美范围内PRP在关节软骨损伤和半月板损伤疾病中的应用远超其在肌腱、韧带和关节唇损伤中的应用，其中尤以PRP治疗KOA的基础及临床研究最多[5]。2008年第一篇高质量关节腔PRP注射治疗KOA的回顾性队列研究问世[6]，自此PRP在KOA临床治疗中的应用日益广泛。既往研究发现，贫白细胞PRP（LP-PRP）较富白细胞PRP（LR-PRP）更加适用于KOA关节腔注射治疗——前者有助于减少炎症级联反应的关键调节因子和炎症相关酶的表达，在抑制炎症反应的同时可改善受损结构的代谢能力，诱导再生，对软骨形成和间充质干细胞的增殖、迁移、分化等有积极作用[7]。

为了进一步规范我国关节腔PRP注射治疗KOA的临床实践，中国医疗保健国际交流促进会骨科分会基于当前最佳证据，制定了《关节腔注射富血小板血浆治疗膝骨关节炎的临床实践指南（2018年版）》，提出6条推荐意见：①在治疗KOA方面，关节腔注射PRP可以缓解关节疼痛（2B）、改善膝关节功能（2B）、提高患者的满意率（2C）；②针对KOA患者，关节腔注射PRP不会增加不良事件发生率，如感染、局部红肿疼痛等（1A）；③关节腔注射PRP更适用于年轻、严重程度轻的KOA患者（2C）；④为提高疗效，多次注射PRP可能会更好地缓解疼痛、改善关节功能（2D），且不会增加不良事件的发生率（2C），若多次注射PRP，建议间隔时间不少于1周，注射次数不少于2次（2C）；⑤伴有关节腔积液的KOA患者可以接受关节腔注射PRP治疗（2C），治疗前建议对量多的积液进行抽吸（2C）；⑥临床决策时，建议同时考虑成本-效益因素、患者的价值观与偏好、医生的经验等（2D）[8]。

迄今为止，已有多项国内外荟萃分析评价了PRP治疗KOA的临床疗效及安全性[9-10]。2016年，Riboh等对6项RCT和3项前瞻性比较试验进行了网络荟萃分析，共纳入1055例患者，结果发现富白细胞PRP和贫白细胞PRP的治疗均可导致终点随访时间点WOMAC平均得分降低，但与安慰剂和透明质酸相比，只有贫白细胞PRP组WOMAC评分显著降低[11]。Dai等研究发现，以12个月的随访为终点，PRP治疗组与单独使用透明质酸组相比，疼痛评分和功能评分分别降低2.83分、12.53分，均超过MCID阈值，而在较短的随访时间内（如6个月）并没有发现上述显著变化[10]。2017年，Shen等在一项纳入4项RCT、共计1423位患者的RCT研究中发现，和对照组相比，即使在较短的随访时间内（如3个月、6个月）PRP治疗组的WOMAC评分改善也呈现出显著性差异[12]。需要强调的是，上述两项荟萃分析均报告了其结果的显著异质性。

中山大学孙逸仙纪念医院康复医学科团队于2020年发表了一项临床回顾性研究，分析了超声引导下PRP注射对不同严重程度KOA的疗效及疗效差异，受试者依据Kellgren-Lawrence（K-L）分级标准分为0、Ⅰ、Ⅱ、Ⅲ、Ⅳ级组，各组患者均接受4次PRP关节腔注射治疗，注射间期为1周，并分别于治疗前、治疗后3个月、治疗后6个月完成VAS评分、WOMAC评分的疗效评估和不良反应评价。结果显示：Ⅰ、Ⅱ、Ⅲ级组患者VAS评分和WOMAC评分均随时间变化而明显改善（$P<0.001$）；各组治疗后3个月、6个月与治疗前相比，VAS评分、WOMAC评分均改善明显（$P<0.05$）；Ⅰ级组治疗后3个月、6个月的WOMAC评分比较，差异无统计学意义（$P>0.05$），但Ⅱ、Ⅲ级组治疗后3个月的WOMAC评分均优于治疗后6个月（$P<0.05$），Ⅳ级组患者随访至治疗后3个月、6个月时，VAS评分和WOMAC评分均无明显变化（$P>0.05$），提示超声引导下关节腔注射PRP可有效缓解轻、中度KOA疼痛，改善患者功能障碍[13]。

综上所述，基于对目前大多数RCT研究等循证学依据可得出结论，关节腔内PRP注射是KOA的安全、有效治疗方法[14-15]。不同研究结论存在

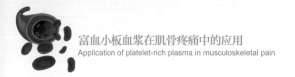
的潜在差异可能与研究设计不同、PRP制备标准不统一、注射次数不同及随访时间不同等异质性因素有关。

3. PRP治疗膝骨关节炎的基础研究进展

PRP包含多种生长因子，可在复杂多样的化学介质环境中发挥作用，与关节内各种内源性细胞及组织成分相互影响。PRP在KOA体外细胞实验和动物模型中均被证实有良好效果，研究还认为PRP激活后持续释放的多种生长因子可能是改善KOA症状和预后的关键因素。此外，局部炎症调节因子可能具有保护软骨细胞、促进软骨愈合和减轻关节内炎症的作用。在分子水平上的体外研究发现，PRP的应用可刺激软骨细胞和滑膜细胞产生软骨基质，同时下调作为炎症反应介质的关键分子，如IL-1和TNF-α等[3, 16]。但各项研究中PRP的制备方法不统一、血小板及细胞因子含量报告不详细等因素容易造成研究结论偏倚。

2020年，Hahn等呼吁标准化PRP生长因子浓度、应用频率等关键因素，他们认为这是基础研究质量控制的前提，因此他们探讨应用特殊制备的标准化PRP冻干粉末、基于不同PRP浓度（0.5%、1%、5%）和刺激频率（2×、3×、6×）对人原代软骨细胞体外增殖、细胞活性以及细胞外基质（Ⅰ型/Ⅱ型前胶原蛋白、硫酸蛋白聚糖和糖胺聚糖）合成的影响，该研究报告了用于细胞培养的PRP原液蛋白定量浓度和生长因子浓度［VEGF（379.3pg/mL），TGF-β1（78 048.0pg/mL），PDGF（3 395.8pg/mL），FGF（30.1pg/mL），IGF-Ⅰ（591.9pg/mL）］[17]。需指出的是，该研究应用的PRP粉末类似于国际分类中的贫白细胞PRP（LP-PRP），且在人为控制的体外环境中，难以模拟KOA关节内部软骨细胞、滑膜细胞、关节液炎症因子综合作用下的复杂病理机制。

二、髌腱病

髌腱病（patellar tendinopathy，PT），俗称"跳跃膝"，是运动员膝关节前部疼痛的常见原因，约占所有运动相关损伤的14.2%，顾名思义该病是由于重复的跳跃运动及其他类似的动作导致髌腱负荷增加而造成的。

1. 概述

PT在职业运动员和业余运动员中都很常见，特别是从事排球、篮球等对髌腱要求比较高的运动的运动员。除运动种类外，髌骨形状、运动员年龄等内在风险因素以及高强度比赛、训练时间过长、动作失误等外在风险因素均是运动员易患PT的关键因素[18]。流行病学调查显示，患者症状的平均持续时间超过2年，严重者症状可以持续15年以上，超过50%患髌腱病的运动员因膝关节疼痛而终止运动生涯[19]。

既往常用的髌腱病保守治疗方案包括股四头肌强化训练、低强度冲击波治疗和皮质类固醇注射等[20]。近年来，PRP对髌腱病的治疗作用正日益受到关注，其基本机制包括损伤组织在PRP制剂生长因子和纤维支架等活性成分的作用下实现修复重塑，从而缩短愈合时间，其治疗作用在多项临床和基础研究中得到证实[21]。

2. PRP治疗髌腱病的临床研究进展

维多利亚运动学院髌腱病评价标准（Victorian Institute of Sport Assessment scale for patellar tendinopathy，VISA-P）在PT的评估和疗效评价中具有重要意义，该评分系统于1998年开发，具有极好的观察者间信度（0.95）和观察者内部信度（0.99），MCID为13分[22-23]。2018年，Andriolo等纳入70项研究、共2530例病例进行荟萃分析，以比较临床上最常见的非手术治疗方法对髌腱病的疗效，包括离心运动训练、体外冲击波治疗（ESWT）和富血小板血浆（PRP）注射，同时对单次PRP注射和多次PRP注射分别进行评估、统计。其中离心运动训练在短期随访中［<6个月，平均（2.7±0.7）个月］疗效最佳（$P<0.05$），然而多次PRP注射治疗组在较长期随访中［≥6月，平均（15.1±11.3）个月］疗效优于ESWT组和离心运动训练组，且纳入的两项前瞻性病例系列研究均证实，多次PRP注射治疗有利于改善髌腱病预后，其中一项研究发现受试者在随访24个月时临床得分显著改善，大多数受试者恢复到患病前运动水平[24]；另外一项病例系列研究发现，患者在随访6个月时表现出显著的临床改善，平均随访至48.6个月时评分保持稳定[25]。同时上述两项研究均表明，双侧膝关节受累且有长期疼痛史的患者治疗后短期和长期随访结果均较差[26]。尽管如此，症状性髌腱病患者也可从单次PRP注射治疗中获益，Dallaudiere等的回顾性研究证实，393例患者经单次PRP注射后有显著的临床改善，平均随访至20.2个月时患者满意率为88.8%[27]。

在PRP注射治疗与其他非手术治疗的比较研究中，单次和多次PRP注射治疗均显示出更为明显的优势。Filardo报告了多次PRP注射联合物理治疗方法治疗顽固性髌腱病与单纯进行物理治疗的非复杂病例的前瞻性临床试验研究结果：随访6个月时两组患者临床评分均有改善，但PRP组患者运动水平显著提高[28]。

2019年，在一项纳入57例Blazina评分等级为ⅢB的运动员的多点单盲随机对照研究中，患者被随机分为超声引导下富白细胞PRP注射组、贫白细胞PRP注射组和盐水注射组，所有患者均接受单次注射及持续6周、每周3次的康复训练（抗重缓阻力训练，向心和离心运动训练），分别于治疗后6周、12周、6个月和12个月评估VISA-P评分（主要观察指标）、活动期间疼痛评分、整体变化分级（次要观察指标）。研究发现随访12周时，3组VISA-P评分、疼痛评分和整体变化分级均没有显著性差异。1年后各组VISA-P评分均数分别为58、71和80（$P>0.05$），活动期间疼痛评分分别为4.0、2.4和2.0（$P>0.05$），整体变化分级为4.7、5.6和5.7（$P>0.05$）[29]。

3. PRP治疗髌腱病的基础研究进展

慢性髌腱病明显的特征包括组织病理学改变，如胶原纤维紊乱、异常血管和感觉神经数量增加、细胞外基质成分改变，最终导致大量细胞凋亡和细胞外基质降解，既往关于PRP治疗髌腱病的动物实验相对较少。2012年，Dragoo等探讨了两种商品PRP制剂——Biomet GPS Ⅲ富白细胞PRP（LR-PRP）和MTF Cascade贫白细胞PRP（LP-PRP）髌腱内注射各2mL对新西兰兔健康肌腱的影响，观察指标包括各组总白细胞、单个核细胞（巨噬细胞和淋巴细胞）、多形核细胞、血管状况、纤维结构和纤维化情况，结果证实LR-PRP在注射后5天引起的急性炎症反应更明显，但注射后14天，各组组织学炎症反应及细胞数量比较无显著性差异[30]。值得注意的是，该研究虽然在健康动物模型上进行，但对临床实践仍有提示作用：急性期髌腱病患者接受LR-PRP注射后肿胀、疼痛等局部不良反应更加明显，这可能导致患者治疗依从性下降。

三、半月板损伤

膝关节半月板损伤（meniscus injury of knee）是一种以膝关节局限性疼痛，部分患者有打软腿或膝关节交锁现象，股四头肌萎缩，膝关节间隙固定的局限性压痛为主要表现的疾病。

1. 概述

近年来，循证学依据所支持的半月板损伤修复方法仍然有限，如目前临床应用较为广泛的半月板切除术在起治疗作用的同时却增加了软骨表面

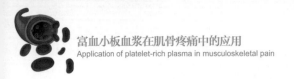
接触应力，增加了骨关节炎进展风险，其他并发症还包括关节软骨损伤、神经血管损伤和术后持续肿胀，而保守治疗方法如物理治疗仅能够缓解轻度损伤患者的临床症状[31]。

一般认为，半月板特殊的解剖结构及损伤部位是影响预后的重要因素。多数研究者习惯将半月板划分为三个区，即红区、红白区及白区。红区有血液供应（约占半月板宽度的30%），撕裂后愈合能力强；白区几乎没有血管及神经分布，愈合能力差；红白区位于红区和白区的交界处，有一定愈合能力。基于半月板损伤后的反应，有学者提出激活损伤局部未分化的间充质干细胞可能是促进组织修复的重要策略。越来越多的国内外学者关注到PRP对半月板损伤的治疗作用。既往研究认为，PRP治疗半月板损伤的积极作用与其持续释放TGF-1β、VEGF和PDGF等生长因子，促进组织增殖和修复密切相关[32]。

2. PRP治疗半月板损伤的临床研究进展

2015年，Fabian Blanke等对10名经MRI证实半月板内病变（Reicher Ⅱ级）的运动员行PRP关节腔非引导下注射治疗，治疗方案为连续注射3次、注射间期为7天，并进行为期6个月的观察，患者于每次注射前行数字分级评分法（numerical rating scale，NRS）评估，观察终点完善MRI评估。结果证实治疗后40%的患者半月板病变改善，60%的患者在观察终点随访时NRS评分改善（从基线的6.9分变为治疗后的4.5分），差异有统计学意义（$P=0.027$）[33]。Ozyalvac等发表的一篇回顾性研究分析了在超声引导下PRP注射对15例症状性2级半月板变性的影响，并分别于注射前及平均治疗32个月后随访患者，评估Lysholm评分和MRI表现，结果提示注射后患者Lysholm评分明显升高，且67%的患者半月板变性改善至1级，作者强调超声引导下注射能够观察到关节镜无法探及的病变部位，可视化、直达损伤部位的注射方式是改善半月板损伤预后的重要保障[34]。

此外，2016年Urzen等报道了一例43岁中年男性经PRP注射治疗后，半月板桶柄样裂（BHMT）显著改善的临床个案。BHMT损伤特点为外伤史、症状均较典型，半月板撕裂部分可移位到髁间窝从而导致膝关节交锁，绝大多数病例需接受手术治疗，但仍有极少数年轻患者存在自发愈合的可能。该患者诊断为BHMT后7个月内接受了3次半月板内侧及外周浸润PRP注射治疗，随访至伤后8个月疼痛症状消失并恢复步行，10个月后的MRI评估及伤后47个月的关节镜检查均显示半月板撕裂完全修复。值得注意的是，作者指出针对BHMT，注射前的手法复位及半月板前后结构完整是损伤修复的必要条件和前提[35]。

3. PRP治疗半月板损伤的基础研究进展

部分基础研究证实单独使用PRP或PRP联合其他生物材料对半月板损伤均有修复作用[36-37]。有学者在动物模型中证实，多种促合成代谢生长因子（FGF、TGF-β1、IGF-I、VEGF、PDGF-AB及表皮生长因子等）有助于半月板组织修复增殖及细胞迁移[38]。但与此同时，部分学者在基础研究中也得出了不同结论。Lee等在兔半月板损伤模型中发现，将兔半月板原代细胞分离，分别在培养基中加入10%的PRP、IL或IL与PRP的混合物，结果PRP组在治疗第1天、第4天和第7天以浓度依赖的方式改善了半月板细胞的活力，但与此同时细胞表现出去分化倾向，即I型胶原合成增加、聚蛋白多糖合成减少，由此推论PRP的去分化作用可能促进了损伤局部的分解代谢、加速了损伤半月板组织的纤维化，而非正常软骨组织的合成[39]。

Zellner等发现，在体外试验中，PRP可在8天内持续释放生长因子，且联合骨形成蛋白-7（bone morphogenetic protein-7，BMP-7）可有效促进体外培养软骨细胞II型胶原蛋白的沉积，但在动物模型3个月的随访观察期，PRP治疗、BMP-7治疗及其联合治疗均未能促进兔半月板白区（无血

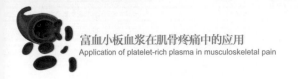

管区）的损伤修复[40]。因此，半月板特殊损伤区域修复的具体机制仍需进一步探讨。

四、前交叉韧带损伤

前交叉韧带（anterior cruciate ligament，ACL）损伤是由膝过伸或过度外展造成的韧带扭伤、撕裂，甚至是韧带完全撕裂和联合性损伤。

1. 概述

ACL损伤多见于运动损伤，损伤机制分接触性损伤和非接触性损伤，前者多由于膝关节受到来自多方向的外力撞击导致，而后者是由于膝关节突然受到扭转应力，如运动跳起后落地不稳所致。对于ACL部分撕裂，可适当选择保守治疗，包括康复治疗、运动训练和富血小板血浆（PRP）注射等[41]。ACL重建是目前绝大多数ACL断裂的治疗金标准，尽管ACL重建术的手术技术日渐完善，但有国外文献数据显示其失败率仍较高[42]。近期，对骨组织尚未完全成熟患者的组织高愈合潜力的观察研究引起了国内外临床工作者对采用生物方法进行初级非手术ACL撕裂修复的兴趣。

2. PRP治疗ACL损伤的临床研究进展

关节腔内PRP注射治疗ACL撕裂及与其他治疗方法的比较RCT研究目前鲜见报道，更多的既往临床研究关注了PRP在ACL重建术后对韧带愈合的促进作用、对重建术后骨隧道位置及宽度的影响以及对供体部位愈合的影响[43-44]。Seijas等探讨了富含生长因子的PRGF-Endoret对ACL部分撕裂运动员的临床疗效，并证实PRP有助于运动员在ACL损伤后缩短恢复运动的时间。该研究纳入19例损伤前Tegner运动水平评分达到9～10分但伴运动损伤后膝关节不稳、需行残余ACL翻修术的受试者，术中将4mL PRGF-Endoret应用于ACL后外侧束较宽部位，同时在手术结束时再次于关节间隙注射6mL PRGF-Endoret，术后配合监护下康复治疗，随访指标包括术后6个月时的前抽屉试验、枢轴移位试验、重返运动时限及MRI表现，结果证实15例9分的患者恢复运动的平均时间为16.2周，3例10分的患者恢复运动的平均时间为12.33周，MRI随访至1年显示解剖结构恢复良好[45]。

此外，中国台湾学者报告了一例25岁右侧ACL部分撕裂的女性患者，其进行了3次超声引导下PRP注射治疗（注射间期为3周）并配合康复训练，6个月后随访，患者右膝关节疼痛、不稳定症状及MRI表现均有显著改善，提示关节腔注射PRP对ACL撕裂可能有积极作用，但未来仍需进行随访时间更长的大样本前瞻性随机对照研究[46]。

3. PRP治疗ACL损伤的基础研究进展

ACL非手术修复的挑战之一在于：ACL在撕裂部位难以形成纤维蛋白血小板凝块（或桥接消失），如果没有这个凝块，两处撕裂的韧带末端之间的级联反应就将停止[47]。因此，PRP与胶原支架联合应用可能为初始ACL的修复提供一种可行方案，胶原蛋白作为一种血小板激活剂，可启动生长因子的释放以促进愈合，并可以保护血小板免受滑膜液纤溶酶的降解作用影响，该方案的可行性已在动物模型中得到证实。在体外培养的人ACL细胞实验证实，富血小板凝块的释放有效促进了细胞的增殖以及Ⅲ型胶原的生成，此外，PRP以剂量依赖和时间依赖的方式增强了ACL细胞的活力[48]。

五、富血小板血浆在侧副韧带损伤中的应用

膝关节的侧副韧带包括内侧副韧带（medial collateral ligament，MCL）和外侧副韧带（lateral collateral ligament，LCL），它们与前、后交叉韧带一样，都是维持膝关节稳定的重要组成部分。侧副韧带损伤通常发

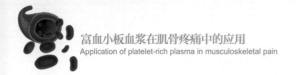

生于复杂的合并伤中。目前尚未见PRP治疗MCL损伤的大样本RCT研究，而PRP治疗LCL损伤的临床研究更为少见。

2012年，Eirale等报道用PRP注射治疗了1例足球运动员的Ⅲ级内侧副韧带损伤。该运动员接受了3次PRP注射，注射间期为1周，随后患者于治疗后第18天顺利恢复体育活动，于治疗后第25天完全恢复竞技运动，随访持续了16个月，疗效满意[49]。Yoshida等报道，3例慢性MCL损伤（Ⅰ～Ⅱ级）愈合欠佳且伴顽固慢性疼痛的患者，通过自体贫白细胞PRP1～2次局部注射治疗后恢复至损伤前的运动水平，随访至观察终点MRI评估显示近端韧带愈合良好[50]。

侯晓东等的前瞻性研究比较了自体PRP注射、激素注射和支具固定治疗急性膝关节内侧副韧带Ⅰ、Ⅱ度损伤的临床效果，该研究共纳入83例单侧膝关节MCL Ⅰ、Ⅱ度运动损伤患者，进一步分为PRP注射组（$n=$37）、激素注射组（$n=35$）、支具固定组（$n=11$），注射组均接受2次注射治疗，注射间期为2周。结果发现3组治疗后1个月、2个月、3个月的疼痛VAS评分均较治疗前明显降低，膝关节功能改良Lysholm评分均较治疗前明显提高（$P<0.05$）；治疗后1个月、2个月、3个月3组疼痛VAS评分比较差异无统计学意义（$P>0.05$），且治疗后2个月、3个月，PRP注射组Lysholm评分明显高于激素注射组和支具固定组，差异有统计学意义（$P<0.05$），作者由此提出PRP注射治疗急性膝关节内侧副韧带Ⅰ、Ⅱ度损伤更具优势[51]。

结语：近年来，随着基础及临床研究循证证据的不断积累，PRP注射疗法正在多种膝关节疾患的治疗中发挥日益重要的作用。既往研究证实，超声引导下PRP注射作为一种精准、安全、有效的治疗手段，值得临床实践进一步推广。然而，PRP相关研究仍面临着制备、激活及储存方案不统一、血小板浓度及白细胞水平（生长因子及细胞因子含量）报告不完善，注射次数、体积及时间间隔不统一等问题。未来仍需学术界共同努力，以期提供更加精准、高效的PRP治疗方案。

（栾烁）

参考文献

[1] 中华医学会骨科分会关节外科学组，吴阶平医学基金会骨科学专家委员会．膝骨关节炎阶梯治疗专家共识：2018年版[J]．中华关节外科杂志（电子版），2019，13（1）：124-130．

[2] TANG X, WANG S F, ZHAN S Y, et al. The prevalence of symptomatic knee osteoarthritis in China: results from the China health and retirement longitudinal study[J]. Arthritis Rheumatol, 2016, 68（3）: 648-653.

[3] ANDIA I, MAFFULLI N. Platelet-rich plasma for managing pain and inflammation in osteoarthritis[J]. Nat Rev Rheumatol, 2013, 9（12）: 721-730.

[4] ZHANG S B, WANG F, KE S J, et al. The effectiveness of ultrasound-guided steroid injection combined with miniscalpel-needle release in the treatment of carpal tunnel syndrome vs. steroid injection alone: a randomized controlled study[J]. Biomed Res Int, 2019（12）: 1-9.

[5] ZHANG J Y, FABRICANT P D, ISHMAEL C R, et al. Utilization of platelet-rich plasma for musculoskeletal injuries: an analysis of current treatment trends in the United States[J]. Orthop J Sports Med, 2016, 4（12）: 1-7.

[6] SANCHEZ M, ANITUA E, AZOFRA J, et al. Intra-articular injection of an autologous preparation rich in growth factors for the treatment of knee OA: a retrospective cohort study[J]. Clin Exp Rheumatol, 2008, 26（5）: 910-913.

[7] SIMENTAL-MENDIA M, VILCHEZ-CAVAZOS J F, PENA-MARTINEZ V M, et al. Leukocyte-poor platelet-rich plasma is more effective than the conventional therapy with acetaminophen for the treatment of early knee osteoarthritis[J]. Arch Orthop Trauma Surg, 2016, 136（12）: 1723-1732.

[8] 中国医疗保健国际交流促进会骨科分会．关节腔注射富血小板血浆治疗膝骨关节炎的临床实践指南：2018年版[J]．中华关节外科杂志（电子版），2018，12（4）：444-448．

[9] BELK J W, KRAEUTLER M J, HOUCK D A, et al. Platelet-rich plasma versus hyaluronic acid for knee osteoarthritis: a systematic review and meta-analysis of randomized controlled trials[J]. Am J Sports Med, 2021, 49（1）: 249-260.

[10] DAI W L, ZHOU A G, ZHANG H, et al. Efficacy of platelet-rich plasma in the treatment of knee osteoarthritis: a meta-analysis of randomized controlled trials[J].

Arthroscopy, 2017, 33（3）：659-670.

[11] RIBOH J C, SALTZMAN B M, YANKE A B, et al. Effect of leukocyte concentration on the efficacy of platelet-rich plasma in the treatment of knee osteoarthritis[J]. Am J Sports Med, 2016, 44（3）：792-800.

[12] SHEN L X, YUAN T, CHEN S B, et al. The temporal effect of platelet-rich plasma on pain and physical function in the treatment of knee osteoarthritis: systematic review and meta-analysis of randomized controlled trials[J]. J Orthop Surg Res, 2017, 12（1）：16.

[13] 栾烁, 栗晓, 林彩娜, 等. 超声引导下关节腔注射富血小板血浆治疗膝骨性关节炎疗效的回顾性研究[J]. 华西医学, 2020, 35（5）：568-573.

[14] PATEL S, DHILLON M S, AGGARWAL S, et al. Treatment with platelet-rich plasma is more effective than placebo for knee osteoarthritis: a prospective, double-blind, randomized trial[J]. Am J Sports Med, 2013, 41（2）：356-364.

[15] SANCHEZ M, FIZ N, AZOFRA J, et al. A randomized clinical trial evaluating plasma rich in growth factors（PRGF-Endoret）versus hyaluronic acid in the short-term treatment of symptomatic knee osteoarthritis[J]. Arthroscopy, 2012, 28（8）：1070-1078.

[16] ZHU Y, YUAN M, MENG H Y, et al. Basic science and clinical application of platelet-rich plasma for cartilage defects and osteoarthritis: a review[J]. Osteoarthritis Cartilage, 2013, 21（11）：1627-1637.

[17] HAHN O, KIEB M, JONITZ-HEINCKE A, et al. Dose-dependent effects of platelet-rich plasma powder on chondrocytes in vitro[J]. Am J Sports Med, 2020, 48（14）：1727-1734.

[18] MALLIARAS P, COOK J, PURDAM C, et al. Patellar tendinopathy: clinical diagnosis, load management, and advice for challenging case presentations[J]. J Orthop Sports Phys Ther, 2015, 45（11）：887-898.

[19] LIAN O, SCOTT A, ENGEBRETSEN L, et al. Excessive apoptosis in patellar tendinopathy in athletes[J]. Am J Sports Med, 2007, 35（4）：605-611.

[20] MUAIDI Q I. Rehabilitation of patellar tendinopathy[J]. J Musculoskelet Neuronal Interact, 2020, 20（4）：535-540.

[21] GOSENS T, DEN OUDSTEN B L, FIEVEZ E, et al. Pain and activity levels before and after platelet-rich plasma injection treatment of patellar tendinopathy: a prospective cohort study and the influence of previous treatments[J]. Int Orthop, 2012, 36（9）：1941-1946.

[22] HERNANDEZ-SANCHEZ S, HIDALGO M D, GOMEZ A. Responsiveness of the VISA-P scale for patellar tendinopathy in athletes[J]. Br J Sports Med, 2014, 48（6）：453-457.

[23] VISENTINI P J, KHAN K M, COOK J L, et al. The VISA score: an index of severity

of symptoms in patients with jumper's knee（patellar tendinosis）. Victorian Institute of Sport Tendon Study Group[J]. J Sci Med Sport, 1998, 1（1）: 22-28.

[24] CHAROUSSET C, ZAOUI A, BELLAICHE L, et al. Are multiple platelet-rich plasma injections useful for treatment of chronic patellar tendinopathy in athletes? a prospective study[J]. Am J Sports Med, 2014, 42（4）: 906-911.

[25] FREDBERG U, BOLVIG L, PFEIFFER J M, et al. Ultrasonography as a tool for diagnosis, guidance of local steroid injection and, together with pressure algometry, monitoring of the treatment of athletes with chronic jumper's knee and Achilles tendinitis: a randomized, double-blind, placebo-controlled study[J]. Scandinavian Journal of Rheumatology, 2004, 33（2）: 94-101.

[26] ANDRIOLO L, ALTAMURA S A, REALE D, et al. Nonsurgical treatments of patellar tendinopathy: multiple injections of platelet-rich plasma are a suitable option: a systematic review and meta-analysis[J]. Am J Sports Med, 2019, 47（4）: 1001-1018.

[27] DALLAUDIERE B, PESQUER L, MEYER P, et al. Intratendinous injection of platelet-rich plasma under US guidance to treat tendinopathy: a long-term pilot study[J]. J Vasc Interv Radiol, 2014, 25（5）: 717-723.

[28] FILARDO G, KON E, DELLA V S, et al. Use of platelet-rich plasma for the treatment of refractory jumper's knee[J]. Int Orthop, 2010, 34（6）: 909-915.

[29] SCOTT A, LAPRADE R F, HARMON K G, et al. Platelet-rich plasma for patellar tendinopathy: a randomized controlled trial of leukocyte-rich PRP or leukocyte-poor PRP versus saline[J]. Am J Sports Med, 2019, 47（7）: 1654-1661.

[30] DRAGOO J L, BRAUN H J, DURHAM J L, et al. Comparison of the acute inflammatory response of two commercial platelet-rich plasma systems in healthy rabbit tendons[J]. Am J Sports Med, 2012, 40（6）: 1274-1281.

[31] MAKRIS E A, HADIDI P, ATHANASIOU K A. The knee meniscus: structure-function, pathophysiology, current repair techniques, and prospects for regeneration[J]. Biomaterials, 2011, 32（30）: 7411-7431.

[32] SCORDINO L E, DEBERARDINO T M. Biologic enhancement of meniscus repair[J]. Clin Sports Med, 2012, 31（1）: 91-100.

[33] BLANKE F, VAVKEN P, HAENLE M, et al. Percutaneous injections of platelet rich plasma for treatment of intrasubstance meniscal lesions[J]. Muscles Ligaments Tendons J, 2015, 5（3）: 162-166.

[34] OZYALVAC O N, TUZUNER T, GURPINAR T, et al. Radiological and functional outcomes of ultrasound-guided PRP injections in intrasubstance meniscal degenerations[J]. J Orthop Surg（Hong Kong）, 2019, 27（2）: 1-4.

[35] URZEN J M, FULLERTON B D. Nonsurgical resolution of a bucket handle meniscal

tear: a case report[J]. PM & R, 2016, 8（11）: 1115–1118.

[36] COOK J L, SMITH P A, BOZYNSKI C C, et al. Multiple injections of leukoreduced platelet rich plasma reduce pain and functional impairment in a canine model of ACL and meniscal deficiency[J]. J Orthop Res, 2016, 34（4）: 607–615.

[37] LIU F, XU H Y, HUANG H. A novel kartogenin-platelet-rich plasma gel enhances chondrogenesis of bone marrow mesenchymal stem cells in vitro and promotes wounded meniscus healing in vivo[J]. Stem Cell Res Ther, 2019, 10（1）: 201.

[38] BHARGAVA M M, ATTIA E T, MURRELL G A, et al. The effect of cytokines on the proliferation and migration of bovine meniscal cells[J]. Am J Sports Med, 1999, 27（5）: 636–643.

[39] LEE H R, SHON O J, PARK S I, et al. Platelet-rich plasma increases the levels of catabolic molecules and cellular dedifferentiation in the meniscus of a rabbit model[J]. Int J Mol Sci, 2016, 17（1）: 120.

[40] ZELLNER J, TAEGER C D, SCHAFFER M, et al. Are applied growth factors able to mimic the positive effects of mesenchymal stem cells on the regeneration of meniscus in the avascular zone? [J]. Biomed Res Int, 2014（5）: 1–10.

[41] BRAUN H J, WASTERLAIN A S, DRAGOO J L. The use of PRP in ligament and meniscal healing[J]. Sports Med Arthrosc Rev, 2013, 21（4）: 206–212.

[42] PRODROMOS C, JOYCE B, SHI K. A meta-analysis of stability of autografts compared to allografts after anterior cruciate ligament reconstruction[J]. Knee Surg Sports Traumatol Arthrosc, 2007, 15（7）: 851–856.

[43] MIRZATOLOOEI F, ALAMDARI M T, KHALKHALI H R. The impact of platelet-rich plasma on the prevention of tunnel widening in anterior cruciate ligament reconstruction using quadrupled autologous hamstring tendon: a randomised clinical trial[J]. Bone Joint J, 2013, 95-B（1）: 65–69.

[44] MAGNUSSEN R A, FLANIGAN D C, PEDROZA A D, et al. Platelet rich plasma use in allograft ACL reconstructions: two-year clinical results of a MOON cohort study[J]. Knee, 2013, 20（4）: 277–280.

[45] SEIJAS R, ARES O, CUSCO X, et al. Partial anterior cruciate ligament tears treated with intraligamentary plasma rich in growth factors[J]. World J Orthop, 2014, 5（3）: 373–378.

[46] YOU C K, CHOU C L, WU W T, et al. Nonoperative choice of anterior cruciate ligament partial tear: ultrasound-guided platelet-rich plasma injection[J]. J Med Ultrasound, 2019, 27（3）: 148–150.

[47] MURRAY M M, SPINDLER K P, ABREU E, et al. Collagen-platelet rich plasma hydrogel enhances primary repair of the porcine anterior cruciate ligament[J]. J Orthop Res, 2007, 25（1）: 81–91.

[48] BISSELL L, TIBREWAL S, SAHNI V, et al. Growth factors and platelet rich plasma in anterior cruciate ligament reconstruction[J]. Curr Stem Cell Res Ther, 2015, 10（1）: 19-25.

[49] EIRALE C, MAURI E, HAMILTON B. Use of platelet rich plasma in an isolated complete medial collateral ligament lesion in a professional football（soccer）player: a case report[J]. Asian J Sports Med, 2013, 4（2）: 158-162.

[50] YOSHIDA M, MARUMO K. An autologous leukocyte-reduced platelet-rich plasma therapy for chronic injury of the medial collateral ligament in the knee: a report of 3 successful cases[J]. Clin J Sport Med, 2019, 29（1）: e4-e6.

[51] 侯晓东，刘洪柏，匡斌. 自体富血小板血浆治疗膝关节内侧副韧带Ⅰ、Ⅱ度损伤的对照研究[J]. 中国骨与关节损伤杂志，2018，33（6）: 619-621.

第六节　富血小板血浆在踝关节疼痛中的应用

足踝疾病可严重影响患者日常生活，导致其生活质量下降。常见的足踝部疼痛性疾病包括踝关节韧带损伤、距骨骨软骨损伤、踝关节骨性关节炎、跟腱疾病、跖筋膜炎、跗骨窦综合征等，另外还包括术后骨不连、关节周围肌肉损伤等。一般情况下，可通过保守治疗如制动、口服非甾体类药物、物理治疗、功能锻炼等方法进行治疗，但对部分顽固性疼痛效果不佳。部分患者虽然可通过手术进行治疗，但手术风险较高，且手术效果也不确切。富血小板血浆（PRP）注射治疗作为一种安全、有效、患者耐受性较好的生物治疗方法，具有简便且无免疫排斥等优势，因此近年来被认为是一种治疗足踝疾病非常有前景的方法。本节主要介绍PRP在常见足踝部疼痛性疾病治疗中的应用。

一、急性跟腱断裂

1. 概述

近年来随着人们健身意识的增强、运动量的增加，跟腱断裂的发病率也显著增加，从2012年的$1.8/10^5$增加到2016年的$2.5/10^5$，每年总发生率为$2.1/10^5$。跟腱断裂常发生于跟腱止点近端2～6cm处，此处血运仅靠腱周组织提供，血供较差，同时此处也是腓肠肌、比目鱼肌纤维交叉处，受拉时应力较大，因此容易发生断裂。急性跟腱断裂的治疗方法分为手术治疗和非手术治疗，采用何种治疗方法，目前尚无统一标准。跟腱保守治疗再次发生断裂的风险较高，而手术治疗有伤口感染和神经损伤等风险[1]。

运动中负荷突然增加是跟腱断裂的直接原因，而外伤、跟腱退行性病变、药物（皮质类固醇和他汀类药物等）不良反应、痛风、甲亢及肥胖等也可增加跟腱断裂的风险。有关急性跟腱断裂的主要理论包括跟腱退化理论、机械损伤理论[2]，跟腱的损伤与机体中胶原有机成分逐渐减少、跟腱弹性减弱密切相关。PRP具有促进胶原再生、血管再生等作用，这为PRP治疗跟腱断裂提供了基础。

2. PRP治疗跟腱断裂的临床研究进展

Sanchez等[3]通过病例对照研究发现，相比于单纯跟腱缝合术，手术联合PRP断端注射能更早恢复踝关节活动度及运动能力、提高跟腱愈合能力。高超等[2]将21例跟腱断裂患者分为PRP组（行改良Kessler缝合术联合PRP注射治疗）和对照组（单纯使用改良Kessler缝合术治疗），在术后3个月、6个月、9个月评估患者的踝背伸角度、VAS评分、维多利亚运动学院足踝运动功能（VISA）评分及美国足踝外科协会踝-后足（AOFAS）评分，结果发现，两组患者在治疗后各随访时间点的跖屈、背伸角度较术前均有改善，PRP组术后踝关节活动度优于对照组，VISA评分及AOFAS评分高于对照组，VAS评分低于对照组，差异均有统计学意义。该研究认为改良Kessler缝合术联合PRP注射是一种安全、实用、可靠的治疗方法。然而，Schepull等[4]进行了一项前瞻性随机对照研究，对PRP的作用提出质疑。该研究将30例接受跟腱缝合术后的急性跟腱断裂患者随机分为2组，试验组在缝合处注射PRP，对照组不注射，以比较单纯手术和手术联合PRP断端注射对跟腱愈合的影响。研究结果表明两组患者跟腱功能结果评分、腱伸长率、弹性模量、力学变量或横向面积等均无显著性差异。研究指出PRP对跟腱断裂的愈合没有显著的积极作用，甚至可能产生负面影响，研究证据等级为2级。值得注意的是，Jeffrey等在2012年发布的一项系统综述里提出，过高血小板浓度（高于基线6倍）的PRP可能造成损伤局部微环境紊乱，产生细胞凋亡、生长因子受体下调和受体脱敏等负面影响，对组织修复有抑制作用[5]。Schepull等的研究中使用的PRP血小板浓度接近基线的17倍，而其他研究中血小板浓度多为基线的3～4倍，不同研究中PRP治疗急性跟腱断裂的疗效差异可能与跟腱损伤程度、PRP制备和保存程序不统一、细胞成分不一致等异质性因素有关。

3. PRP治疗跟腱断裂的基础研究进展

国内外动物研究已表明了外源性生长因子对促进肌腱愈合和功能恢复的重要性。2003年，Zhang等[6]分别对大鼠跟腱缺损模型行改良Kessler缝合术（对照组）和改良Kessler缝合术联合跟腱断端局部注射VEGF治疗（实验组），并在术后1周、2周取材进行拉力试验，结果显示实验组跟腱拉力明显高于对照组，提示VEGF可以促进跟腱愈合。2004年，Kashiwagi等[7]证实在大鼠跟腱断端局部予TGF-β1注射治疗后可以提高Ⅰ、Ⅲ型胶原纤维mRNA的表达，同时可提高跟腱的韧性和强度。有研究显示TGP-$β_1$几乎参与了跟腱愈合的整个过程，通过刺激蛋白酶、胶原、细胞基质的合成，在组织损伤后第3周表达TGP-β₁的mRNA仍然是增高的。PRP在损伤局部被生理性激活后，可释放多种生长因子（如VEGF、PDGF、TGP-β₁、IGF等），共同促进成纤维细胞再生、新生血管形成，产生趋化作用，并刺激成纤维细胞增殖和胶原合成。2011年，Lyras等[8]进行了兔跟腱断裂模型随机对照试验，其中实验组接受PRP注射，对照组注射生理盐水，在注射后每周随机抽取动物进行病理切片，并采用免疫组织化学法检测跟腱组织的病理变化，结果发现实验组在肌腱愈合的炎症期和增殖期血管形成明显增多，与对照组比较，跟腱胶原纤维的排列更接近自然水平，因此作者认为PRP能促进新生血管形成，缩短损伤跟腱的愈合时间，促进瘢痕愈合及形成组织质量较好的瘢痕组织。

二、慢性跟腱病

1. 概述

慢性跟腱病是一种与运动密切相关的疾病，好发于运动人群，据报道，其在经常跑步的人群中每年的发病率为7%～9%，占所有运动损伤的6%～18%[9]。常见发病原因为运动中腓肠肌和跟腱承受压力过大而造成跟腱内纤维发生慢性损伤。慢性跟腱病包括滑囊炎、腱鞘炎、起止点炎和肌腱炎，其临床表现为疼痛、肿胀和运动障碍。研究已证实跟腱病的病理改变并不是炎症，而是黏类蛋白的退变以及较差的自我愈合能力[10]。

目前没有治疗慢性跟腱病的金标准，常见治疗方式包括负荷调整、口服非甾体抗炎药、理疗、功能锻炼等，对于顽固病例，可采取冲击波疗法、注射疗法和手术治疗。临床上多采用保守治疗，但部分病例效果不佳。局部激素注射短期疗效显著，但复发率高，并且可能引起肌腱萎缩、脆性增加，甚至导致跟腱断裂。

　　跟腱损伤愈合的过程包括炎症期、增生期和修复期。在炎症期，局部损伤促使炎症细胞聚集、活化，以及释放白细胞介素–1、白细胞介素–6、肿瘤坏死因子–α等多种炎症介质，介导早期炎症反应。随后，局部形成的血凝块分泌多种细胞因子，启动并促进修复进程。在修复早期，以Ⅲ型胶原蛋白修复为主，此时组织排列紊乱，机械性能较低。随着适当负重和拉伸等机械刺激的增加，Ⅲ型胶原蛋白逐渐向Ⅰ型胶原蛋白转化。Ⅰ型胶原蛋白是跟腱细胞中的主要成分，其在正常跟腱细胞中的含量为65%～80%，具有较高的强度和韧性。随着修复的继续，跟腱的强度和韧性逐渐增强。此过程中，Ⅳ型胶原蛋白和Ⅴ型胶原蛋白在维持Ⅰ型胶原蛋白结构的有序和稳定中起着关键作用。针对跟腱损伤的修复机制，国内外学者提出，PRP在生理性激活后可释放多种组织修复所需的生长因子，有效改善损伤局部微环境，对跟腱损伤的预后具有积极作用。在炎症期，PRP中的白细胞发生聚集和活化，释放大量细胞因子，对大肠杆菌、金黄色葡萄球菌等产生一定的抑制作用，同时通过受体–配体结合，调控细胞内信号传导通路；纤维蛋白在损伤部位形成的纤维网状结构，发挥着"临时支架和生物活性分子载体"的作用，有利于血小板、白细胞的吸附和稳定。在增生期，高浓度的血小板释放TGF-β、PDGF、VEGF、IGF-Ⅰ等生长因子，在新生血管形成、细胞再生等方面发挥关键作用。综上所述，在跟腱损伤后，PRP可通过释放白细胞、纤维蛋白及生长因子在不同阶段发挥促进损伤修复的作用[11-12]。

2. PRP治疗慢性跟腱病的临床研究进展

　　Boesen等[9]在一项双盲随机对照试验中，将60例男性慢性跟腱病（病程＞3个月）患者随机分为3组，分别进行大容量注射（high-volume injection，HVI）、PRP注射和安慰剂注射治疗，并在治疗前及治疗后6周、12周、24周时进行疼痛和功能评估，检查肌腱厚度和腱内超声彩色多普勒信号改善情况。结果发现，与安慰剂组相比，PRP组患者在疼痛、活动水平、肌腱厚度和腱内血流信号密度等方面改善更显著，说明PRP有促进跟腱愈合的潜力。Filardo等[13]在一项前瞻性的临床研究中对27例患者进行了3次跟腱内PRP注射（注射间期为2周），经过平均54.1个月（最少30个月）的随访观察，结果发现，患者的运动功能评分显著改善，提示多次注射PRP在治疗跟腱病上总体中期疗效较好。Guelfi等[14]对73例患者进行单次PRP注射治疗并进行了平均50.1个月的随访观察，随访期间未发现跟腱断裂发生，跟腱相关功能评分及基线满意度指数较前明显改善，提示单次注射PRP对慢性跟腱病的长期疗效较好，能够降低不良反应的发生率，是治疗慢性跟腱病的新方向。但也有部分研究不支持上述结论，认为PRP注射并不能改善慢性跟腱病的疼痛和功能评分[15-16]。De Jonge等[16]在一项研究中比较了PRP和安慰剂单次注射对54例慢性肌腱炎患者的疗效，结果发现，PRP和安慰剂治疗均未能有效缓解疼痛、改善功能。De Vos等[17]在一项双盲随机对照试验中，对54例慢性跟腱炎患者给予PRP治疗，结果显示PRP注射未能改变损伤跟腱超声回声结构和新生血管形成评分。对于不同研究中出现的疗效差异，Boesen等学者提出，既往大多数研究采用的不是理想的肌腱炎模型，并且在不同研究中患者接受PRP注射的次数和间隔时间不同，上述异质性因素可能导致了PRP对慢性肌腱损伤的疗效差异。该团队认为，多次PRP注射可提高其对跟腱病的治疗作用，单次PRP注射在短期内可提高损伤肌腱的恢复能力，但随着时间的推移，PRP的治疗效果逐渐消失[18-19]，而多次注射可延长跟腱对生长因子的反应时间，有利于跟腱组织的恢复。值得注意的是，目前国内外专家对PRP的治疗方法暂无定论，最佳治疗方案仍需进一步探讨。

3. PRP治疗慢性跟腱病的基础研究进展

Fedato等[20]将41只慢性跟腱炎模型大鼠随机分为4组，实验组分别接

受干细胞（SC）、PRP、SC联合PRP注射治疗，对照组只接受离心训练
（eccentric training，ET）。4周后，对模型大鼠的跟腱进行生物力学和组
织学分析。生物力学评估结果显示，PRP组大鼠跟腱最大变形和弹性模量
明显优于其他各组。弹性模量是评估跟腱的重要指标，肌腱弹性是构成
适当生理功能的基础，此研究提示PRP在跟腱病的治疗中具有积极作用。
Shah等[21]研究评估了重组人血小板源性生长因子（rhPDGF-BB）在大鼠
胶原酶诱导的肌腱病变模型中的作用。结果表明，经rhPDGF-BB处理的肌
腱的生物力学强度有持续性改善，此结果支持生长因子对大鼠肌腱病变模
型有修复作用这一观点，即PRP衍生的生长因子可改善受伤肌腱的生物力
学特性，在病理条件下可刺激新组织形成。Yan等[22]将24只慢性跟腱病模
型兔分为3组，分别注射贫白细胞PRP（LP-PRP）、富白细胞PRP（LR-
PRP）和生理盐水，4周后采用MRI扫描比较跟腱愈合情况，并通过免疫
组织化学法、基因表达分析法和透射电镜（TEM）测定跟腱相关分子表
达差异。结果发现，与生理盐水组相比，LP-PRP组Ⅰ型胶原蛋白表达明
显增加，LP-PRP和LR-PRP两组较生理盐水组基质金属蛋白酶MMP-1和
MMP-3的表达水平显著降低，表明PRP对跟腱愈合有促进作用。研究结果
还表明，LP-PRP可以通过促进细胞外基质的成熟来促进肌腱愈合。

三、跖筋膜炎

1. 概述

跖筋膜炎（PF）是引起足跟疼痛最常见的原因之一，好发于长期运动
和久坐的人群，一般人群的患病率为3.6%～7%，约占所有跑步相关损伤
的8%[23]。其临床表现为足跟部疼痛不适，压痛点常位于足底近足跟处，
MRI可表现为足底腱膜增厚。目前跖筋膜炎的治疗仍以保守治疗为主，包

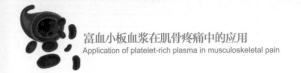
括应用非甾体类药物、牵拉锻炼及足跟垫保护等措施，据Wolgin等对跖筋膜炎患者的统计研究，80%以上的保守治疗对跖筋膜炎有效。然而，对于顽固性跖筋膜炎，保守治疗效果不佳。以往认为类固醇局部注射是治疗顽固性跖筋膜炎的有效方法，事实上，研究已表明，激素更适用于跖筋膜炎的短期镇痛治疗，其在短期内可明显减轻疼痛，同时影像学检查可见跖筋膜的厚度显著下降。但局部注射激素的长期疗效尚不明确，反复注射还可能引起注射点疼痛、骨质疏松、内分泌紊乱、跖筋膜断裂等不良反应，因此，尽管激素注射起效迅速，曾被作为跖筋膜炎的首选治疗方案，但上述不良反应限制了其在临床上的应用[10, 24]。

　　跖筋膜炎通常被认为是足底筋膜（或筋膜前结构）止点的炎症反应，反复的过度活动、牵拉、挤压可使跟骨止点筋膜长期承受过度应力，足底前部负重增加，导致连接跟骨与跖骨表面的致密结缔组织发生缺血和慢性纤维组织炎症，进而形成骨刺，引起拇展肌、趾短屈肌和跖筋膜内侧张力增加，或引起滑膜囊炎，从而出现足跟痛[10]。然而，组织学研究却发现跖筋膜炎是一种非炎性退变过程，在节律性应力的反复牵引下，局部筋膜发生微创伤，出现巨噬细胞、淋巴细胞和浆细胞浸润，组织破坏，新生血管形成和纤维化等炎症与修复共存现象。正常的筋膜组织被未成熟的血管和增生的成纤维细胞所取代，并且向周围组织延伸，局部血液供应不足、损伤部位参与修复的细胞减少、局部生长因子浓度降低等因素共同导致退变筋膜修复能力减弱，形成一个慢性退化循环[25]。已证实PRP对其他慢性退行性病变如软骨变性、骨关节炎、肌腱损伤等具有积极作用，将其注射到损伤部位后，能显著增加局部生长因子浓度，理论上解决了跖筋膜炎中胶原变性、供血不足等潜在病理生理学问题，可有效改善患者足部疼痛及活动受限[25-26]。

2. PRP治疗跖筋膜炎的临床研究进展

2019年，Shetty等[26]报道了一项包含90例慢性跖筋膜炎患者的随机对照试验，该研究中3组患者分别接受PRP、类固醇激素和安慰剂注射，并在不同时间点进行VAS评分、R&M评分和SF-12健康情况评估，结果发现PRP和类固醇激素在短期（<1个月）和长期（6～18个月）均能显著改善VAS和R&M评分；短期内类固醇激素缓解疼痛和改善功能的效果优于PRP，而PRP长期缓解疼痛和改善功能的效果优于类固醇激素，表明PRP注射可有效缓解疼痛，且具有更持久的效果。研究者提出，PRP和类固醇激素都是治疗慢性跖筋膜炎安全有效的方法，但PRP效果持久，再注射和/或手术率更低，对于慢性跖筋膜炎的治疗具有更好的前景。同年，Peerbooms等[27]进行了一项比较PRP与皮质类固醇注射治疗慢性跖筋膜炎的多中心随机对照试验，115例患者经随机分组，分别给予PRP（试验组）或类固醇激素（对照组）注射，并进行了长达1年的随访。1年后，试验组疼痛评分明显低于对照组，试验组中症状改善的患者比例高达84.4%，显著高于对照组的55.6%，试验组的FFI残疾评分也明显低于对照组。该研究证实单次注射PRP比注射类固醇激素更能改善跖筋膜炎的疼痛和活动功能障碍，证据等级为1级。魏芳远等[25]在一项临床研究中纳入了19例顽固性跖筋膜炎患者。患者在PRP治疗前均接受过保守治疗，包括小腿肌肉牵拉锻炼、口服非甾体抗炎药等，但疗效不佳，其中6例曾接受过足跟部皮质类固醇注射治疗，2例接受了3次以上的注射。研究者在实施单次跖筋膜穿刺注射PRP后分别记录患者治疗前及治疗后6个月、12个月的VAS评分、AOFAS评分。结果显示，与治疗前比较，注射PRP后患者的VAS评分显著下降，AOFAS评分显著上升，且未出现严重不良反应，提示PRP注射治疗顽固性跖筋膜炎是安全有效的，能有效改善患者足部疼痛及活动受限。2020年，Hurley等[28]对PRP或类固醇激素注射治疗跖筋膜炎的9个随机对照研究进

行了荟萃分析，共纳入239例PRP注射患者与240例类固醇激素注射患者，结果发现，治疗后短期内（1～3个月）AOFAS评分无差异，而长期随访中（6～12个月）PRP与类固醇激素注射的AOFAS评分存在差异，临床证据显示PRP对慢性跖筋膜炎患者疼痛和功能障碍的改善优于类固醇激素，且暂未发现PRP注射相关严重不良反应，目前的临床证据推荐PRP用于跖筋膜炎的治疗，推荐等级为A级。

四、距骨骨软骨损伤

1. 概述

距骨骨软骨损伤（OCLTs）包括距骨表面软骨和/或距骨软骨下骨的损伤，是踝关节慢性疼痛的主要病因之一，占急性踝关节损伤的50%以上。OCLTs常发生于运动量较大的人群（如运动员等），无明显性别差异，大多数OCLTs患者有明确的踝关节创伤或关节不稳相关病史，或因无明显特异性诱因的踝关节深部疼痛就诊，多与负重相关。结合病史、症状、体格检查和影像学检查一般可诊断OCLTs，X线主要用于筛查和早期诊断，CT对于诊断和手术方案的设计具有极其重要的意义，而MRI可早期发现软骨病变并可对预后进行评估[29]。目前临床上对于OCLTs的治疗分为非手术治疗和手术治疗两大类，非手术治疗主要针对的是临床症状较轻且无明显移位的病变，治疗方法包括减少活动、减轻负重、使用石膏和行走靴等支具，以及使用非类固醇类抗炎药等。手术治疗包括清创、骨髓刺激术、内固定术、自体软骨移植、同种异体软骨移植、自体软骨细胞移植、关节腔注射生物制剂等。

大多数OCLTs与外伤相关，如踝关节扭伤和骨折，其他致病因素包括血管功能不全、滑膜损伤、软组织撞击、慢性踝关节不稳、遗传易感性和内分泌或代谢异常等，由于距骨软骨组织血供少，损伤后修复能力差，而胫距关节为重要承重关节，因此长期承受巨大应力、发生软骨损伤后，滑膜炎症会造成软骨周围微环境改变，使金属蛋白酶组织抑制因子与金属蛋白酶（MMP-13等）失衡，导致损伤局部炎症瀑布效应及软骨细胞变性凋亡，尤其是血管闭塞导致距骨软骨下骨囊性变，最终可能发展成距骨病理性骨折。在局部炎性物质及多种细胞因子相互作用下，病变范围会逐渐扩大，若不进行及时有效的治疗，可能导致继发性踝关节骨性关节炎[30]。

关于OCLTs的分期，目前最常用的是由Hepple等[31]在1999年提出的MRI修正分期系统。根据Hepple分期，对于Ⅰ、Ⅱ期及慢性距骨骨软骨损伤的初始治疗大多选择保守治疗[32]。手术治疗适用于有症状的Ⅲ、Ⅳ、Ⅴ期患者及灶性OCLTs非手术治疗失败者，或有急性撕脱碎片的患者[33]。距骨骨软骨损伤后自行修复能力有限，而PRP可促进软组织和骨组织的再生并可用于治疗骨折的并发症等。PRP中高浓度血小板激活后可释放用于组织修复的生长因子，激活细胞内信号通路，诱导蛋白的再生过程；同时PRP中的纤维蛋白、纤维连接蛋白、黏连蛋白等可连接细胞，填充组织缺损，促进软骨组织的修复和再生，在OCLTs的治疗中有良好的应用前景。

2. PRP治疗OCLTs的临床研究进展

2012年，Mei-Dan等[34]在一项随机对照试验中比较了PRP与透明质酸（HA）在缓解距骨剥离性骨软骨炎（OCD）所致疼痛和改善踝关节功能等方面的近期疗效与安全性。研究中纳入了32例OCD患者，随机分组后，对照组行关节腔内HA注射治疗，试验组行关节腔内PRP注射治疗，两组患者均接受3次注射，随访时间为28周。研究发现两组患者的AOFAS评分、VAS评分、关节僵硬程度、踝关节功能以及主观整体功能评分均有改善且持续至少6个月，组间比较发现PRP效果优于HA，由此研究者提出，对于

Ⅰ～Ⅲ级距骨骨软骨损伤患者踝关节腔注射PRP可有效减少疼痛和僵硬、改善功能，且安全性高，因此建议将关节腔注射PRP作为OCLTs的一线治疗选择，证据等级为2级。2013年，Lee等[35]将49例早期退行性软骨缺损患者（年龄40～50岁）分为两组，对照组仅行微骨折手术，治疗组行微骨折手术联合PRP注射，随访2年发现两组患者临床情况均有明显改善，关节镜检查结果显示治疗组患者软骨弹性较好，提示PRP可以促进软骨损伤修复。同年，Ahmet等[36]比较了单纯微骨折手术与微骨折手术联合PRP注射对OCLTs患者预后的影响，平均随访16个月，经对两组患者进行AOFAS评分、足踝关节能力测量和VAS评分的比较分析，研究者提出PRP联合微骨折手术比单纯微骨折手术有更好的中期效果，证据等级为2级。随后在2015年，Ahmet等[37]报道了一项病例对照研究，该研究纳入了54例OCLTs患者，以比较关节镜下微骨折手术、微骨折手术联合PRP注射和镶嵌成形术三种不同治疗方式治疗距骨骨软骨损伤的预后。研究结果显示，与基线水平相比，三组的AOFAS评分和足踝功能评分均有改善，但组间比较结果显示微骨折手术联合PRP未显现出明显优势，证据等级为2级。

2020年初，Boffa等[38]进行了一项评价踝关节腔注射治疗距骨骨软骨病变（包括距骨骨软骨损伤和踝关节炎）临床证据的荟萃分析，共纳入24项研究，涵盖HA、PRP、生理盐水、类固醇激素、A型肉毒杆菌毒素、间充质干细胞（mesenchymal stem cells，MSCs）注射治疗和增生疗法。作者在分析后发现，关节腔注射PRP治疗踝关节OA和OCLTs是安全的，但仍缺乏等级较高的临床证据证明其有效性。目前大部分国内外临床研究和荟萃分析都显示PRP治疗膝关节骨性关节炎有良好的效果，然而，与PRP治疗膝关节疾病相关文献相比，踝关节疾病相关文献明显缺乏。临床上关于距骨骨软骨病变的治疗方法大多源于膝关节病变的治疗，值得注意的是，膝关节和距骨关节软骨有较大的差别，损伤后可能会表现出不同的病理状况以及不同的关节内环境和治疗反应，因此，PRP治疗踝关节病变不应依赖于膝关节治疗经验的推断，而应进行更多踝关节软骨病变相关的高水平随机对照研究。

3. PRP治疗OCLTs的基础研究进展

2013年，Bergen等[39]在16只成年山羊的距骨中建立了标准化的6mm软骨缺损模型，随机分组后，对照组山羊接受安慰剂治疗，实验组山羊接受自体PRP或PRP联合脱钙骨基质（DBM）注射治疗。24周后，取距骨标本进行宏观评估、显微计算机断层扫描（microCT）检查、骨组织形态计量学测定和荧光显微镜分析，以评估软骨缺损的改善情况。研究结果显示，DBM没有改善修复，PRP没有增强DBM的再生能力。为了观察PRP对距骨软骨内基质细胞衍生因子SDF-1/CxC趋化受体CxCR4信号通路、糖胺聚糖（GAG）、基质金属蛋白酶-13（MMP-13）表达的影响，并探讨PRP治疗距骨骨软骨损伤的作用机制，2015年魏远芳等[30]比较了16例OCLTs患者关节镜术前及注射PRP前关节液样本中SDF-1及GAG的水平，并于关节镜术中取距骨病灶区软骨样本，经预处理后将距骨软骨细胞接种于培养板中，随机分为PRP治疗组及空白对照组，分别经PRP及不含PRP的人血清处理后比较两组细胞培养液中SDF-1、CxCR4、MMP-13及GAG的水平。研究结果表明，距骨骨软骨损伤时，软骨细胞内SDF-1/CxCR4信号通路可能参与了软骨细胞的退变及降解过程，PRP可能通过抑制该通路来抑制软骨细胞的退变及降解，从而促进距骨骨软骨损伤的修复。

五、跗骨窦综合征

1. 概述

跗骨窦综合征（STS）是常见的足踝部损伤之一，多由踝关节扭伤引

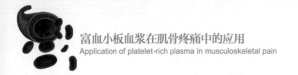
起，临床表现为跗骨窦区域的长期持续性疼痛，有时伴有肿胀，活动后加重，甚至出现整个足踝部的不适。其发病机制尚不明确，可能与韧带撕裂、关节纤维化、关节去神经化等改变有关。STS的治疗分为非手术治疗和手术治疗，临床上多采用口服药物、超声波治疗、局部类固醇激素注射等保守治疗方法，当踝关节不稳、反复扭伤或保守治疗无效时可予关节镜术治疗。

STS多由外伤引起，其中踝内翻扭伤致跗骨窦内软组织旋出引起的占70%以上；足极度旋前或撞击导致的跗骨窦内软组织旋入也较为常见，占比为20%～30%，此型病变常合并窦内韧带损伤；外侧韧带尤其是跟腓韧带的损伤也可引起STS。目前对STS的诊断暂无统一标准，主要参照以下3个方面：跗骨窦区域疼痛，诊断性局部激素注射后缓解，合并后足不稳。足踝外伤后的影像学检查首选X线，MRI的软组织分辨率高，在诊断STS方面具有重要价值。关节镜也是重要的诊断方法，但因其有创，一般不作为首选[40]。

2. PRP治疗STS的临床研究进展

目前仍缺乏分析PRP注射治疗STS疗效的随机对照试验。2012年，庄汝杰等[41]报道了一项关于PRP注射结合超声波治疗STS的临床研究，22例患者接受跗骨窦内PRP弥散注射联合超声波治疗，在注射后15个月随访时发现，VAS评分从治疗前的7.5分减少至2.4分，踝-后足功能评分从治疗前的39.3分提高至87.8分，提示PRP注射结合超声波治疗STS有减轻疼痛和改善功能的效果，且远期疗效确切，因此PRP或可用于STS的治疗。该研究为STS的保守治疗带来新的启示，但值得注意的是，该研究样本量较小，且未设对照组，要探讨PRP在STS治疗中可能发挥的积极作用，未来仍需进行随访时间更长、样本量更大的前瞻性随机对照研究。

六、踝关节炎

1. 概述

踝关节炎是一种慢性退行性病变，占骨性关节炎的13%左右。踝关节炎多由外伤、运动过度或慢性劳损导致，在亚洲人群中，由胫骨跖板内翻或盘腿等不良姿势引起的原发性踝内翻性关节炎也很常见。目前常见的踝关节炎保守治疗方法包括制动、口服非甾体类药物、物理治疗等，短期内可缓解症状，但长期效果不佳[42]。已证实，PRP激活后释放的多种生长因子在维持关节腔内环境稳态和促进关节愈合等过程中发挥了关键性作用。近年来，关节腔内PRP注射已广泛用于关节炎的治疗，其在踝关节炎中的应用也越来越多[43]。

2. PRP治疗踝关节炎的临床研究进展

2017年，Fukawa等[42]对20例内翻型踝关节炎患者予关节腔内PRP注射治疗，在治疗后4周、12周和24周进行疗效和不良事件评估。结果显示，患者在VAS评分、日本足外科学会（JSSF）踝关节/后脚量表和足部评估问卷（SAFE-Q）等方面的评估均较治疗前有显著改善，且随访期间未见严重不良反应，初步显示了关节腔内PRP注射治疗踝关节炎的安全性和有效性。同年，Repetto等[44]报道了20例踝关节炎患者接受关节腔内PRP注射后的中期临床结果（平均随访17.7个月），结果发现，PRP对踝关节炎患者的疼痛（$P<0.01$）和关节功能（$P<0.01$）有明显的积极作用，患者满意度调查显示"非常满意"的比例高达80%，仅2例患者治疗后效果不佳，最终需要接受手术治疗。该研究表明，PRP注射可显著改善踝关节炎的疼痛程度和关节功能，且能够延缓或避免手术。值得注意的是，目前分析PRP对OA的临床疗效RCT研究多数仍是关于膝、髋等关节的，PRP在踝

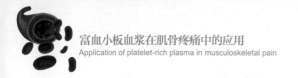
关节炎中的安全性和有效性仍有待进一步探讨。

3. PRP治疗踝关节炎的基础研究进展

大量基础研究已表明PRP在细胞再生和软骨修复中有积极作用，但目前关于PRP和踝关节炎的基础研究仍较少。2021年，Ragab等[45]使用碘乙酸单钠（MIA）建立大鼠踝关节炎模型，探究PRP对踝关节炎症、软骨损伤及氧化应激的治疗效果。30只大鼠被随机分为3组，其中1组为正常对照组，另2组为模型大鼠。建模成功后，2组模型大鼠分别接受踝关节腔内生理盐水注射或PRP注射。治疗后观察关节肿胀程度、大鼠体重、白细胞计数、踝关节形态学及组织学的改变，并检测血清脂质过氧化物、谷胱甘肽和谷胱甘肽-转移酶等氧化应激生物标志物，以及肿瘤坏死因子-α、白细胞介素-17、白细胞介素-4等血清炎症指标，并进行关节软骨MRI检查。结果显示PRP能显著降低踝关节炎大鼠的氧化应激水平和炎症水平，形态学观察、组织学分析和MRI显示PRP注射后大鼠关节软骨破坏程度改善，提示PRP可能是通过抑制炎症因子表达和降低氧化应激水平来发挥治疗作用的。

结语：总体来说，PRP制备简单、经济、安全性高、副作用少，在足踝部疾病的治疗中被认为具有积极作用，且PRP临床试验未出现严重不良反应或并发症，说明其治疗具有安全性和有效性。因此，PRP在足踝损伤领域有着广阔的发展前景，未来可能会替代传统疗法成为足踝部疾病的首选保守治疗方法。当然，在PRP被广泛应用于临床前也有许多亟待解决的问题，例如PRP应用于足踝部疾病的适应证、PRP细胞成分及其作用、PRP标准制备方法、激活剂的选择以及注射的剂量和次数等，都需要更多的基础实验和高质量临床随机对照试验来探讨。

（王少玲）

参考文献

［1］ 王振宇，姜良勇，李强．急性闭合性跟腱断裂治疗方法的研究进展［J］．山东化工，2020，49（20）：52-53．

［2］ 高超，张航，陈凯文，等．富血小板血浆在急性跟腱断裂治疗中的应用［J］．中华创伤骨科杂志，2020，22（1）：38-44．

［3］ SANCHEZ M，ANITUA E，AZOFRA J，et al．Comparison of surgically repaired Achilles tendon tears using platelet-rich fibrin matrices［J］．Am J Sports Med，2007，35（2）：245-251．

［4］ SCHEPULL T，KVIST J，NORRMAN H，et al．Autologous platelets have no effect on the healing of human achilles tendon ruptures：a randomized single-blind study［J］．Am J Sports Med，2011，39（1）：38-47．

［5］ DELONG J M，RUSSELL R P，MAZZOCCA A D．Platelet-rich plasma：the PAW classification system［J］．Arthroscopy：The Journal of Arthroscopic & Related Surgery，2012，28（7）：998-1009．

［6］ ZHANG F，LIU H，STILE F，et al．Effect of vascular endothelial growth factor on rat Achilles tendon healing［J］．Plast Reconstr Surg，2003，112（6）：1613-1619．

［7］ KASHIWAGI K，MOCHIZUKI Y，YASUNAGA Y，et al．Effects of transforming growth factor-beta 1 on the early stages of healing of the Achilles tendon in a rat model［J］．Scand J Plast Reconstr Surg Hand Surg，2004，38（4）：193-197．

［8］ LYRAS D N，KAZAKOS K，GEORGIADIS G，et al．Does a single application of PRP alter the expression of IGF-Ⅰ in the early phase of tendon healing？［J］．J Foot Ankle Surg，2011，50（3）：276-282．

［9］ BOESEN A P，HANSEN R，BOESEN M I，et al．Effect of high-volume injection，platelet-rich plasma，and sham treatment in chronic midportion achilles tendinopathy：a randomized double-blinded prospective study［J］．Am J Sports Med，2017，45（9）：2034-2043．

［10］ 宋国勋，余伟林，施忠民．富血小板血浆在足踝外科临床应用中的研究进展［J］．国际外科学杂志，2014，41（8）：562-566．

［11］ 高超，程宇，张洪涛．富血小板血浆在治疗跟腱损伤中的作用机制及研究进展［J］．足踝外科电子杂志，2019，6（1）：55-59．

［12］ SNEDEKER J G，FOOLEN J．Tendon injury and repair：a perspective on the basic mechanisms of tendon disease and future clinical therapy［J］．Acta Biomater，2017，63：18-36．

［13］ FILARDO G，KON E，DI MATTEO B．Platelet-rich plasma injections for the treatment of refractory Achilles tendinopathy：results at 4 years［J］．Blood Transfus，2014，12（4）：533-540．

[14] GUELFI M, PANTALONE A, VANNI D, et al. Long-term beneficial effects of platelet-rich plasma for non-insertional Achilles tendinopathy[J]. Foot Ankle Surg, 2015, 21（3）: 178-181.

[15] ZHANG Y J, XU S Z, GU P C, et al. Is platelet-rich plasma injection effective for chronic Achilles tendinopathy? A meta-analysis[J]. Clin Orthop Relat Res, 2018, 476（8）: 1633-1641.

[16] DE JONGE S, DE VOS R J, WEIR A, et al. One-year follow-up of platelet-rich plasma treatment in chronic Achilles tendinopathy: a double-blind randomized placebo-controlled trial[J]. Am J Sports Med, 2011, 39（8）: 1623-1629.

[17] DE VOS R J, WEIR A, VAN SCHIE H, et al. Platelet-rich plasma injection for chronic Achilles tendinopathy a randomized controlled trial[J]. The Journal of the American Medical Association, 2010, 303（2）: 144-149.

[18] DRAGOO J L, WASTERLAIN A S, BRAUN H J, et al. Platelet-rich plasma as a treatment for patellar tendinopathy: a double-blind, randomized controlled trial[J]. Am J Sports Med, 2014, 42（3）: 610-618.

[19] ANDIA I, SANCHEZ M, MAFFULLI N. Tendon healing and platelet-rich plasma therapies[J]. Expert Opinion on Biological Therapy, 2010, 10（10）: 1415-1426.

[20] FEDATO R A, FRANCISCO J C, SLIVA G, et al. Stem cells and platelet-rich plasma enhance the healing process of tendinitis in mice[J]. Stem Cells Int, 2019（5）: 1-9.

[21] SHAH V, BENDELE A, DINES J S, et al. Dose-response effect of an intra-tendon application of recombinant human platelet-derived growth factor-BB（rhPDGF-BB）in a rat Achilles tendinopathy model[J]. J Orthop Res, 2013, 31（3）: 413-420.

[22] YAN R J, GU Y J, RAN J S, et al. Intratendon delivery of leukocyte-poor platelet-rich plasma improves healing compared with leukocyte-rich platelet-rich plasma in a rabbit Achilles tendinopathy model[J]. Am J Sports Med, 2017, 45（8）: 1909-1920.

[23] RATHLEFF M S, MOLGAARD C M, FREDBERG U, et al. High-load strength training improves outcome in patients with plantar fasciitis: a randomized controlled trial with 12-month follow-up[J]. Scand J Med Sci Sports, 2015, 25（3）: e292-e300.

[24] UDEN H, BOESCH E, KUMAR S. Plantar fasciitis—to jab or to support? A systematic review of the current best evidence[J]. J Multidiscip Healthc, 2011, 4: 155-164.

[25] 魏芳远, 曲峰, 王显军, 等. 富含血小板血浆治疗慢性跖筋膜炎疗效分析[J]. 中国医学前沿杂志, 2019, 11（5）: 43-46.

[26] SHETTY S H, DHOND A, ARORA M, et al. Platelet-rich plasma has better long-term results than corticosteroids or placebo for chronic plantar fasciitis: randomized control trial[J]. J Foot Ankle Surg, 2019, 58（1）: 42-46.

[27] PEERBOOMS J C, LODDER P, DEN OUDSTEN B L, et al. Positive effect of platelet-rich plasma on pain in plantar fasciitis: a double-blind multicenter randomized

controlled trial[J]. Am J Sports Med, 2019, 47（13）: 3238-3246.

[28] HURLEY E T, SHIMOZONO Y, HANNON C P, et al. Platelet-rich plasma versus corticosteroids for plantar fasciitis: a systematic review of randomized controlled trials[J]. Orthop J Sports Med, 2020, 8（4）: 1-8.

[29] 韩宇, 常非, 姜振德, 等. 距骨软骨损伤: 病因、诊断、治疗及前景[J]. 中国组织工程研究, 2019, 23（15）: 2443-2449.

[30] 魏芳远, 曲峰, 王显军, 等. 富含血小板血浆通过抑制基质细胞衍生因子-1/CxC趋化因子受体4通路治疗距骨软骨损伤的作用机制[J]. 中国临床医生杂志, 2019, 47（7）: 834-837.

[31] HEPPLE S, WINSON I G, GLEW D. Osteochondral lesions of the talus: a revised classification[J]. Foot Ankle Int, 1999, 20（12）: 789-793.

[32] MURAWSKI C D, KENNEDY J G. Operative treatment of osteochondral lesions of the talus[J]. J Bone Joint Surg Am, 2013, 95（11）: 1045-1054.

[33] 谢盼盼, 叶方, 叶积飞. 距骨软骨损伤的诊疗进展[J]. 中国骨伤, 2018, 31（9）: 880-884.

[34] MEI-DAN O, CARMONT M R, LAVER L, et al. Platelet-rich plasma or hyaluronate in the management of osteochondral lesions of the talus[J]. Am J Sports Med, 2012, 40（3）: 534-541.

[35] LEE G W, SON J H, KIM J D, et al. Is platelet-rich plasma able to enhance the results of arthroscopic microfracture in early osteoarthritis and cartilage lesion over 40 years of age?[J]. Eur J Orthop Surg Traumatol, 2013, 23（5）: 581-587.

[36] GUNEY A, AKAR M, KARAMAN I, et al. Clinical outcomes of platelet rich plasma （PRP）as an adjunct to microfracture surgery in osteochondral lesions of the talus[J]. Knee Surg Sports Traumatol Arthrosc, 2015, 23（8）: 2384-2389.

[37] GUNEY A, YURDAKUL E, KARAMAN I, et al. Medium-term outcomes of mosaicplasty versus arthroscopic microfracture with or without platelet-rich plasma in the treatment of osteochondral lesions of the talus[J]. Knee Surgery, Sports Traumatology, Arthroscopy, 2015, 24（4）: 1293-1298.

[38] BOFFA A, PREVITALI D, DI LAURA F G, et al. Evidence on ankle injections for osteochondral lesions and osteoarthritis: a systematic review and meta-analysis[J]. Int Orthop, 2020, 45: 1-55.

[39] VAN BERGEN C J, KERKHOFFS G M, OZDEMIR M, et al. Demineralized bone matrix and platelet-rich plasma do not improve healing of osteochondral defects of the talus: an experimental goat study[J]. Osteoarthritis Cartilage, 2013, 21（11）: 1746-1754.

[40] 刘金来, 崔树森, 王彦清. 跗骨窦综合征MRI评分与AOFAS踝-后足功能评分的相关性研究[J]. 中国中西医结合影像学杂志, 2020, 18（5）: 512-515.

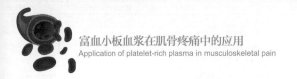
[41] 庄汝杰，童培建，张晓冬，等．富血小板血浆注射结合超声波治疗跗骨窦综合征疗效观察[J]．中医正骨，2012，24（5）：10-12．

[42] FUKAWA T, YAMAGUCHI S, AKATSU Y, et al．Safety and efficacy of intra-articular injection of platelet-rich plasma in patients with ankle osteoarthritis[J]．Foot Ankle Int，2017，38（6）：596-604．

[43] VANNABOUATHONG C, DEL FABBRO G, SALES B, et al．Intra-articular injections in the treatment of symptoms from ankle arthritis：a systematic review[J]．Foot Ankle Int，2018，39（10）：1141-1150．

[44] REPETTO I, BITI B, CERRUTI P, et al．Conservative treatment of ankle osteoarthritis：can platelet-rich plasma effectively postpone surgery？[J]．J Foot Ankle Surg，2017，56（2）：362-365．

[45] RAGAB G H, HALFAYA F M, AHMED O M, et al．Platelet-rich plasma ameliorates monosodium iodoacetate-induced ankle osteoarthritis in the rat model via suppression of inflammation and oxidative stress[J]．Evid Based Complement Alternat Med，2021（1）：1-13．

第七节　富血小板血浆在盘源性疼痛中的应用

由于椎间盘退变刺激纤维环中的伤害性感受器所产生的疼痛称为"盘源性疼痛"。研究表明，椎间盘退行性病变引起的盘源性疼痛与局部促炎细胞因子、神经营养因子表达增强以及椎间盘内部破裂等相关。此外，已退变椎间盘会出现细胞外基质降解、髓核蛋白多糖和水分丢失、纤维环胶原变性、Ⅱ型胶原减少而Ⅰ型胶原增多等改变，这些退行性病变可引起椎间盘内部破裂，具体表现为径向和周向撕裂、开裂、产生裂隙，进而刺激椎间盘内的伤害性感受器。此外，椎间盘破裂后的异常组织重塑，包括血管化肉芽组织和伤害性神经纤维的长入都与疼痛相关。

1. 概述

盘源性疼痛的治疗方法多样，大致分为非手术治疗和手术治疗。非手术治疗包括药物治疗、物理治疗、核心肌群训练、手法治疗、针灸、心理治疗、注射治疗和介入治疗等。药物治疗主要包括非甾体抗炎药、肌松药、抗焦虑药等的应用。介入治疗包括硬膜外糖皮质激素注射、椎间盘内热疗、脊髓电刺激、化学溶盘等[1]。手术治疗包括椎间盘融合和全椎间盘置换等。

2. 富血小板血浆在盘源性疼痛中的临床应用

富血小板血浆（PRP）作为一种通过离心分离血液而获得的血小板浓度高于生理基线的自体血，已被广泛应用于骨科疾病的治疗，包括膝骨关节炎、肩袖损伤、跟腱疾病等，近年来，PRP也逐渐被应用于盘源性疼痛的治疗，其治疗机制与血小板释放生长因子和抗菌蛋白显著相关。PRP所含的血小板浓度是全血的3～8倍，随着血小板浓度的升高，PRP含有的生长因子和细胞因子的浓度也更高，如上皮生长因子、胰岛素样生长因子、血小板源性生长因子、转化生长因子及血管内皮生长因子等。高浓度的生长因子被释放到胶原损伤或变性的部位，可刺激参与再生的细胞聚集、增殖和分化，增加胶原含量，从而促进愈合。

在临床研究方面，越来越多的证据提示PRP可用于治疗盘源性疼痛，并可明显改善盘源性疼痛的疼痛程度及功能损害。2016年，Tuakli-Wosornu等纳入47例保守治疗无效的慢性中重度腰椎间盘源性疼痛患者，进行了一项双盲随机对照临床研究。其中29例患者给予单次椎间盘内PRP注射作为试验组，另18例患者进行常规治疗作为对照组，采用NRS评分评估疼痛程度，采用功能等级指数（FRI）评估功能改善情况，采用改良的北美脊柱外科协会结果问卷评估患者的满意度。结果显示：治疗结束8周后，试验组在疼痛、功能及满意度方面较对照组有明显的改善，并且试验组在1年的随访过程中功能改善均较对照组有明显提高；在安全性方面，未发现椎间盘间隙感染、神经损伤等不良反应[2]。

2016年，Levi等探讨了椎间盘内PRP注射对盘源性腰痛患者的治疗效

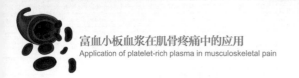
果，采用VAS评分评估疼痛改善情况，采用Oswestry伤残指数（Oswestry disability index，ODI）评估功能改善情况。治疗后6个月随访时发现，47%的患者报告疼痛改善至少50%，ODI评分改善30%[3]。

2017年，Akeda等进行了一项前瞻性探索性临床研究，对14例3个月以上不伴下肢痛的慢性腰痛患者进行椎间盘内PRP注射治疗，治疗1个月后发现患者VAS评分较治疗前显著减低，并且此效果在1年的随访过程中一直存在，且在治疗过程中未发现不良事件[4]。

2019年，Cheng等对19例病程在6个月以上、经保守治疗无效的慢性下腰痛患者给予椎间盘内PRP注射治疗，在注射5～9年后，约71%的患者的疼痛和功能较基线水平有明显改善，其余29%的患者需要手术干预[5]。

2020年，Rawson报道，2例有症状的腰椎间盘突出症患者在接受腰椎PRP注射和硬膜外浓缩血小板裂解物衍生的生长因子注射治疗后4周，疼痛减轻50%，并且步行能力改善；在第二次注射后4周，患者疼痛消失，功能几乎完全改善，并且腰椎MRI显示有良好的腰椎间盘突出再吸收效果，只残留有轻微的腰椎间盘突出，未压迫到脊神经，继续随访6个月，疼痛和功能改善仍然显著存在[6]。

3. PRP在盘源性疼痛治疗中的基础研究

在基础研究方面，对人椎间盘标本注射PRP后发现，细胞的增殖和分化及Ⅱ型胶原和蛋白多糖的合成增加[7]，从PRP分离的可溶性因子可促进猪椎间盘细胞的基质代谢[8]。在动物实验中，椎间盘内注射PRP可使实验性损伤的椎间盘正常细胞结构和椎间盘高度得到恢复[9-10]。

针对盘源性疼痛患者，自体PRP注射相较于手术治疗更安全，且对于保守治疗无效的患者也可显著改善疼痛和功能，尤其适用于有糖皮质激素使用禁忌证的患者。PRP注射治疗在盘源性疼痛方面可能是一个安全且有较好疗效的治疗方法，但仍需要更多的RCT来探讨和支持。

（许珍）

参考文献

[1] MOHAMMED S, YU J. Platelet-rich plasma injections: an emerging therapy for chronic discogenic low back pain[J]. Journal of spine surgery（Hong Kong），2018，4（1）：115-122.

[2] TUAKLI-WOSORNU Y A, TERRY A, BOACHIE-ADJEI K, et al. Lumbar intradiskal platelet-rich plasma（PRP）injections: a prospective, double-blind, randomized controlled study[J]. Pm&R, 2016, 8（1）：1-10.

[3] LEVI D, HORN S, TYSZKO S, et al. Intradiscal platelet-rich plasma injection for chronic discogenic low back pain: preliminary results from a prospective trial[J]. Pain Med, 2016, 17（6）：1010-1022.

[4] AKEDA K, OHISHI K, MASUDA K, et al. Intradiscal injection of autologous platelet-rich plasma releasate to treat discogenic low back pain: a preliminary clinical trial[J]. Asian spine journal, 2017, 11（3）：380-389.

[5] CHENG J, SANTIAGO K A, NGUYEN J T, et al. Treatment of symptomatic degenerative intervertebral discs with autologous platelet-rich plasma: follow-up at 5-9 years[J]. Regen Med, 2019, 14（9）：831-840.

[6] RAWSON B. Platelet-rich plasma and epidural platelet lysate: novel treatment for lumbar disk herniation[J]. J Am Osteopath Assoc, 2020, 120（3）：201-207.

[7] CHEN W H, LO W C, LEE J J, et al. Tissue-engineered intervertebral disc and chondrogenesis using human nucleus pulposus regulated through TGF-beta1 in platelet-rich plasma[J]. J Cell Physiol, 2006, 209（3）：744-754.

[8] AKEDA K, AN H S, PICHIKA R, et al. Platelet-rich plasma（PRP）stimulates the extracellular matrix metabolism of porcine nucleus pulposus and anulus fibrosus cells cultured in alginate beads[J]. Spine（Phila Pa 1976），2006，31（9）：959-966.

[9] GULLUNG G B, WOODALL J W, TUCCI M A, et al. Platelet-rich plasma effects on degenerative disc disease: analysis of histology and imaging in an animal model[J]. Evid Based Spine Care J, 2011, 2（4）：13-18.

[10] OBATA S, AKEDA K, IMANISHI T, et al. Effect of autologous platelet-rich plasma-releasate on intervertebral disc degeneration in the rabbit anular puncture model: a preclinical study[J]. Arthritis Res Ther, 2012, 14（6）：1-11.

第八节　富血小板血浆在骨组织修复中的应用

富血小板血浆（PRP）在骨组织修复中的应用主要涉及的疾病包括骨不连和骨坏死。

一、骨不连

骨不连又称为骨折不愈合，是指创伤性骨折后愈合过程的中断，是骨折端受到某些因素影响后愈合功能降低的表现，美国食品和药物监督管理局（FDA）对骨不连的定义为：超过9个月骨折不愈合且连续动态观察3个月未见到骨折有明显的愈合迹象。

1. 概述

骨不连是创伤性骨折常见的严重并发症之一。根据感染情况可将骨不连分为非感染性骨不连和感染性骨不连。非感染性骨不连与血液供应、骨折断端距离和固定的稳定性等因素有关；感染性骨不连常伴有慢性骨髓炎，往往与开放性骨折或外科手术有关，典型症状是红、肿、热、痛，可能伴有脓性物渗出等症状。据统计，骨折后骨不连的总体发生率达5%～10%，平均风险为1.9%。骨不连不仅严重影响患者的生活质量，也增加了医疗资源的负担[1]。

PRP是自体来源的富含血小板的血浆制品，含有许多在骨骼修复过程中发挥重要作用的细胞因子和生长因子，包括血小板源性生长因子（PDGF）、血管内皮生长因子（VEGF）、转化生长因子（TGF-β1和TGF-β2）和胰岛素样生长因子（IGF）等。血小板活化后释放的生长因子能促进细胞增殖、基质合成、类骨质生成及胶原合成[1]。目前，应用PRP修复骨组织在体外细胞实验和动物模型中均展现出较好的愈合效果，但是在临床应用中疗效不一，仍缺乏高质量、前瞻性的临床试验。

2. PRP在骨不连治疗中的临床研究

Say等单独应用PRP治疗下肢骨不连患者22例，方法是在手术后6～8个月内将氯化钙活化后的PRP注入骨折线，每周1次，共注射3次，并进行8～12个月的临床检查和X线片随访，结果6例患者在15周左右骨折愈合，11例患者不愈合，3例患者骨折愈合不确定[2]。

Marhotra等进行了一项PRP治疗长骨骨不连的前瞻性研究，共纳入94例骨不连的患者（涉及胫骨35例、股骨30例、肱骨11例、桡骨4例、尺骨12例、桡骨合并尺骨2例）。研究者在骨不连部位注入15～20mL PRP，并进行了4个月的随访，发现在4个月后有82例患者骨折愈合，有12例患者未显示有任何骨折愈合的迹象[3]。

Tawfik等对20例长骨骨不连患者应用PRP治疗，随访至17周时，有17例患者可见骨痂形成，随访至24周，其余3例患者仍未愈合[4]。上述研究表明PRP在单独应用时效果不一。

此外，也有许多PRP结合其他手段治疗骨不连的临床尝试，如联合自体骨移植、内固定或间质干细胞等。Tarallo等对10例尺骨骨不连的患者行骨移植术，使用动态钢板固定并联合注射PRP进行治疗，结果9例患者平均4个月可达到骨愈合标准，1例患者治疗失败。虽然该研究表现出较好的结果，但缺乏对照，因此无法说明PRP的作用[5]。

Peerbooms在一项前瞻性研究中纳入了41例行高位胫骨截骨术的患者，分组后一组在骨折端添加PRP和骨碎屑，另一组只加入骨碎屑，12周后发现应用PRP没有使患者在胫骨愈合中获益[6]。

Ghaffarpasand等在一项为期12个月的双盲RCT中纳入了75例长骨（股

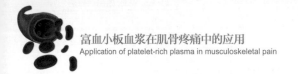

骨、胫骨、肱骨和尺骨）骨折后不愈合的患者，所有患者进行自体骨移植，并根据具体情况选择髓内钉或切开复位内固定，试验组注射5mL PRP，对照组注射同剂量生理盐水作为安慰剂，经过9个月的随访，发现PRP组的治愈率更高，愈合时间更短，疼痛评分更低[7]。

张松等在一项RCT中探讨了骨髓间充质干细胞联合PRP应用于长骨骨折后不愈合的治疗效果，该研究共纳入47例患者，其中试验组患者采用骨髓间充质干细胞联合PRP注射，对照组只采用骨髓间充质干细胞注射，随访3个月后发现，试验组患者的骨折愈合率和功能恢复水平均高于对照组[8]。

目前的研究表明，PRP治疗骨不连有一定的效果，证据级别是Ⅳ级，仍缺乏Ⅱ级和Ⅲ级（临床试验）证据[1]。大部分研究存在样本量小或缺乏严格对照等问题，不同试验也存在PRP制备方法以及激活方式的差异，因此仍需要大样本、高质量的临床试验提供可靠的证据。

3. PRP在骨不连治疗中的基础研究

成骨细胞和内皮细胞培养实验发现，PRP衍生物（如生长因子）具有剂量依赖性的刺激血管生成的能力，补充PRP衍生物可以显著增强成骨细胞的增殖，而添加低体积百分比的PRP衍生物能使内皮细胞培养物中的小管形成显著增加[9]。在体外培养中，PRP凝胶膜联合骨髓来源的间充质干细胞（BMSCs）可显著诱导人内皮细胞迁移，并增加骨形成蛋白-2（BMP-2）的表达，这些细胞还可分泌大量可溶性促血管生成因子，例如PDGF-BB、VEGF和白细胞介素-8（IL-8）。而在小鼠和兔子的骨缺损模型中，PRP/BMSCs凝胶膜也展现出类似促进骨膜增强、骨再生的能力[10]。此外，已有研究证明将PRP与不同来源（骨髓或脂肪组织）的MSCs结合使用可促进细胞增殖、软骨特异性基因和蛋白质的表达以及软骨下骨再生[11]。

目前研究较多的动物模型是小型动物如大鼠和兔子，与人类最接近的动物模型如狗、羊、小型猪因成本和愈合周期等原因相对使用较少[12]。Canbeyli等研究PRP治疗兔子股骨干骨折时发现，PRP能促进成纤维细胞的增殖，使成熟的骨组织增多而编织骨减少，但没有发现PRP对BMP-2和VEGF的影响[13]。

Gunay在兔子肋骨骨折模型中发现，应用PRP能促进成纤维细胞增殖和毛细血管生成，PRP组的愈伤组织和髓内区域更加明显[14]。Szponder将活化的PRP和β-三磷酸钙注入兔子胫骨粉碎性骨折的缺损中，在实验组中观察到了正确的骨结合，同时，在其他小型动物模型的实验中，超过91%的动物观察到了骨结合[15]。Jungbluth等在小型猪的胫骨近端干骺部骨折的研究中发现，使用PRP和磷酸钙复合物能促进骨骼再生，但不能使愈合的骨融合得更牢固[16]。

局部缺氧是骨愈合受限的因素之一，Schneppendahl在兔子自体骨移植的研究中证明，额外应用高压氧联合PRP能显著增加骨缺损（中心区和皮质区）处新骨和周围血管的形成，提高骨再生能力[17]。

动物种类、健康状况、血小板、生长因子和白细胞浓度以及骨不连的类型都会影响PRP促进骨折愈合的效果。总体而言，PRP在动物模型中表现出可促进骨折愈合的积极效果，为其临床应用提供了有力的证据。此外，许多研究探讨了PRP联合其他治疗手段如自体（异体）骨移植和应用生物活性玻璃、自体支架、矿化的胶原蛋白基质、磷酸钙颗粒、羟基磷灰石等的效果，也得到了不错的结果，可以预见PRP联合疗法在骨折不愈合的治疗中有很好的应用前景[12]。

二、骨坏死

骨坏死是骨质血供丧失而导致的一种疾病，表现为缺乏血液供应的骨

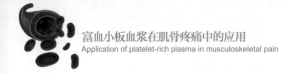
髓质、骨皮质和骨髓逐步变性坏死。

1. 概述

根据病因可将骨坏死分为创伤性骨坏死、非创伤性骨坏死和感染性骨坏死。创伤性骨坏死可能由血管机械性阻断、血栓形成和栓塞、血管壁压力升高以及静脉阻塞导致；非创伤性骨坏死的发病机制尚不明确，可能与不良嗜好、疾病及治疗方法有关，如酗酒、吸烟、血液凝固障碍疾病、肾脏疾病、大剂量皮质激素的使用等；感染性骨坏死是炎性病变的结果与表现。骨坏死早期可无明显症状，随着病情进展可出现关节疼痛及功能受限，在负重下疼痛加剧。临床上以负重的股骨头坏死最为常见，颌骨坏死也不在少数，如双膦酸盐相关性颌骨坏死（BRONJ）等，而发生在其他小关节非负重骨的坏死则较少[18-19]。

骨坏死的治疗是骨科棘手的问题，临床上常见的治疗方法可分为保守治疗和手术治疗两类。保守治疗种类繁多，如药物、高压氧、物理因子、干细胞、生长因子、运动训练等的治疗，这些治疗手段疗效不一，大部分很难持续改善坏死骨的功能，最终还需要进行手术治疗[19]。

作为拥有超生理浓度血小板的PRP，在骨坏死治疗方面表现出积极的作用。PRP含有多种丰富的生长因子和细胞因子，能促进血管的生成，增强坏死骨的成骨作用。有研究表明PRP能调节炎性细胞因子浓度，总体下调炎症反应，从而抑制股骨头坏死的进展，并可通过中断关节的炎症损伤过程来减轻疼痛[20]。而与PRP类似的PRGF能通过多种生长因子的共同作用来促进组织血管的生成。与PRP和PRGF相比，PRF的生产技术简单，成本较低，并且不需要进行多次吸液分离。PRF含有大量的纤维蛋白、血小板和白细胞，其致密的纤维蛋白网络为血管生成提供了有利于组织细胞存储和附着的天然支架。

PRP在骨坏死中的应用主要涉及颌骨坏死和股骨头坏死。其中股骨头坏死详见本章第四节。

2. PRP在颌骨坏死治疗中的临床应用

Bocanegra-Perez等报道了应用PRP治疗BRONJ的研究，他们对8例诊断为BRONJ的患者进行手术创口清理和坏死骨清除，局部敷PRP后缝合伤口，接受定期的临床和放射学随访检查。结果显示，治疗后2～4周所有患者创口均闭合良好，在平均14个月的随访期间没有骨坏死暴露的迹象[21]。

Martins等对21例发生BRONJ的癌症患者进行治疗，其中2例进行药物治疗，5例进行药物联合外科治疗，14例进行PRP联合综合治疗（包括药物治疗、外科治疗和激光治疗），经过1个月的随访观察评估发现，PRP联合综合治疗组患者颌骨坏死创口愈合率达到86%，明显高于药物治疗组（0%）和药物联合外科治疗组（40%）[22]。

Longo等评估了72例BRONJ患者的非手术治疗（如口服环丙沙星）、手术治疗以及手术联合PRP治疗对颌骨坏死伤口愈合的效果，其中非手术治疗组如治疗2周后无好转迹象即进行手术。结果23例患者经非手术治疗后完全愈合，15例接受手术治疗的患者8例完全愈合、7例部分愈合，34例接受手术联合PRP治疗的患者32例完全愈合、2例部分愈合。PRP在改善颌骨坏死伤口愈合方面显示出良好的效果[23]。

除了应用PRP联合手术治疗颌骨坏死外，也有许多临床医生探究了PRGF和PRF联合手术治疗的效果。Mozzati等应用PRGF治疗BRONJ时发现，PRGF可能会增强骨和上皮组织的血管生成与再生，该研究纳入了32例ⅡB级BRONJ患者，手术切除感染的坏死骨后敷用PRGF凝胶膜并进行缝合，在术后6个月、1年以及48～50个月的随访中每年进行影像学和临床检查，结果发现所有患者黏膜闭合完好，临床和影像学评估均无残留感染坏死的骨[24]。

Szentpeteri等在一项研究中纳入了101例药物相关的颌骨坏死（MRONJ）患者，进行传统外科手术与PRF辅助手术治疗效果的比较，术后进行体格检查和影像学检查，如观察到伤口愈合且未出现骨坏死迹象即表明治愈。在术后4周的检查中发现，传统外科手术组的73例患者中38例康复（52.05%）、30例伤口愈合不良（41.10%），应用PRF辅助手术治疗的28例患者中23例治疗效果较好（82.14%）、5例伤口愈合不良（17.86%）。在随访中也发现传统外科手术组的复发率显著高于PRF辅助手术治疗组。一方面，PRF通过减少骨重塑、减弱血管生成和抑制免疫机制来阻断骨坏死的进程；另一方面，PRF可以为骨坏死的修复提供稳定的支架，充当牙槽骨和口腔之间的屏障膜，防止伤口愈合并发症的发生，为MRONJ患者闭合骨暴露的创口提供快速、简便和有效的替代手段[25-26]。

尽管PRP及其类似衍生物联合手术等其他疗法在颌骨坏死的治疗中表现出积极的效果，但缺乏PRP（或其类似衍生物）对照或单独应用的临床研究。总体而言，目前这方面的临床研究差异性较大，质量不高，提供的证据级别有限。

3. PRP在骨坏死治疗中的基础研究

双膦酸盐常用于骨转移疾病或骨质疏松症的抗吸收治疗，其在抑制破骨细胞功能的同时，也会对成骨细胞和成纤维细胞的增殖产生负面影响，易导致颌骨坏死[27]。PRP、PRF和PRGF含有高浓度的PDGF、TGF和IGF等生长因子，在颌骨坏死局部应用时可促进成骨细胞和成纤维细胞的黏附、增殖和迁移。

Steller等研究应用PRP和PRF对唑来膦酸（ZA）处理的成骨细胞和口腔成纤维细胞的增殖、迁移及存活能力的影响。研究中使用ZA处理成纤维细胞和成骨细胞后，分别加入PRP和PRF培养，用实时细胞分析仪（RTCA）分析细胞增殖，用划痕实验和MTT测量分析细胞的迁移和生存能力，结果表明，PRP和PRF能在24h内增强细胞活力，降低ZA对细胞迁移的负面影响，且PRF的作用比PRP更为显著。这表明PRF和PRP可能对BRONJ的治疗有积极作用[28]。另有研究表明，ZA可通过调节连接蛋白43（Cx43）干扰成骨细胞的代谢，而PRP和PRF中存在的TGF-β1会改变Cx43的表达，这可能是PRP和PRF调节ZA对成骨细胞的作用机制之一[29]。此外，蛋白质酪氨酸磷酸酶也是ZA作用的目标之一，而PRF和PRP可能通过调节相关的离子通道对抗ZA诱导的骨丢失[27]。

Cardoso在大鼠拔牙部位使用双膦酸盐诱导形成BRONJ，然后分两组分别进行手术治疗（BRONJ边缘切除）和PRP联合手术治疗，在术后14天、28天和42天后进行取样评估。显微断层扫描结果表明，两组之间无显著性差异，而组织形态计量学分析显示，在术后28天和42天时，PRP联合手术治疗组比手术治疗组有更多的新骨和更大的血管形成，以及更高的VEGF表达，这表明使用PRP可以有效改善大鼠BRONJ局部组织的修复[30]。

Toro等采用大鼠模型研究PRP预防MRONJ的有效性，大鼠被分为唑来膦酸盐治疗并拔牙（ZOL）组和唑来膦酸盐治疗并拔牙后局部施用PRP（PRP-ZOL）组，并在术后28天对大鼠拔牙部位的组织学切片进行组织学和免疫组化分析。结果显示，PRP-ZOL组比ZOL组有较高的新生骨组织百分比和较低的非重要骨组织百分比，以及针对TNF-α和IL-1β的更低免疫标记，证明PRP能提高大鼠拔牙部位的组织修复能力并防止拔牙后发生MRONJ[31]。Barba-Recreo等的研究也表明，在MRONJ的预防方面，PRP和脂肪衍生干细胞可能有协同作用，联用BMP-2可以进一步改善效果[32]。

（袁泽）

参考文献

[1] ANDERSEN C, NICHOLAS M W, SHARIATZADEH M, et al. The use of platelet-rich plasma (PRP) for the management of non-union fractures[J]. Curr Osteoporos Rep, 2021, 19 (suppl 2): 1-14.

[2] SAY F, TÜRKELI E, BÜLBÜL M. Is platelet-rich plasma injection an effective choice in cases of non-union? [J]. Acta Chir Orthop Traumatol Cech, 2014, 81 (5): 340-345.

[3] MALHOTRA R, KUMAR V, GARG B, et al. Role of autologous platelet-rich plasma in treatment of long-bone nonunions: a prospective study[J]. Musculoskelet Surg, 2015, 99 (3): 243-248.

[4] TAWFIK A, KAMEL N. Assessment of autologous platelet gel injection in nonunited long bones[J]. The Egyptian Journal of Haematology, 2017, 42 (1): 31.

[5] TARALLO L, MUGNAI R, ADANI R, et al. Treatment of the ulna non-unions using dynamic compression plate fixation, iliac bone grafting and autologous platelet concentrate[J]. Eur J Orthop Surg Traumatol, 2012, 22 (8): 681-687.

[6] PEERBOOMS J C, COLARIS J W, HAKKERT A A, et al. No positive bone healing after using platelet rich plasma in a skeletal defect. An observational prospective cohort study[J]. Int Orthop, 2012, 36 (10): 2113-2119.

[7] GHAFFARPASAND F, SHAHREZAEI M, DEHGHANKHALILI M. Effects of platelet rich plasma on healing rate of long bone non-union fractures: a randomized double-blind placebo controlled clinical trial[J]. Bull Emerg Trauma, 2016, 4 (3): 134-140.

[8] ZHANG S, ZHANG T, FU G H, et al. Therapeutic effect of autologous platelet rich plasma combined with bone marrow mesenchymal stem cell transplantation on long shaft fracture bone nonunion[J]. Chinese Journal of Tissue Engineering Research, 2017, 21 (29): 4716-4721.

[9] MOOREN R E, HENDRIKS E J, VAN DEN BEUCKEN J J, et al. The effect of platelet-rich plasma in vitro on primary cells: rat osteoblast-like cells and human endothelial cells[J]. Tissue Eng Part A, 2010, 16 (10): 3159-3172.

[10] EL BACKLY R M, ZAKY S H, MURAGLIA A, et al. A platelet-rich plasma-based membrane as a periosteal substitute with enhanced osteogenic and angiogenic properties: a new concept for bone repair[J]. Tissue Eng Part A, 2013, 19 (1-2): 152-165.

[11] VAN PHAM P, BUI K H, NGO D Q, et al. Activated platelet-rich plasma improves adipose-derived stem cell transplantation efficiency in injured articular cartilage[J]. Stem Cell Res Ther, 2013, 4 (4): 91.

[12] MARCAZZAN S, WEINSTEIN R L, DEL FABBRO M. Efficacy of platelets in bone healing: A systematic review on animal studies[J]. Platelets, 2018, 29 (4): 326-

337.

[13] CANBEYLI I D, AKGUN R C, SAHIN O, et al. Platelet-rich plasma decreases fibroblastic activity and woven bone formation with no significant immunohistochemical effect on long-bone healing: An experimental animal study with radiological outcomes[J]. J Orthop Surg（Hong Kong）, 2018, 26（3）: 1-10.

[14] GUNAY S, CANDAN H, YILMAZ R, et al. The efficacy of platelet-rich plasma in the treatment of rib fractures[J]. Thorac Cardiovasc Surg, 2017, 65（7）: 546-550.

[15] SZPONDER T, WESSELY-SZPONDER J, SOBCZYNSKA-RAK A, et al. Application of platelet-rich plasma and tricalcium phosphate in the treatment of comminuted fractures in animals[J]. In Vivo, 2018, 32（6）: 1449-1455.

[16] JUNGBLUTH P, WILD M, GRASSMANN J P, et al. Platelet-rich plasma on calcium phosphate granules promotes metaphyseal bone healing in mini-pigs[J]. J Orthop Res, 2010, 28（11）: 1448-1455.

[17] SCHNEPPENDAHL J, JUNGBLUTH P, SAGER M, et al. Synergistic effects of HBO and PRP improve bone regeneration with autologous bone grafting[J]. Injury, 2016, 47（12）: 2718-2725.

[18] MANKIN H J. Nontraumatic necrosis of bone（osteonecrosis）[J]. N Engl J Med, 1992, 326（22）: 1473-1479.

[19] 杨述华, 吴星火. 骨坏死临床研究的现状、进展与前景[J]. 中华关节外科杂志（电子版）, 2008, 2（1）: 53-56.

[20] HAN J, GAO F Q, LI Y J, et al. The use of platelet-rich plasma for the treatment of osteonecrosis of the femoral head: a systematic review[J]. BioMed Research International, 2020（10）: 1-11.

[21] BOCANEGRA-PEREZ S, VICENTE-BARRERO M, KNEZEVIC M, et al. Use of platelet-rich plasma in the treatment of bisphosphonate-related osteonecrosis of the jaw[J]. Int J Oral Maxillofac Surg, 2012, 41（11）: 1410-1415.

[22] MARTINS M A, MARTINS M D, LASCALA C A, et al. Association of laser phototherapy with PRP improves healing of bisphosphonate-related osteonecrosis of the jaws in cancer patients: a preliminary study[J]. Oral Oncol, 2012, 48（1）: 79-84.

[23] LONGO F, GUIDA A, AVERSA C, et al. Platelet rich plasma in the treatment of bisphosphonate-related osteonecrosis of the jaw: personal experience and review of the literature[J]. Int J Dent, 2014（3）: 1-7.

[24] MOZZATI M, GALLESIO G, ARATA V, et al. Platelet-rich therapies in the treatment of intravenous bisphosphonate-related osteonecrosis of the jaw: a report of 32 cases[J]. Oral Oncol, 2012, 48（5）: 469-474.

[25] SZENTPETERI S, SCHMIDT L, RESTAR L, et al. The effect of platelet-rich fibrin membrane in surgical therapy of medication-related osteonecrosis of the jaw[J]. J Oral

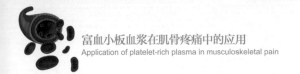

Maxillofac Surg, 2020, 78（5）：738-748.

[26] INCHINGOLO F, CANTORE S, DIPALMA G, et al. Platelet rich fibrin in the management of medication-related osteonecrosis of the jaw: a clinical and histopathological evaluation[J]. J Biol Regul Homeost Agents, 2017, 31（3）：811-816.

[27] SAVINO S, TOSCANO A, PURGATORIO R, et al. Novel bisphosphonates with antiresorptive effect in bone mineralization and osteoclastogenesis[J]. Eur J Med Chem, 2018, 158: 184-200.

[28] STELLER D, HERBST N, PRIES R, et al. Positive impact of platelet-rich plasma and platelet-rich fibrin on viability, migration and proliferation of osteoblasts and fibroblasts treated with zoledronic acid[J]. Sci Rep, 2019, 9（1）：1-11.

[29] CHELLINI F, TANI A, VALLONE L, et al. Platelet-rich plasma prevents in vitro transforming growth factor-beta1-induced fibroblast to myofibroblast transition: involvement of vascular endothelial growth factor（VEGF）-A/VEGF receptor-1-mediated signaling（dagger）[J]. Cells, 2018, 7（9）：142.

[30] CARDOSO C L, CURRA C, CURI M M, et al. Treatment of bisphosphonate-related osteonecrosis using platelet-rich plasma: microtomographic, microscopic, and immunohistochemical analyses[J]. Braz Oral Res, 2019, 33（9）：1-12.

[31] TORO L F, DE MELLO-NETO J M, SANTOS F, et al. Application of autologous platelet-rich plasma on tooth extraction site prevents occurence of medication-related osteonecrosis of the jaws in rats[J]. Sci Rep, 2019, 9（1）：22.

[32] BARBA-RECREO P, DEL CASTILLO PARDO DE VERA J L, GEORGIEV-HRISTOV T, et al. Adipose-derived stem cells and platelet-rich plasma for preventive treatment of bisphosphonate-related osteonecrosis of the jaw in a murine model[J]. J Craniomaxillofac Surg, 2015, 43（7）：1161-1168.

第四章

富血小板血浆在软组织修复中的应用

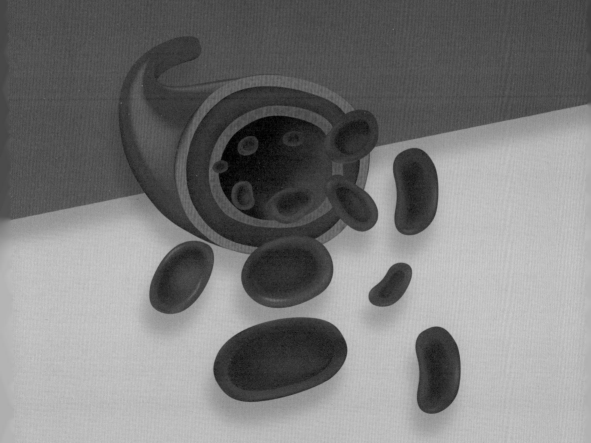

第一节　富血小板血浆在肌腱修复中的应用

肌腱是一种结构复杂的组织，成熟的肌腱组织是由散布在肌腱细胞中的胶原纤维和非胶原分子网络组成的。肌腱最小的结构单位是胶原原纤维，然后逐渐聚集为微原纤维、原纤维、纤维，纤维束通过薄的疏松结缔组织束缚在一起，这些组织称为腱膜，分为腱内膜和腱外膜。腱膜一方面能减少纤维束之间滑动时产生的摩擦，另一方面可通行与肌腱组织相关的血管和神经。肌腱的主要功能是将力从肌肉传递到骨骼，将肌肉收缩转化为关节运动。肌腱的刚度介于肌肉和骨骼之间，可以充当缓冲器，防止因肌肉与骨骼直接连接而导致的应力集中，在运动中起保护骨骼和肌肉的作用[1-2]。

一、概述

由于衰老、氧化应激、过度负荷及外伤等因素，慢性或急性的肌腱损伤在生活中非常常见。因所在部位和所参与运动的差异，某些肌腱比其他肌腱更容易发生损伤变性，如跟腱、髌腱及前臂伸肌和肩袖肌群等的肌腱。此外，手和手指的伸肌腱及屈肌腱也易发生直接撕裂伤。有研究表明，所有运动损伤中有30%～50%涉及肌腱损伤，总人口中有16%患有肩袖相关的肩痛，这一数据在老年人群中达到21%，在体育界更高。因肌腱在人体力学中的关键作用，肌腱的损伤或退化不仅让患者饱受疼痛的困扰，而且会造成运动功能的严重损害甚至残疾，增加患者和社会的医疗负担[2]。

肌腱损伤后的愈合可分为三个有部分重叠的阶段：第一阶段是炎症反应期，发生在损伤后几天内，表现为损伤部位被红细胞、白细胞和血小板浸润，形成血纤蛋白凝块填充，巨噬细胞则会消化坏死的组织碎片，肌腱细胞被募集到受伤区域并发生增殖；第二阶段是增生修复期，发生在损伤后两周左右，此时生物活性物质开始合成，巨噬细胞开始转变角色，释放多种生长因子及募集细胞，肌腱细胞主要合成Ⅲ型胶原蛋白；第三阶段是重塑期，发生在损伤后1～2个月，持续时间可超过一年，此期Ⅰ型胶原蛋白逐渐占主导地位，胶原纤维束开始恢复有序的排列，但很难恢复损伤前的生物力学特性[1]。肌腱的血管化较差，成熟的肌腱组织几乎无血管结构，发生变性时难以逆转，因此肌腱的愈合能力低下，发生损伤时难以修复[3]。

临床上肌腱损伤常用的治疗方式有保守治疗（休息、冷疗、药物治疗、加压和抬高患肢）、手术缝合和肌腱移植等。口服非甾体类药物、物理治疗、局部注射皮质类固醇等保守治疗一般很难恢复肌腱原来的结构和功能水平，而且应用皮质类固醇治疗时常伴有肌腱萎缩和脆性增加等不良反应。有研究表明，干细胞疗法、基因疗法可作为肌腱修复的新疗法，但目前尚处于临床前探索和开发阶段。

随着对组织康复中生长因子疗法研究的深入，使用富血小板血浆（PRP）作为丰富的生长因子来源治疗运动损伤的研究日益受到关注。PRP是自体来源的富含高浓度血小板的血浆，含有丰富的生长因子，如VEFG、TGF-β、PDGF、IGF和EGF等，这些生长因子能诱导细胞信号传导，从而刺激组织血管生成，促进肌腱细胞的增殖、分化以及新基质的形成，对肌腱细胞的胶原蛋白合成、内源性生长因子的产生有积极的影响。除生长因子以外，PRP还含有白细胞介素、趋化因子、蛋白酶、蛋白酶抑制剂、鞘脂、血栓素、5-羟色胺等，可在肌腱损伤的早期阶段发挥抗炎等

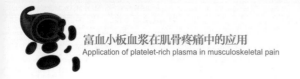

作用[2, 4]。

PRP制备简单且成本低，目前已应用于肱骨外上髁炎、跟腱损伤、慢性跟腱炎、肩袖损伤等常见肌腱损伤变性的治疗，展现了一定的临床疗效。近年来在肌腱修复领域应用PRP的实验和临床研究逐渐增多，应用PRP有望成为肌腱修复的新疗法。

二、PRP在跟腱损伤中的应用

跟腱由腓肠肌和比目鱼肌部分远端肌腱合并形成，是人体最大最强的肌腱，担负着重要的功能。近些年由于运动潮流的兴起，急性跟腱断裂越发常见，严重损害患者的行动能力。这种损伤能持续非常长的一段时间，即使在跟腱损伤愈合后，正常的运动功能也会受到不同程度的影响[5]。

1. 概述

急性跟腱断裂主要有手术治疗和非手术治疗两种选择，接受非手术治疗的患者恢复的时间更长。最近的研究发现，没有证据表明这两种治疗方式在患者跟腱的再断裂率以及功能结局方面存在差异[6]。因此考虑到医疗资源的限制以及患者的负担，非手术治疗无疑是一个合理的选择。

由于PRP在大部分实验研究中均显示出对肌腱愈合的积极的细胞和组织方面的作用，因此现已广泛用于运动医学和骨科医学中，具有广阔的市场前景。但由于PRP制备的标准不同以及临床试验的异质性，不同的临床试验中PRP治疗跟腱断裂的疗效不一，甚至有高质量临床试验证明PRP无效[7]。目前的证据仅支持PRP作为手术治疗的有效辅助手段[8]。

2. PRP治疗跟腱损伤的临床研究

英国一项多中心临床随机对照试验研究了PRP治疗跟腱断裂的效果。该研究纳入了19家医院共230例急性跟腱断裂的患者，其中114例患者接受

PRP注射，另外116例患者接受安慰剂注射，两组患者均进行标准的康复护理。结果显示，在治疗后24周进行脚跟抬起耐力测试以评估跟腱的功能时，两组主要结局指标——肢体对称指数没有差异，次要结局指标——跟腱完全断裂评分（ATRS）、VAS评分、患者特定功能评分和不良事件均不存在差异，这表明注射PRP并没有改善急性跟腱断裂后的客观肌腱功能、患者报告功能和生活质量，即PRP对急性跟腱断裂的患者无益处[7]。

Boesen等的研究也有类似的结果。他们的研究纳入了40例发生急性跟腱断裂的男性患者，所有患者均配戴矫形器，在第1天即进行负重训练，并每隔14天进行PRP或安慰剂（生理盐水，<0.5mL）注射，共注射4次，从第9周开始，所有患者均接受相同的运动训练。在第3、6、12周进行治疗效果的测量评估（包括ATRS、脚跟抬高、肌腱伸长、小腿围和脚踝背屈运动范围），随访38个月。结果发现两组之间的ATRS在任何时间点均无显著性差异（随访12个月时，PRP组为90.1分，安慰剂组为88.8分），所有功能结局指标也无差异。与未受伤的下肢相比，患侧在12个月时未恢复正常的功能，表明PRP在急性跟腱断裂保守治疗中没有给患者带来任何临床和功能的改善[9]。

虽然在急性跟腱断裂后单独应用PRP的研究大部分显示无效，但研究也显示PRP作为一种辅助手段与手术联用时有较好的临床疗效。邹健等研究了PRP作为急性跟腱断裂术后生物增强剂的效果。该研究纳入了36例患者，随机分成PRP组（16例）和对照组（20例），PRP组除修复缝合断裂的跟腱外，还将PRP注射到副腱鞘和破裂的组织周围。术后3个月、6个月、12个月和24个月时进行等速肌力评估，术后6个月、12个月和24个月时评估踝部ROM、小腿围、Leppilahti评分和SF-36评分。与对照组相比，3个月时PRP组的等速肌力评估结果较好，在6个月和12个月时PRP组也获得了较高的SF-36评分和Leppilahti评分，在24个月时PRP组的踝关节活动

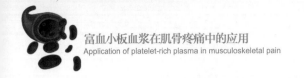
范围有所改善，表明PRP可以作为急性跟腱断裂修复的生物增强剂，改善短期和中期功能结局[10]。

3. PRP治疗跟腱损伤的基础研究

大量研究表明，PRP中的生长因子对肌腱组织的修复有多方面的生物学效应，包括促进血管生成、细胞增殖及趋化、生物合成、免疫调节、消炎、抗纤维化等[5]。有研究发现在PRP处理后的跟腱中Ⅰ型胶原蛋白合成的基因表达增加，而基质金属蛋白酶MMP-1和MMP-3的表达降低[11]。Cross也发现贫白细胞PRP可以刺激正常的胶原蛋白基质合成，并减少与基质降解和炎症相关的细胞因子，如MMP-9、MMP-13和IL-1β[12]。

Kaux等用大鼠跟腱断裂模型研究PRP能否促进肌腱愈合，他们在切断大鼠跟腱后立即注射PRP（60只）和生理盐水（60只），结果发现在第15天和第30天PRP组大鼠跟腱组织机械强度的增加比生理盐水组更明显，在第30天PRP组Ⅰ型胶原蛋白的增加更多，表明应用PRP能促进跟腱断裂早期愈合并增加愈合跟腱的机械强度[13]。Çirci等研究了跟腱损伤后在不同时间注射PRP对大鼠跟腱愈合的影响，结果发现损伤后第1天注射与第3天注射相比，炎症程度、成纤维细胞的密度和表面厚度、胶原纤维的合成均明显增加，说明跟腱损伤后应立即注射PRP[14]。Kimura等在家兔跟腱断裂模型中研究PRP的作用，其在不同时间点获取肌腱组织进行组织学检查和定量评估，结果显示在损伤后1周和2周，PRP组的成纤维细胞数量和新血管形成程度均高于对照组，成纤维细胞数量和CD31阳性细胞的面积比在损伤后2周达到峰值后降低，在损伤后6周，PRP组的成纤维细胞数量明显减少，胶原纤维束在一个方向上平行于肌腱的长轴排列。这些结果表明PRP在肌腱愈合的早期能促进成纤维细胞的迁移、增殖及新血管的形成，使重塑阶段更早开始。Kimura的研究还表明，与低浓度的PRP（基线浓度的3.8倍）相比，高浓度的PRP（基线浓度的12.8倍）在促进兔子跟腱组织愈合和改善跟腱机械性能方面更具有优势[15]。

4. 小结

尽管PRP因其独特吸引力成为跟腱损伤修复治疗的关注点，但其应用仍处于早期阶段，需要更多的基础研究探索PRP治疗跟腱损伤的机制，进而发掘PRP治疗的潜力。同时，标准化PRP制剂的制备方法将使PRP的研究变得更加有序。目前，PRP在临床研究中大多数未能表现出与实验研究预期相符的治疗效果，因此，在跟腱损伤的保守治疗中应慎重考虑是否使用PRP。

（袁泽）

参考文献

［1］ VOLETI P B，BUCKLEY M R，SOSLOWSKY L J．Tendon healing：repair and regeneration［J］．Annu Rev Biomed Eng，2012，14（1）：47-71．

［2］ DOCHEVA D，MULLER S A，MAJEWSKI M，et al．Biologics for tendon repair［J］．Adv Drug Deliv Rev，2015，84：222-239．

［3］ BENJAMIN M，RALPHS J R．Tendons and ligaments—an overview［J］．Histol Histopathol，1997，12（4）：1135-1144．

［4］ RAJABI H，SHEIKHANI S H，NOROUZIAN M，et al．The healing effects of aquatic activities and allogenic injection of platelet-rich plasma（PRP）on injuries of Achilles tendon in experimental rat［J］．World J Plast Surg，2015，4（1）：66-73．

［5］ MAFFULLI N，PERETTI G M．Treatment decisions for acute Achilles tendon ruptures［J］．Lancet，2020，395（10222）：397-398．

［6］ OCHEN Y，BEKS R B，VAN HEIJL M，et al．Operative treatment versus nonoperative treatment of Achilles tendon ruptures：systematic review and meta-analysis［J］．Bmj，2019，364：k5120．

［7］ KEENE D J，ALSOUSOU J，HARRISON P，et al．Platelet rich plasma injection for acute Achilles tendon rupture：PATH-2 randomised，placebo controlled，superiority trial［J］．Bmj，2019，367：1-11．

［8］ PADILLA S，SANCHEZ M，VAQUERIZO V，et al．Platelet-rich plasma applications for Achilles tendon repair：a bridge between biology and surgery［J］．Int J Mol Sci，2021，22（2）：824．

［9］ BOESEN A P，BOESEN M I，HANSEN R，et al．Effect of platelet-rich plasma on nonsurgically treated acute Achilles tendon ruptures：a randomized，double-blinded prospective study［J］．Am J Sports Med，2020，48（9）：2268-2276．

［10］ ZOU J，MO X L，SHI Z M，et al．A prospective study of platelet-rich plasma as biological augmentation for acute Achilles tendon rupture repair［J］．Biomed Res Int，2016（1）：1-8．

［11］ YAN R J，GU Y J，RAN J S，et al．Intratendon delivery of leukocyte-poor platelet-rich plasma improves healing compared with leukocyte-rich platelet-rich plasma in a rabbit Achilles tendinopathy model［J］．Am J Sports Med，2017，45（8）：1909-1920．

［12］ CROSS J A，COLE B J，SPATNY K P，et al．Leukocyte-reduced platelet-rich plasma normalizes matrix metabolism in torn human rotator cuff tendons［J］．Am J Sports Med，2015，43（12）：2898-2906．

［13］ KAUX J F，DRION P V，COLIGE A，et al．Effects of platelet-rich plasma（PRP）on the healing of Achilles tendons of rats［J］．Wound Repair Regen，2012，20（5）：748-756．

［14］ ÇIRCI E，AKMAN Y E，ŞÜKÜR E，et al．Impact of platelet-rich plasma injection timing on healing of Achilles tendon injury in a rat model［J］．Acta Orthop Traumatol Turc，2016，50（3）：366-372．

［15］ KIMURA S，YAMAGUCHI S，SADAMASU A，et al．Effect of platelet rich plasma concentration on tendon healing in a rabbit achilles tendon transection model［J］．Chiba Medical Journal，2020，96E：47-54．

第二节　富血小板血浆在韧带修复中的应用

　　韧带是关节上连接骨与骨的致密结缔组织。不同韧带的大小、形状、方向和位置各不相同。韧带表面覆有一层结缔组织，与韧带实质部分相似，并与韧带附着部位周围的骨膜融合。在结缔组织下是紧密平行排列的胶原纤维束，沿韧带长轴排列，并有波纹状或卷曲状结构，这种结构扮演着重要的生物力学角色，在韧带的负荷增加时，其允许韧带延长从而保护韧带免受损伤。在显微镜下可见被基质包围的成纤维细胞，这些细胞负责合成韧带的组成基质。韧带具有维持关节稳定、引导关节在正常范围内活动的功能，此外还有助于维持关节内稳态以及组成关节本体感觉系统[1-2]。

一、概述

韧带的损伤通常是由外部创伤或运动引起的急性或慢性损伤。当韧带承受的负荷超过其最大弹性限度时，容易造成结构的改变。急性韧带损伤一般由意外创伤和剧烈运动引起，可造成韧带破裂、部分断裂或全部断裂。慢性韧带损伤可能是由于年龄增长或长期的超负荷作用而引起韧带变性，还可能与急性韧带损伤后出现的慢性不稳定、胶原纤维的过度拉伸或撕裂及关节松弛有关，可能还伴有炎症反应[3]。随着生活方式的转变，越来越多的人开始参与各种各样的运动，伴随而来的肌腱、韧带损伤也越来越常见。

韧带损伤后的愈合过程与肌腱类似，可分为部分重叠的急性反应期、增生期和重塑期三个阶段。由于结构和功能的差异，不同韧带的损伤的概率不同。在经常参与体育运动的年轻人群中，前交叉韧带（ACL）和内侧副韧带（MCL）的损伤占膝关节所有韧带损伤的90%。不同的韧带愈合能力也不同，如ACL破裂后几乎难以愈合，需要进行手术缝补，而MCL损伤后有很强的自愈倾向，这可能与膝关节的内环境有关[4]。此外，损伤的韧带虽然能愈合，但往往不能完全恢复到正常韧带的形态、组成和生物力学水平。目前已有许多策略用于提高韧带的愈合质量，如关节控制运动、生化调节、手术修复、移植、基因治疗和组织工程等[1]。

富血小板血浆（PRP）及其衍生物富含多种生长因子和细胞因子，对组织修复有积极的作用。这些生长因子不仅能使成纤维细胞和其他炎性细胞迁移到韧带损伤部位，而且还能刺激成纤维细胞的增殖以及胶原蛋白（Ⅰ型、Ⅲ型和Ⅴ型）和非胶原蛋白（如蛋白聚糖）的合成。PDGF和TGF-β是伤口愈合调节领域被研究最多的生长因子，其对炎症细胞和成纤维细胞具有趋化作用和促进增殖作用。TGF-β可以使细胞表面的PDGF受体数量增加，并通过诱导PDGF-BB的表达来促进细胞的增殖，EGF除了对成纤维细胞具有趋化作用和促进增殖作用，还能刺激非胶原蛋白和糖胺聚糖的合成，bFGF能将成纤维细胞吸引到伤口部位并刺激其复制[5]。目前PRP已经广泛应用于肌肉骨骼系统损伤的修复，有关PRP治疗韧带损伤的用法及机制也在进一步研究中。以下介绍PRP在比较常见的ACL损伤中的研究与应用现状。

二、PRP在ACL损伤中的应用

ACL断裂是最常见的与运动有关的韧带损伤，占膝关节运动损伤的50%以上。流行病学显示，在美国有20多万人受此影响，每年产生的直接和间接费用超过70亿美元，其中参加高水平比赛的青少年具有最高的损伤风险。40%的ACL断裂是由非接触性行为造成的，包括旋转和跳跃等。此外，ACL损伤与一些危险因素相关，如性别（女性的风险是男性的3倍）、年龄（发病高峰期在16～18岁）和运动的强度及频率（剧烈和频繁的运动易致损伤）等，骨形态、神经肌肉控制、遗传特征和激素环境的变化也可能有影响[6]。

1. 概述

由于大多数ACL损伤患者为运动活跃的青年，所以他们对功能恢复有较高的期望。ACL重建手术是目前恢复ACL断裂后膝关节稳定和功能的金标准，已发展形成多种成熟的技术。尽管在中长期的随访中，ACL重建手术的临床疗效总体良好，但并非所有的患者都能恢复其损伤前的运动功能水平，许多因素都会影响临床结果，如移植物的类型和术前的处理等。膝盖松弛是ACL重建术后最常见的问题，对于特殊的人群如职业运动员而言，这足以影响他们的职业生涯[7]。因此，需要新的治疗手段来增强ACL重建后的恢复效果，其中PRP作为一种生物增强剂在这一方面可能具有很大的潜力。

在手术部位施用PRP能减少促炎因子的释放，减轻术后的炎症反应，加速组织修复和伤口愈合。PRP在ACL重建中可能有助于改善移植物的融合，将移植物更好地整合到骨隧道内，使移植物更好更快地韧带化。此外，PRP的施用可能会降低移植物供体部位的发病率[7]。目前国内外已有许多学者进行相关的研究，探讨PRP在ACL重建中是否能改善患者的预后，恢复其损伤前的功能水平。

2. PRP治疗ACL损伤的临床研究

You等报道了一例超声引导下注射PRP治疗ACL部分撕裂的病例。患者为25岁女性，MRI诊断为ACL部分撕裂，经3次超声引导下注射PRP后，患者膝关节疼痛和不稳定的症状均得到改善，MRI显示ACL损伤减轻，提示PRP在ACL撕裂的治疗中具有一定潜力[8]。Berdis开展了一项包括143例21岁及以下年龄的ACL损伤患者的回顾性研究，患者均接受了ACL重建手术并使用PRP和多孔胶原蛋白载体进行辅助治疗，平均随访时间为52个月，结果有132例患者（92%）恢复到损伤前的水平，仅7例患者（5%）因再次损伤需进行二次手术，这表明应用PRP辅助治疗可能会降低ACL再损伤的风险[9]。纪庆明等进行了PRP是否能增强ACL重建效果的临床研究。该研究纳入42例进行关节镜下ACL重建手术的患者，其中17例患者的移植物使用PRP进行浸泡（试验组），19例患者的移植物常规处理（对照组），采用K-L分级、VAS评分、Lysholm评分和国际膝关节文献委员会（IKDC）活动评分进行效果评估，随访3~12个月。结果发现，术后3个月试验组各项评分均优于对照组，但在术后12个月，两组评分比较无显著性差异[10]。

ACL损伤重建中，自体骨–肌腱–骨移植物（BPTP）具有最强的愈合潜力，Cervellin等进行了PRP联合BPTP技术治疗ACL损伤的临床研究，将40例进行了BPTP手术的年轻运动员随机分成PRP组（20例）和对照组（20例），PRP凝胶也同时应用于移植物获取的部位。治疗后随访12个月，其间使用VAS评分和VISA评分进行评估。结果发现，虽然VAS评分没有显著性差异，但接受PRP治疗的患者VISA评分显著更高，表明在BPTP手术中应用PRP能够减轻膝关节疼痛[11]。然而，Walters等进行的相似研究却得出不同的结果，他们的研究纳入了50例进行BPTP手术的ACL损伤患者，并随机分为PRP组（27例）和对照组（23例），术后12周、6个月、1年和2年时进行评估，结果显示两组的跪姿和日常活动性疼痛评分以及IKDC评分均无差异，术后6个月时，MRI显示两组供体部位的愈合情况无差异[12]。此外，Vadalà等进行的研究评估了应用PRP对ACL重建后股骨与胫骨隧道拓宽的影响，这项前瞻性研究纳入了40例男性患者，并随机分为PRP组（20例）和对照组（20例），随访时间为10～16个月。结果显示，PRP组的骨隧道直径从（9.0±0.1）mm增加到（9.8±0.3）mm，对照组的骨隧道直径从（9.0±0.1）mm增加到（9.4±0.5）mm，表明PRP并不能有效地防止骨隧道扩大，而体格检查和膝关节相关的功能量表评估也显示两组并无差异[13]。

虽然有部分PRP改善ACL损伤预后的病例报道及研究，但大多数高质量的临床试验表明在ACL损伤重建中，应用PRP进行治疗并不能改善临床和影像学结果。最近的一篇关于PRP在ACL损伤中应用的系统综述表明，目前的Ⅰ级证据不支持使用PRP可改善移植部位的愈合、降低供体部位的发病率、减轻术后疼痛或改善ACL重建后的功能结局。该综述纳入了13项RCT，涉及765名患者[14]。此外，Beyzadeoglu等研究了PRF在ACL重建中的效果。该研究纳入了44例单纯ACL损伤且接受了关节镜下半腱肌移植术的患者，其中PRF组（23例）在移植物表面喷洒PRF，对照组（21例）不做处理。术后第5个月的MRI检查显示，PRF的应用使ACL移植物近端三分之一处具有优越的移植物整合和成熟度，但两组的移植物中间或胫骨远端的MRI信号强度无显著性差异。研究还发现，PRF的应用显著降低了术后需要抽吸的关节血肿的发生率[15]。Schurholz等研究了经动态韧带内固定术（DIS）后采用胶原蛋白包裹韧带和应用PRF进行增强修复的效果。该研究共纳入117例患者，其中58例使用胶原蛋白包裹韧带并局部应用PRF，随访5年，结果表明使用胶原蛋白包裹韧带和局部应用PRF不能提高ACL的DIS修复成功率[16]。

3. PRP治疗ACL损伤的基础研究

Fallouh等研究了PRP对损伤ACL的细胞活力和胶原合成的影响，他们使用PRP和PPP培养4例患者行ACL重建术后的ACL残留物，结果显示，两者对Ⅰ型胶原基因表达的影响并没有显著性差异。与PPP凝块释放物相比，PRP的凝块释放物可使体外处理后的ACL细胞数量显著增加、总胶原蛋白生产量显著提高，表明自体PRP可以增强ACL细胞的体外存活力和功能[17]。Krismer等研究了不同的PRP制剂对人ACL细胞体外培养的影响，结果表明极低浓度PRP中的可溶性因子在有或没有白细胞的情况下都可刺激细胞的增殖和线粒体的活性，而MMP的表达情况则与白细胞数量有关，白细胞浓度低时MMP-3的表达增强，白细胞浓度高时MMP-13的表达增强[18]。Krismer等研究了LR-PRP和纯PRP对体外胶原膜片上培养的人ACL细胞的影响，结果显示，与空白对照组相比，LR-PRP和纯PRP处理组ACL细胞的增殖显著增加，但细胞外基质的产量没有增加。此外，添加白细胞虽然没有促进细胞增殖，但增加了分解代谢基因的选择性表达[19]。

Bozynski等在狗ACL损伤模型中比较了不同疗法的治疗效果。他们将27只狗随机分为三组：常规治疗组（休息和使用非甾体抗炎药）、生理盐水冲洗组和LP-PRP组，在术前、术后当天以及治疗后第1、2、4、7周，对每只狗进行骨科检查以评估膝关节ROM、疼痛和积液情况、临床跛行情况及功能水平。结果显示，与常规治疗组相比，生理盐水冲洗组和LP-PRP组的跛行、疼痛和积液情况更少见，功能和活动范围更大，其中LP-PRP组显示出最好的治疗效果[20]。Li等研究了热敏水凝胶与PRP的结合物治疗大鼠ACL损伤的效果，他们将150只大鼠分成正常对照组、病变对照组、纯热敏水凝胶组和治疗组（热敏水凝胶+PRP），在不同时间点对病变对照组（术后0、2、6周）、纯热敏水凝胶组及治疗组（术后2、6周）进行生物力学测试、组织学分析（H&E和免疫组织化学染色）和评分。结果显示，与病变对照组相比，治疗组的ACL生物力学性能明显更好，但尚未恢复至正常水平。此外，ACL损伤部位的成熟度指数在任何时间点都没有显著的组间差异，但检测到治疗组VEGF和Ⅰ型胶原蛋白的表达增加[21]。Zhang则研究了PRP与明胶海绵（GS）联合治疗对兔子ACL损伤重建后肌腱及骨愈合的影响，研究者将18只兔子随机分为3组（无PRP的自体移植组、PRP组和PRP-GS组）进行半腱肌自体移植ACL重建手术，术后8周进行MRI扫描、生物力学测试和组织学评估。结果显示，使用PRP的两组均有较低的MRI信号，表明有纤维软骨形成；与PRP组相比，PRP-GS组的组织学染色显示肌腱-骨连接处具有更大的纤维软骨过渡区，且组织学评分更高。此外，PRP-GS组ACL的最大破坏载荷和刚度均高于其他2组。实验结果还表明，PRP联合GS可以延长PRP的生物活性时间，促进BMSCs的增殖和成骨基因的表达[22]。

Hexter等报道了在大型动物ACL重建模型中，BMSCs和PRP对同种异体肌腱移植物成熟的影响。研究者将15只进行ACL重建术的绵羊随机分为三组：第一组给予1000万同种异体的BMSCs（辅以2mL的纤维蛋白封闭剂），第二组注入12mL PRP至移植物和骨隧道中，第三组（对照组）不进行任何辅助治疗。治疗12周后的结果显示，与对照组相比，BMSCs组和PRP组具有更高的移植物成熟度评分，说明BMSCs和PRP在ACL重塑模型中可增强同种异体移植的愈合[23]。而Teng等的研究则表明PRP和BMSCs联用能增强兔ACL重建模型中的腱-骨愈合，具有临床应用潜力[24]。此外，Han等在大鼠ACL重建模型的研究中发现，与单一疗法相比，骨形态发生蛋白-2持续释放装置联合PRF使用可使大鼠ACL损伤重建后腱-骨的愈合具有更好的效果。这种联合疗法有效地提高了受伤部位VEGF的水平，减轻了炎症反应，并促进了与骨形成和肌腱再生有关的信号的产生与传递[25]。

4. 小结

目前的动物实验和体外细胞实验表明PRP对于ACL损伤重建可能有潜在的治疗价值。从现有的临床证据来看，使用PRP是一种安全的治疗手段，且有部分研究证明，PRP在自体移植重建ACL的情况下，能有效促进韧带的愈合，并随时间的推移对移植物的成熟有积极的作用，但大部分研究显示PRP对于ACL损伤的愈合无明显的益处[7]。不同研究使用的PRP有不同的血小板浓度、白细胞浓度，其激活方式、应用部位、保留和持续时间、介质释放的速率以及应用的频率等也不同，这可能是导致研究结果出现差异的原因[26]。此外，PRP的治疗效果还取决于个体因素，如年龄、性别、运动水平和基因型等。因此，需要更多高质量的研究来确定PRP在ACL损伤重建过程中的作用。

（袁泽）

参考文献

[1] FRANK C B. Ligament structure, physiology and function[J]. J Musculoskelet Neuronal Interact, 2004, 4（2）: 199-201.

[2] LEONG N L, KATOR J L, CLEMENS T L, et al. Tendon and ligament healing and

current approaches to tendon and ligament regeneration[J]. J Orthop Res, 2020, 38（1）: 7-12.

[3] PAOLONI J, DE VOS R J, HAMILTON B, et al. Platelet-rich plasma treatment for ligament and tendon injuries[J]. Clin J Sport Med, 2011, 21（1）: 37-45.

[4] WOO S L, DEBSKI R E, ZEMINSKI J, et al. Injury and repair of ligaments and tendons[J]. Annu Rev Biomed Eng, 2000, 2（1）: 83-118.

[5] HOGAN M V, KAWAKAMI Y, MURAWSKI C D, et al. Tissue engineering of ligaments for reconstructive surgery[J]. Arthroscopy, 2015, 31（5）: 971-979.

[6] MUSAHL V, KARLSSON J. Anterior cruciate ligament tear[J]. N Engl J Med, 2019, 380（24）: 2341-2348.

[7] ANDRIOLO L, DI MATTEO B, KON E, et al. PRP Augmentation for ACL reconstruction[J]. Biomed Res Int, 2015（1）: 1-15.

[8] YOU C K, CHOU C L, WU W T, et al. Nonoperative choice of anterior cruciate ligament partial tear: ultrasound-guided platelet-rich plasma injection[J]. J Med Ultrasound, 2019, 27（3）: 148-150.

[9] BERDIS A S, VEALE K, FLEISSNER P R JR. Outcomes of anterior cruciate ligament reconstruction using biologic augmentation in patients 21 years of age and younger[J]. Arthroscopy, 2019, 35（11）: 3107-3113.

[10] 纪庆明, 杨育晖, 陈昊, 等. 富血小板血浆辅助前交叉韧带重建治疗的临床疗效分析[J]. 中国修复重建外科杂志, 2017, 31（4）: 410-416.

[11] CERVELLIN M, DE GIROLAMO L, BAIT C, et al. Autologous platelet-rich plasma gel to reduce donor-site morbidity after patellar tendon graft harvesting for anterior cruciate ligament reconstruction: a randomized, controlled clinical study[J]. Knee Surg Sports Traumatol Arthrosc, 2012, 20（1）: 114-120.

[12] WALTERS B L, PORTER D A, HOBART S J, et al. Effect of intraoperative platelet-rich plasma treatment on postoperative donor site knee pain in patellar tendon autograft anterior cruciate ligament reconstruction: a double-blind randomized controlled trial[J]. Am J Sports Med, 2018, 46（8）: 1827-1835.

[13] VADALÀ A, IORIO R, DE CARLI A, et al. Platelet-rich plasma: does it help reduce tunnel widening after ACL reconstruction? [J]. Knee Surg Sports Traumatol Arthrosc, 2013, 21（4）: 824-829.

[14] DAVEY M S, HURLEY E T, WITHERS D, et al. Anterior cruciate ligament reconstruction with platelet-rich plasma: a systematic review of randomized control trials[J]. Arthroscopy, 2020, 36（4）: 1204-1210.

[15] BEYZADEOGLU T, PEHLIVANOGLU T, YILDIRIM K, et al. Does the application of platelet-rich fibrin in anterior cruciate ligament reconstruction enhance graft healing and maturation? A comparative MRI study of 44 cases[J]. Orthop J Sports Med, 2020, 8

（2）：1-7.

[16] SCHURHOLZ K, LIECHTI E, KOHL S, et al. Collagen wrapping and local PRF do not improve the survival rates of ACL repair with dynamic intraligamentary stabilization. A retrospective study with a minimum follow-up of 5-years[J]. Swiss Med Wkly, 2020：S30.

[17] FALLOUH L, NAKAGAWA K, SASHO T, et al. Effects of autologous platelet-rich plasma on cell viability and collagen synthesis in injured human anterior cruciate ligament[J]. J Bone Joint Surg Am, 2010, 92（18）：2909-2916.

[18] KRISMER A, CABRA R, MAY R, et al. In the regenerative effects of two common platelet-rich plasma production methods on human anterior cruciate ligamentocytes[R]. Proceedings of the ORS, 2017.

[19] KRISMER A, CABRA R, MAY R, et al. Biologic response of human anterior cruciate ligamentocytes on collagen-patches to platelet-rich plasma formulations with and without leucocytes[J]. J Orthop Res, 2017, 35（12）：2733-2739.

[20] BOZYNSKI C C, STANNARD J P, SMITH P, et al. Acute management of anterior cruciate ligament injuries using novel canine models[J]. J Knee Surg, 2016, 29（7）：594-603.

[21] LI Y, FU S C, CHEUK Y C, et al. The effect of thermosensitive hydrogel platelet-rich-plasma complex in the treatment of partial tear of anterior cruciate ligament in rat model[J]. J Orthop Translat, 2020, 24：183-189.

[22] ZHANG M Y, ZHEN J, ZHANG X, et al. Effect of autologous platelet-rich plasma and gelatin sponge for tendon-to-bone healing after rabbit anterior cruciate ligament reconstruction[J]. Arthroscopy, 2019, 35（5）：1486-1497.

[23] HEXTER A T, SANGHANI-KERAI A, HEIDARI N, et al. Mesenchymal stromal cells and platelet-rich plasma promote tendon allograft healing in ovine anterior cruciate ligament reconstruction[J]. Knee Surg Sports Traumatol Arthrosc, 2020, 29（11）：1-11.

[24] TENG C, ZHOU C H, XU D F, et al. Combination of platelet-rich plasma and bone marrow mesenchymal stem cells enhances tendon-bone healing in a rabbit model of anterior cruciate ligament reconstruction[J]. J Orthop Surg Res, 2016, 11（1）：96.

[25] HAN L, HU Y G, JIN B, et al. Sustained BMP-2 release and platelet rich fibrin synergistically promote tendon-bone healing after anterior cruciate ligament reconstruction in rat[J]. Eur Rev Med Pharmacol Sci, 2019, 23（20）：8705-8712.

[26] HOHMANN E. Editorial commentary：platelet-rich plasma or profit-rich placebo：variability of composition, concentration, preparation, and many other yet-unknown factors determine effectiveness[J]. Arthroscopy, 2019, 35（10）：2885-2886.

第三节　富血小板血浆在创面修复中的应用

创面修复是外科医生经常面对的问题，根据损伤愈合的时间，可把创面分为急性伤口和慢性伤口。急性伤口的常见原因有意外创伤、手术及烧伤等，严重的急性伤口常伴随疼痛、感染等问题，如烧伤最严重的并发症就是危及生命的全身感染。慢性伤口是指不愈合或愈合时间长且容易破裂的伤口，是创面修复的棘手问题，常见的慢性伤口有压疮、小腿静脉性溃疡、动脉溃疡、神经营养性溃疡和足溃疡[1]。这种慢性损伤迁延不愈，不仅严重影响患者的生活质量，还造成了沉重的医疗护理负担。

一、概述

伤口愈合的过程与肌腱、韧带的愈合类似，也包括三个阶段：炎症期、增生期和重塑期。当急性伤口愈合过程中断时，即形成慢性伤口。通常导致伤口愈合不良的风险因素有局部原因（如伤口感染、组织缺氧、反复创伤及碎片或坏死组织的存在）、全身性疾病（如糖尿病、免疫缺陷或营养不良）和某些药物因素（如皮质类固醇）等。慢性伤口的处理措施有切除坏死或感染的组织、负压治疗、压迫疗法、维持伤口湿润、预防或治疗感染、减少伤口与周围环境的摩擦、伤口清洁以及饮食管理等[1-2]。此外，慢性伤口的治疗还需结合病因进行，如脊髓损伤患者的压疮需要经常翻身，糖尿病相关的压疮需要控制血糖，对于慢性静脉疾病或缺血性血管疾病，可能需要血管外科手术介入等[1]。尽管进行了治疗管理，但还是会有许多的慢性伤口长时间不愈合或在愈合后复发[3]。

富血小板血浆（PRP）是从血液离心过程中获得的血小板浓缩液，其浓度是血小板生理浓度的3～5倍。PRP富含纤维蛋白和多种生长因子，如PDGF、TGF-α、TGF-β、IGF、FGF、VEGF和EGF等，这些生长因子在组织修复过程中都有特定的生物分子功能（表3），其分泌后与靶区细胞的跨膜受体结合，可介导细胞生长、有丝分裂及趋化作用，促进细胞外基质形成，在伤口愈合过程中发挥重要作用[4]。PRP能发挥生理状态下血小板在凝血过程中的作用，促进血凝块的形成，进而有助于创面的愈合。此外PRP还可以促进角质形成细胞和成纤维细胞的增殖、胶原蛋白和弹性蛋白的合成以及血管的生成和肉芽组织的产生，加速组织的修复，且自体PRP无免疫原性[5]。另有研究显示PRP作用于局部能杀死微生物，改变基质金属蛋白酶和细胞因子的表达，从而促进溃疡愈合[6]。随着相关研究的开展，PRP改善伤口症状和提高自愈率的研究报道也在增多，因此应用PRP有望成为创面修复的新的辅助疗法。

表3 PRP中的成分在创面修复中的作用

成 分	作 用
表皮生长因子（EGF）	·刺激表皮上皮细胞、成纤维细胞和胚胎细胞的增殖 ·是成纤维细胞和上皮细胞的趋化因子 ·刺激上皮再生，促进血管生成 ·影响细胞外基质的合成
血小板源性生长因子（PDGF）	·A、B亚型是成纤维细胞、动脉平滑肌细胞、软骨细胞以及上皮和内皮细胞的有效促分裂原 ·是造血和间充质细胞、成纤维细胞和肌肉细胞的强化学趋化因子 ·激活TGF-β，刺激中性粒细胞、巨噬细胞、成纤维细胞和平滑肌细胞的有丝分裂，促进胶原蛋白的合成，增强胶原酶活性和血管生成功能

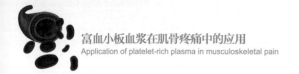
续表

成 分	作 用
转化生长因子-α（TGF-α）	·类似于EGF，可结合相同的受体 ·刺激间质细胞、上皮细胞和内皮细胞的生长，刺激内皮细胞的趋化性，控制表皮发育 ·刺激内皮细胞的增殖，比EGF更有效 ·促进成骨细胞的生成，在成骨过程中影响成骨细胞与骨基质的结合 ·通过抑制胶原蛋白的合成和钙的释放来影响骨骼的形成与重塑
转化生长因子-β（TGF-β）	·刺激成纤维细胞的趋化性和增殖，刺激胶原蛋白的合成 ·减少皮肤瘢痕 ·是上皮细胞、内皮细胞、成纤维细胞、神经元、造血细胞和角质形成细胞的生长抑制剂 ·拮抗EGF、PDGF、aFGF和bFGF的生物活性
角化细胞生长因子（KGF或FGF-7）	·是促进皮肤角化细胞生成的最有效的生长因子，可在皮肤受伤后的组织修复中发挥作用 ·通过促进细胞的增殖分化、血管生成、细胞迁移加速伤口愈合 ·作为有丝分裂原可作用于许多上皮细胞，但不适用于成纤维细胞和内皮细胞
酸性纤维母细胞生长因子（aFGF或FGF-1）	·参与细胞的增殖分化、血管生成、细胞迁移 ·是皮肤源性角化细胞、真皮成纤维细胞和血管内皮细胞的有丝分裂原
碱性纤维母细胞生长因子（bFGF或FGF-2）	·刺激成纤维细胞、成肌细胞、成骨细胞、神经细胞、内皮细胞、角质形成细胞和软骨细胞的生长 ·刺激血管生成、内皮细胞增殖、胶原合成、伤口收缩、基质合成、上皮化和KGF产生
血管内皮生长因子（VEGF/ VEP）	·刺激大血管内皮细胞增殖 ·作为强血管生成蛋白诱导新生血管形成 ·诱导金属蛋白酶的合成，降解Ⅰ型、Ⅱ型、Ⅲ型胶原
结缔组织生长因子（CTGF）	·诱导血管内皮细胞的增殖、迁移、小管形成和血管生成 ·有效刺激成骨细胞的增殖分化，促进基质矿化

续表

成 分	作 用
粒细胞-巨噬细胞集落刺激因子（GM-CSF）	·促进成骨细胞的增殖分化 ·与促红细胞生成素协同促进骨髓祖细胞增殖 ·对中性粒细胞具有趋化作用
胰岛素样生长因子（IGF）	·是正常成纤维细胞的生长因子，可用于多种中胚层细胞的体外有丝分裂 ·促进成纤维细胞胶原酶和前列腺素E_2的合成 ·刺激骨细胞合成胶原和基质，调节关节软骨代谢
肿瘤坏死因子-α（TNF-α）	·是成纤维细胞的生长因子 ·促进血管生成
白细胞介素-1β（IL-1β）	·抑制内皮细胞和肝细胞的生长 ·激活破骨细胞，抑制新骨形成，低浓度时促进新骨生长 ·增强炎症反应和胶原酶活性
白细胞介素-8（IL-8）	·促进血管生成 ·促进表皮细胞有丝分裂

注：本表引自 "P. Rozman and Z. Bolta，Use of platelet growth factors in treating wounds and soft-tissue injuries"。

二、PRP在创面修复中的临床研究

目前应用PRP治疗急性伤口的临床研究虽然不多，但大部分显示有较好的疗效。Kazakos等评估了自体PRP凝胶治疗肢体软组织急性伤口的益处，59例急性伤口（开放性或闭合性骨折伴皮肤坏死、摩擦伤和烧伤）患者被随机分为两组，A组（32例）采用常规敷料治疗，B组（27例）采用PRP凝胶治疗。治疗后每7天进行一次伤口表面积测量和疼痛评估，同时记录组织再生至足以进行整形手术所需的时间。结果显示，B组在第1、2、3周的伤口愈合速度明显更快，组织再生至足以进行整形手术所需的时间平均为21.26天，而A组为40.6天。此外B组患者疼痛评分低于A组，且未观察到不良反应或感染迹象。该研究表明PRP凝胶可为急性伤口的治疗提供有效的帮助[7]。Mohamadi等研究了PRP对毛发性窦性鼻窦炎术后伤口的影响，110例患者被随机分为治疗组和对照组，术后对照组进行常规伤口敷料护理，治疗组则使用PRP凝胶治疗。研究过程中记录伤口愈合所需时间、抗生素使用时间及疼痛持续时间，在伤口完全愈合前3～5天进行伤口活检以评估血管的生成。结果显示，对照组和治疗组伤口愈合所需的平均时间分别为8.3周和4.8周，疼痛持续时间分别为3.4周和1.3周，抗生素使用时间分别为1.74周和0.57周，微血管计数平均值分别为53.0和68.3。该研究表明，与传统的敷料相比，PRP凝胶在加速伤口愈合方面更成功[8]。

Yeung等研究了冷冻干燥PRP粉末对严重二级烧伤创面的治疗效果。患者被随机分成PRP组（$n=15$）和对照组（$n=12$），将用PRP粉末配制成的PRP溶液和安慰剂溶液以喷雾形式均匀喷至创面，每天1次并持续4天，分别在治疗后2周和3周时测量伤口闭合率和细菌清除率。结果发现PRP组在2周时的伤口闭合率达到近80%，并在3周内突破了90%，对照组在2周和3周内的伤口闭合率分别为60%和80%，PRP组的感染率（26.67%）低于对照组（33.33%），表明PRP粉末可有效促进伤口愈合[9]。

Marck等研究了自体PRP对需要使用网状裂口皮肤移植物（SSG）进行手术的烧伤创面愈合的影响。52例不同区域深部真皮至全层烧伤的患者接受了SSG手术，在患者烧伤部位选择可比较的区域A和区域B，随机分为治疗组（SSG联合PRP）和对照组（单独使用SSG）进行治疗。在术后第5～7天评估上皮形成情况和移植物存活率，结果发现治疗组和对照组之间并无差异，在非预定的分析中PRP则表现出较小的益处。术后3个月、6个月、12个月采用POSAS问卷、皮肤光谱仪和测量仪来评估瘢痕的质量，结果显示两组并无统计学差异，表明PRP似乎并不能显著改善急性烧伤的伤口愈合或瘢痕形成[10]。最近一篇荟萃分析结果显示，经PRP治疗的烧伤创面愈合速度明显更快，瘢痕质量也更好，但在上皮化、感染率和不良事件发生率方面与对照创面相比没有差异。需要注意的是，相关研究的设计类型、样本量、伤口类型和PRP制备方案等的差异都可能对研究结果产生影响[11]。

　　慢性不愈合的溃疡多发生于下肢，是导致非创伤性下肢截肢的主要原因。Suthar等进行了应用PRP治疗慢性不愈合溃疡效果的研究，共纳入24例不同病因的慢性溃疡患者，如压力性溃疡、静脉性溃疡、动脉性溃疡和糖尿病足溃疡等。在清除所有坏死和感染的组织且清洁伤口区域后，根据伤口的大小，从6mL已制备的PRP溶液中分出2～3mL制成凝胶敷于创口处，其余3～4mL皮下注射至创面周边，随访24周。结果所有患者均显示出创面愈合的迹象，溃疡面积减小，愈合的平均时间为8.2周，在此期间无不良反应发生。这项研究证明PRP治疗慢性非愈合性溃疡有潜在的安全性和有效性[12]。Jaseem等在一项回顾性研究中也得到类似结果。该研究纳入了20例持续时间超过4周的慢性非愈合性溃疡患者（14例糖尿病，4例周围动脉疾病，2例静脉功能不全），所有患者均接受自体来源的PRP治疗并随访20周。治疗前的平均溃疡面积和体积分别为13.72cm^{2}和20.17cm^3，完成治疗后的平均面积和体积分别为1.98cm^{2}和2.92cm^3，溃疡愈合的平均持续时间为11.25周，结果80%的患者溃疡面积缩小超过75%[13]。

　　Ahmed等研究了PRP治疗糖尿病足溃疡的效果。该研究纳入了56例慢性糖尿病足溃疡患者并分成两组，对照组使用抗菌药膏敷料治疗（每天1次），PRP组使用PRP凝胶治疗（每周2次），每周在外科门诊对患者进行两次检查。结果显示，对照组的治愈率为68%，PRP组中有86%的患者实现了完全治愈，治愈率在前8周较高，此后开始下降。此外，使用PRP凝胶降低了伤口感染率。研究表明，在糖尿病足溃疡的治疗和预防感染方面，

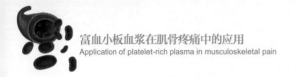
PRP凝胶比局部抗菌敷料更有效[14]。

　　Ramos-Torrecillas等报道了一例使用PRP治疗压疮的病例，患者为86岁女性，其右脚跟上有Ⅲ级压疮，经过4个月的治疗未见愈合迹象。提取该患者20mL外周血制成PRP，用10%的氯化钙激活并形成凝胶，施用于压疮部位，每3天进行一次随访，共随访8周，至第54天发现压疮完全愈合[15]。Singh等研究了局部应用PRP治疗脊髓损伤患者压疮的效果，共纳入25例至少有两个压疮伤口的脊髓损伤患者，并分为PRP组和生理盐水对照组。PRP组均选择Ⅳ级压疮（25个），生理盐水对照组的压疮有Ⅱ级11个、Ⅲ级4个、Ⅳ级10个，通过测量创口的表面积、应用压疮愈合量表（PUSH）、活检和临床检查来评估治疗效果。5周后两组PUSH得分均降低，PRP组压疮面积明显减小，有更多良好的肉芽组织和上皮形成，24个（96%）改善，1个恶化，而对照组中17个（68%）有所改善，7个恶化，1个无变化[16]。Volakakis等也进行了PRP治疗压疮的研究，共纳入36例患者，共计64个压疮，对患者进行4周的常规治疗后根据情况清创，然后每周在创口表面和边缘注射PRP，持续4周。结果显示，与常规治疗相比，PRP治疗后创口表面积的减少（63% vs 41%）、最大直径的减少（33% vs 20%）及中位周长的减少（38% vs 21%）均更显著，表明PRP可以加速压疮的愈合[17]。

　　笔者团队应用PRP凝胶治疗外伤术后难愈性创面，临床观察效果满意。见图4-1至图4-3。

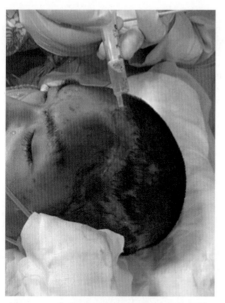

图4-1　应用PRP凝胶治疗外伤术后难愈性创面（1）

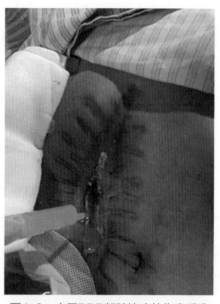

图4-2　应用PRP凝胶治疗外伤术后难愈性创面（2）

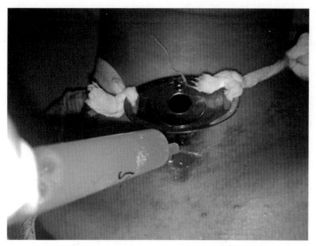

图4-3　应用PRP凝胶治疗外伤术后难愈性创面（3）

三、PRP在创面修复中的基础研究

伤口从出现到愈合将经历凝血、炎症、细胞迁移、细胞增殖和重塑的过程，其中角质形成细胞的迁移或增殖是加速伤口愈合的关键步骤，这一过程受到各种细胞周期调节蛋白的精确调控。慢性皮肤溃疡的细胞可因细胞周期阻滞而出现增殖率降低，如在糖尿病足溃疡或下肢静脉溃疡中，角质形成细胞的增殖和迁移受到损害，可导致上皮细胞形成缓慢[18]。有研究报道，PRP可通过上调周期蛋白E（cyclin E）和周期蛋白依赖性激酶4（CDK4）诱导成纤维细胞的增殖和迁移，使Ⅰ型胶原蛋白和MMP-1的表达增加，从而加速伤口愈合过程[19]。Kim等利用PRP处理的人永生化角质形成细胞（HaCaT细胞）进行了一系列分子研究，发现PRP的处理可使HaCaT细胞的增殖和迁移增加，而HaCaT细胞经低浓度（0.5%）PRP处理后，cyclin A和CDK4的表达显著增加。在同期进行的PRP治疗急性和慢性溃疡的研究中，11例慢性溃疡（包括瘀血溃疡、糖尿病足溃疡、下肢静脉溃疡和外伤性溃疡等）中有9例在15天左右出现90%～100%的上皮化，5例急性伤口（包括裂开、开放创面和烧伤创面）在4～20天内上皮化达到80%～100%。研究结果表明PRP可能通过上调cyclin A和CDK4而使急性伤口和慢性皮肤溃疡的上皮形成过程显著加速[18]。Guo在糖尿病模型大鼠中的研究则表明PRP释放的胞外体可能通过激活Erk和Akt信号通路来促进血管生成，并发现PRP能激活转录共激活因子（YAP），实现诱导上皮再生的过程[20]。

Ostvar等利用兔子急性伤口模型进行了PRP疗效的实验研究，研究中在兔子的背外侧（双侧）皮肤上手术建立一个大小为3cm的伤口，并将兔子随机分为PRP组和对照组（未治疗）。在第7、14、21天时，PRP组的伤口面积小于对照组；在第14、21天时，与对照组相比，PRP组的伤口平均血管密度显著增加[21]。Farghali等在5只犬的胸部对称地建立直径为3cm的双侧急性全层皮肤伤口，用激活的PRP溶液浸润右侧伤口，左侧伤口作为对照。在第3周对伤口皮肤进行活检时发现，与对照伤口相比，PRP处理的伤口上皮化百分比显著增加，胶原蛋白组织良好，Ⅰ型胶原蛋白A1的表达和Ⅰ型胶原蛋白A2的强度显著增加，丙二醛浓度显著降低，MMP-9活性明显较高，表明PRP的浸润增强了伤口上皮的形成并减少了瘢痕组织的形成[22]。Jee等也进行了类似的犬类动物实验，发现采用PRP处理后的急性伤口有更快的上皮形成和更多的肉芽生成以及胶原沉积[23]。Huber等在大鼠急性伤口模型上比较了冻干PRP和新鲜PRP的治疗效果，发现与新鲜PRP组相比，冻干PRP组伤口处成纤维细胞的数量和血管密度明显增加，但两者无统计学差异。尽管PRP在冷冻干燥后生长因子浓度增加，但未观察到与使用新鲜PRP时存在愈合动力学方面的差异[24]。

Maciel等研究了马的深二度（dSD）烧伤创面模型中PRP的治疗效果，实验组分别接受1次PRP（G1组）和2次PRP（G2组）处理，而对照组用盐溶液处理。在第25天，与对照组相比，G1组的胶原纤维比例更高，G2组的愈合伤口类似未损伤的组织；在第40天，G1组的创面类似于完整的组织，G2组则表现为致密的组织，所有的实验组均无感染并发症出现。该结果表明PRP能促进马的dSD烧伤创面的修复、诱导纤维化并可能有抗菌活性[25]。Venter等在大鼠实验中研究了PRP对dSD、糖尿病相关的深二度（dSDD）和三度（TD）烧伤创面的治疗效果。研究者在第21天进行皮肤活检时发现，用PRP处理的dSD和dSDD创面早期血管增生显著，能更快地进入创面愈合的后期阶段，而PRP处理的dSDD和TD创面，肉芽组织的增生较少。结果表明PRP可以加速dSD和dSDD创面的愈合过程，但对于TD创面的效果有限[26]。然而，Singer等在猪的烧伤模型中发现，PRP的治疗效果不尽如人意。他们在10只猪的背部和侧腹部皮肤共建立了120处烧伤，在有无进行皮肤移植、有无使用PRP和不同时期进行皮肤移植及使用PRP的治疗选择中，组合了6种治疗方法。结果表明：进行早期皮肤移植的烧伤再上皮化最快，瘢痕最薄；未进行皮肤移植的烧伤再上皮化最慢，瘢

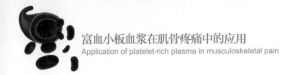
痕形成量最大；PRP的应用对再上皮化、瘢痕深度、瘢痕收缩情况均无影响[27]。

Dionyssiou等研究了兔子耳朵全层缺损模型中PRP治疗非愈合性慢性伤口的有效性，结果显示：PRP组的20只兔子中有19只平均在24.9天内治愈；对照组的20只兔子中有7只平均在26.7天内治愈，在第28天还有7只没有治愈，有6只还存在全层的缺损[28]。在术后第3、7、14天，与对照组相比，PRP组的伤口闭合率较高、羟脯氨酸的含量较多、Ⅰ型和Ⅲ型胶原的比例较高，且排列较整齐密集，其mRNA都有较高的表达。该研究表明，PRP可能通过增强胶原蛋白合成来促进伤口的愈合[29]。

Morimoto等研究了PRP治疗犬的压疮的效果。该研究纳入了18只双侧大转子或肩关节突起部位存在压疮的犬，每只犬的创面随机归入PRP凝胶组和石蜡纱布敷料组进行治疗，每5天进行1次治疗，共治疗5次。治疗开始时比较伤口愈合情况和伤口面积，然后每隔5天评估1次，直到第25天治疗结束。结果显示：第一次治疗后至研究结束时PRP凝胶组的愈合效果均优于石蜡纱布敷料组；在第25天时，PRP凝胶组和石蜡纱布敷料组的伤口面积平均减少93.5%和13.2%[30]。Yu等研究了PRF生物活性膜治疗压力性溃疡（PU）的可行性，研究者把形成PU的大鼠随机分为治疗组（PRF生物活性膜治疗）和对照组（正常护理），每3天进行1次治疗。在第3天和第7天，治疗组的PU面积明显小于对照组；在治疗14天后，治疗组的PU全部愈合。此外，免疫组织化学和蛋白质分析结果表明，PRF生物活性膜可通过增加再生表皮的厚度和上调VEGF的表达来诱导伤口愈合[31]。

四、小结

值得注意的是，因为慢性伤口的难治愈性，PRP在此类创面中有更大的临床价值，但可能由于动物实验成本或技术的问题，采用PRP治疗慢性创面的动物实验较少，较多的是急性创伤伤口的动物实验，因此在临床转化应用时，必须考虑伤口的正常愈合潜力[32]。此外，尽管在烧伤创面的治疗中使用PRP已被证明是安全的，但无论是在临床研究中还是在动物实验中，PRP的治疗效果都尚不能令人满意，因此，临床上选择PRP治疗烧伤创面时应慎重考虑。大部分研究表明，PRP可加快组织修复的速度，在创面修复中有较大的价值，尽管如此，仍需要进行更多的研究来标准化PRP制剂及其使用方法，进而更好地认识其在创面修复中的作用机制和临床疗效，为临床医生使用PRP治疗急性或慢性伤口提供合适、高质量的治疗策略。

（袁泽）

参考文献

[1] MARTINEZ-ZAPATA M J, MARTI-CARVAJAL A J, SOLA I, et al. Autologous platelet-rich plasma for treating chronic wounds[J]. Cochrane Database Syst Rev, 2016, 5（5）：CD006899.

[2] JONES R E, FOSTER D S, LONGAKER M T. Management of chronic wounds-2018[J]. JAMA, 2018, 320（14）：1481-1482.

[3] RODRIGUES I, MÉGIE M F. Prevalence of chronic wounds in Quebec home care：an exploratory study[J]. Ostomy Wound Manage, 2006, 52（5）：46-48, 50, 52-57.

[4] GENTILE P, GARCOVICH S. Systematic review-the potential implications of different platelet-rich plasma（PRP）concentrations in regenerative medicine for tissue repair[J]. Int J Mol Sci, 2020, 21（16）：1-22.

[5] MERCHÁN W H, GÓMEZ L A, CHASOY M E, et al. Platelet-rich plasma, a powerful tool in dermatology[J]. J Tissue Eng Regen Med, 2019, 13（5）：892-901.

[6] HESSELER M J, SHYAM N. Platelet-rich plasma and its utility in medical dermatology：a systematic review[J]. J Am Acad Dermatol, 2019, 81（3）：834-846.

[7] KAZAKOS K, LYRAS D N, VERETTAS D, et al. The use of autologous PRP gel as an aid in the management of acute trauma wounds[J]. Injury, 2009, 40（8）：801-805.

[8] MOHAMADI S, NOROOZNEZHAD A H, MOSTAFAEI S, et al. A randomized

controlled trial of effectiveness of platelet-rich plasma gel and regular dressing on wound healing time in pilonidal sinus surgery: role of different affecting factors[J]. Biomed J, 2019, 42（6）: 403-410.

[9] YEUNG C Y, HSIEH P S, WEI L G, et al. Efficacy of lyophilised platelet-rich plasma powder on healing rate in patients with deep second degree burn injury: a prospective double-blind randomized clinical trial[J]. Ann Plast Surg, 2018, 80（2S Suppl 1）: S66-S69.

[10] MARCK R E, GARDIEN K L, STEKELENBURG C M, et al. The application of platelet-rich plasma in the treatment of deep dermal burns: a randomized, double-blind, intra-patient controlled study[J]. Wound Repair Regen, 2016, 24（4）: 712-720.

[11] ZHENG W, ZHAO D L, ZHAO Y Q, et al. Effectiveness of platelet rich plasma in burn wound healing: a systematic review and meta-analysis[J]. J Dermatolog Treat, 2020, 33（2）: 1-25.

[12] SUTHAR M, GUPTA S, BUKHARI S, et al. Treatment of chronic non-healing ulcers using autologous platelet rich plasma: a case series[J]. J Biomed Sci, 2017, 24（1）: 16.

[13] JASEEM M, ALUNGAL S, WARAN D, et al. Effectiveness of autologous PRP therapy in chronic nonhealing ulcer: a 2-year retrospective descriptive study[J]. J Family Med Prim Care, 2020, 9（6）: 2818-2822.

[14] AHMED M, REFFAT S A, HASSAN A, et al. Platelet-rich plasma for the treatment of clean diabetic foot ulcers[J]. Ann Vasc Surg, 2017, 38: 206-211.

[15] RAMOS-TORRECILLAS J, DE LUNA-BERTOS E, GARCÍA-MARTÍNEZ O, et al. Use of platelet-rich plasma to treat pressure ulcers: a case study[J]. J Wound Ostomy Continence Nurs, 2013, 40（2）: 198-202.

[16] SINGH R, ROHILLA R K, DHAYAL R K, et al. Role of local application of autologous platelet-rich plasma in the management of pressure ulcers in spinal cord injury patients[J]. Spinal Cord, 2014, 52（11）: 809-816.

[17] VOLAKAKIS E, PAPADAKIS M, MANIOS A, et al. Platelet-rich plasma improves healing of pressure ulcers as objectively assessed by digital planimetry[J]. Wounds, 2019, 31（10）: 252-256.

[18] KIM S A, RYU H W, LEE K S, et al. Application of platelet-rich plasma accelerates the wound healing process in acute and chronic ulcers through rapid migration and upregulation of cyclin A and CDK4 in HaCaT cells[J]. Mol Med Rep, 2013, 7（2）: 476-480.

[19] CHO J W, KIM S A, LEE K S. Platelet-rich plasma induces increased expression of G1 cell cycle regulators, type I collagen, and matrix metalloproteinase-1 in human skin fibroblasts[J]. Int J Mol Med, 2012, 29（1）: 32-36.

[20] GUO S C, TAO S C, YIN W J, et al. Exosomes derived from platelet-rich plasma promote the re-epithelization of chronic cutaneous wounds via activation of YAP in a diabetic rat model[J]. Theranostics, 2017, 7（1）: 81-96.

[21] OSTVAR O, SHADVAR S, YAHAGHI E, et al. Effect of platelet-rich plasma on the healing of cutaneous defects exposed to acute to chronic wounds: a clinico-histopathologic study in rabbits[J]. Diagn Pathol, 2015, 10: 85.

[22] FARGHALI H A, ABDELKADER N A, KHATTAB M S, et al. Evaluation of subcutaneous infiltration of autologous platelet-rich plasma on skin-wound healing in dogs[J]. Biosci Rep, 2017, 37（2）: 1-13.

[23] JEE C H, EOM N Y, JANG H M, et al. Effect of autologous platelet-rich plasma application on cutaneous wound healing in dogs[J]. J Vet Sci, 2016, 17（1）: 79-87.

[24] HUBER S C, JUNIOR J, SILVA L Q, et al. Freeze-dried versus fresh platelet-rich plasma in acute wound healing of an animal model[J]. Regen Med, 2019, 14（6）: 525-534.

[25] MACIEL F B, DEROSSI R, MÓDOLO T J, et al. Scanning electron microscopy and microbiological evaluation of equine burn wound repair after platelet-rich plasma gel treatment[J]. Burns, 2012, 38（7）: 1058-1065.

[26] VENTER N G, MARQUES R G, SANTOS J S, et al. Use of platelet-rich plasma in deep second- and third-degree burns[J]. Burns, 2016, 42（4）: 807-814.

[27] SINGER A J, TOUSSAINT J, CHUNG W T, et al. The effects of platelet rich plasma on healing of full thickness burns in swine[J]. Burns, 2018, 44（6）: 1543-1550.

[28] DIONYSSIOU D, DEMIRI E, FOROGLOU P, et al. The effectiveness of intralesional injection of platelet-rich plasma in accelerating the healing of chronic ulcers: an experimental and clinical study[J]. Int Wound J, 2013, 10（4）: 397-406.

[29] LIU C, ZHANG H W, XU N. Allogeneic platelet-rich plasma promotes wound collagen synthesis in diabetic rats[J]. Chinese Journal of Tissue Engineering Research, 2014, 18（39）: 6329-6334.

[30] TAMBELLA A M, ATTILI A R, DINI F, et al. Autologous platelet gel to treat chronic decubital ulcers: a randomized, blind controlled clinical trial in dogs[J]. Vet Surg, 2014, 43（6）: 726-733.

[31] YU Y J, SHEN J, FANG G Z, et al. Use of autologous platelet rich fibrin-based bioactive membrane in pressure ulcer healing in rats[J]. J Wound Care, 2019, 28（Sup4）: S23-S30.

[32] TAMBELLA A M, ATTILI A R, DUPRÉ G, et al. Platelet-rich plasma to treat experimentally-induced skin wounds in animals: a systematic review and meta-analysis[J]. PLoS One, 2018, 13（1）: 1-26.

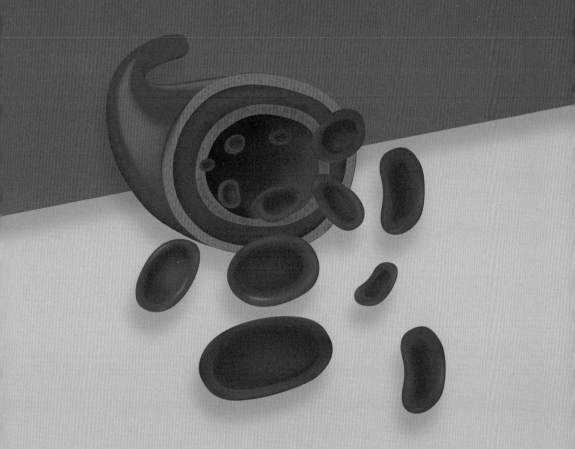

第五章

富血小板血浆在神经修复中的应用

第一节　富血小板血浆在根性神经痛中的应用

根性神经痛（radicular pain）在生理上是由背根神经节或者其他神经节发出的异常放电所引起的，其中神经炎症是其关键的病理生理过程。正常的神经根受到挤压只会引起短暂放电，但是发炎的背根神经节受挤压会引起Aβ、Aδ和C纤维放电。

1. 概述

在探讨根性神经痛之前，首先需要清楚根性神经痛的定义。根性神经痛在定义上不同于伤害性腰痛（nociceptive back pain）、牵涉痛（referred pain）或者神经根病（radiculopathy）。

伤害性腰痛是由于腰椎结构的伤害性刺激引起的疼痛，棘间韧带、腰椎关节突关节、骶髂关节等受到伤害性刺激时都可引发腰部的隐痛，这些类型的疼痛称为伤害性腰痛。牵涉痛是指伤害性刺激在引起腰痛之外，还可刺激脊髓结构内的神经末梢，进一步传入脊髓二级神经元，再传至该二级神经元支配的下肢末端区域，引起下肢的疼痛，由于躯体性疼痛并不涉及刺激压迫神经根，因而没有神经受损的麻木、乏力等症状。牵涉痛一旦建立，位置相对固定，并且疼痛范围边界不清，通过刺激腰椎关节突关节或者椎间盘可以诱发牵涉痛，阻滞关节突关节可缓解牵涉痛。神经根病是指因脊神经或者脊神经根的传导受阻而出现的麻木、乏力、反射减弱等症状或体征[1]。

在严格定义下，根性神经痛的患病率大概为12%[2]，椎间盘突出症是引起根性神经痛的主要原因。

根性神经痛的治疗包括保守治疗和手术治疗，保守治疗包括休息、药物治疗、牵引、运动疗法、整脊、心理治疗等，其中药物治疗所用药物包括非甾体抗炎药、肌松剂、类固醇类、阿片类。此外，硬膜外类固醇注射也被广泛应用，但此技术的风险有感染、瘫痪、头痛、出血或者血肿，不良事件包括感染性或者无菌性脑膜炎、脊髓栓塞；类固醇本身还会产生副作用，包括库欣综合征、肾上腺抑制、肌病、绝经后妇女骨质丢失、血糖升高等。因此，仍需为根性神经痛探寻其他的治疗方法。

2. PRP治疗根性神经痛的临床应用

PRP在肌腱疾病、骨性关节炎疾病的治疗中具有明显的疗效和较高的安全性，因此已经成为疼痛管理的重要手段。PRP也被应用于椎间盘、小关节、韧带以及神经根病中，其机制与高浓度的生长因子对组织愈合的修复作用相关，且与抗炎蛋白α2-巨球蛋白、白细胞介素受体拮抗剂、金属蛋白酶组织抑制剂等的释放关系密切[3-4]，这正好贴合了根性神经痛的神经炎症机制。

2016年，Bhatia等纳入10例病程持续4周以上的根性神经痛患者，在荧光透视引导下将5mL的自体PRP通过硬膜外注射至受累神经根处，采用VAS评分、直腿抬高试验、改良Oswestry残疾问卷（MODQ）进行随访，结果显示在接受治疗3个月后患者情况持续好转，VAS评分从5分以上降到3～4分，MODQ由操作前的严重功能障碍转为轻度或者中度功能障碍，直腿抬高试验也提升到70°，未见注射相关的并发症[5]。

2017年，Centeno等纳入470例腰椎根性神经痛患者给予硬膜外血小板裂解物注射治疗。血小板裂解物是将血小板裂解并去除细胞碎片而产生的富含生长因子的注射剂。采用数字疼痛评分（numeric pain score，NPS）、FRI评分、改良单次数字评估（modified single assessment numeric evaluation rating，SANE）进行随访评估，结果显示NPS评分由基线状态的5.1分降至注射1个月后的2.6分，并且此疼痛的改善效果延续至24个月时；SANE在24

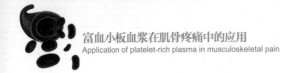
个月的随访中从35.9%增至49%，表明患者自我感觉在注射后病情出现了改善；FRI评分在治疗1个月后从基线状态的52.6分均升高超过9分，评分改善均超过FRI的最小临床重要差异度。此外，29例患者报告了不良反应，其中与疼痛相关的不良反应包括疼痛、炎症、酸痛、肌肉紧绷、僵硬、麻木，与硬膜穿刺相关的不良反应有恶心、呕吐伴体位性头痛和头晕，以及皮肤反应（红肿）。所有不良反应都是自限性的，可在1～6个月内恢复[6]。

2020年，Bise等进行了一项非随机对照研究，征集了60例持续性（＞6周）腰椎根性神经痛的患者，将其分为两组，分别接受CT引导下硬膜外PRP注射和CT引导下硬膜外激素注射，采用NRS评分和ODI评分进行后续随访。结果显示，两组在治疗后6周NRS评分均较基线明显下降。PRP组平均NRS评分从基线状态的6.3分（±2.2分）降至3.7分（±2.3分），激素组平均NRS评分从基线状态的5.2分（±2.4分）降至3.4分（±2.4分）；ODI评分也较基线状态降低，PRP组平均ODI评分从基线状态的29.8分（±9.4分）降至23分（±12分），激素组平均ODI评分从基线状态的30分（±13分）降至20分（±14分）。两组之间NRS评分和ODI评分的下降无显著性差异，未发现严重并发症，提示硬膜外注射PRP和硬膜外注射激素的疗效相当[7]。

中山大学孙逸仙纪念医院康复医学科团队于2021年发表了一篇随机对照临床研究，征集了124例持续3周以上的腰椎根性神经痛患者，随机分成超声引导下激素注射组与超声引导下PRP注射组，并在治疗前以及治疗后1周、1个月、3个月、6个月和12个月分别采用VAS评分、压力疼痛感觉阈值（pressure pain threshold，PPT）、ODI评分和SF-36量表中的生理功能（physical function，PF）和躯体疼痛（bodily pain，BP）部分评估记录患者的疼痛及功能改善情况，并在治疗前和治疗后12个月分别评估患者患侧F波的潜伏期和出现率，以反映神经近端功能改善情况。结果显示：在治疗后1个月，两组的VAS、PPT、ODI、PF、BP评估结果均较治疗前有明显改善（$P<0.05$），并且其效果可持续12个月；在治疗后12个月，两组的患侧F波潜伏期和出现率均较治疗前有显著改善（$P<0.05$）。超声引导下激素治疗组与超声引导下PRP治疗组之间的治疗效果未见显著性差异（$P>0.05$）。在12个月的随访过程中，两组均未见不良事件发生。这提示超声引导下PRP注射与超声引导下激素注射对慢性腰椎根性神经痛的疼痛及功能改善程度相当，且安全性高，并发症少，可作为超声引导下激素注射治疗的一个安全替代疗法，适用于不适合接受激素注射治疗的患者，如感染、严重高血压、严重骨质疏松患者等[8]。

3. PRP治疗根性神经痛的基础研究

基础研究发现，对行L4～L6背根神经节单侧切断术的大鼠注射PRP后，可部分恢复其足爪回缩反射，提示初级传入纤维从背根神经节重新进入脊髓，而不加重神经胶质反应性，此外，有研究表明PRP的治疗具有免疫调节作用[9]。

目前，应用PRP治疗根性神经痛尚属比较新的领域，在这方面的研究不多，仍需后期进一步探索。

（许珍）

参考文献

[1] BOGDUK N. On the definitions and physiology of back pain, referred pain, and radicular pain[J]. Pain, 2009, 147（1-3）：17-19.

[2] DEYO R A, TSUI-WU Y J. Descriptive epidemiology of low-back pain and its related medical care in the United States[J]. Spine（Phila Pa 1976）, 1987, 12（3）：264-268.

[3] CHEN X Y, KONG X B, ZHANG Z Q, et al. Alpha-2-macroglobulin as a radioprotective agent: a review[J]. Chin J Cancer Res, 2014, 26（5）：611-621.

[4] VILLENEUVE J, BLOCK A, LE BOUSSE-KERDILÈS M C, et al. Tissue inhibitors of matrix metalloproteinases in platelets and megakaryocytes: a novel organization for these secreted proteins[J]. Exp Hematol, 2009, 37（7）：849-856.

[5] BHATIA R, CHOPRA G. Efficacy of platelet rich plasma via lumbar epidural route in

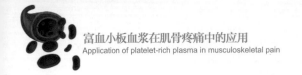
chronic prolapsed intervertebral disc patients：a pilot study［J］. J Clin Diagn Res，2016，10（9）：UC05-UC07.

［6］ CENTENO C，MARKLE J，DODSON E，et al. The use of lumbar epidural injection of platelet lysate for treatment of radicular pain［J］. J Exp Orthop，2017，4（1）：38.

［7］ BISE S，DALLAUDIERE B，PESQUER L，et al. Comparison of interlaminar CT-guided epidural platelet-rich plasma versus steroid injection in patients with lumbar radicular pain［J］. Eur Radiol，2020，30（6）：3152-3160.

［8］ XU Z，WU S L，LI X，et al. Ultrasound-guided transforaminal injections of platelet-rich plasma compared with steroid in lumbar disc herniation：a prospective，randomized，controlled study［J］. Neural Plast，2021（6）：1-11.

［9］ CASTRO M V，SILVA M，CHIAROTTO G B，et al. Reflex arc recovery after spinal cord dorsal root repair with platelet rich plasma（PRP）［J］. Brain Res Bull，2019，152：212-224.

第二节　富血小板血浆在痛性周围神经病中的应用

痛性周围神经病是由躯体感觉系统损伤或疾病导致的疼痛，它不是一种单一的疾病，而是由许多不同疾病和损害引起的综合征，可严重影响患者的生活质量。

1. 概述

痛性周围神经病的病因多种多样，分为先天遗传性和后天获得性。先天遗传性病因包括遗传性感觉神经和自主神经病、家族性淀粉样变性多发性神经病、法布里病、卟啉性神经病、丹吉尔病等。主要的后天获得性病因如下：

（1）代谢性和营养障碍性疾病：最常见的为糖代谢异常，如糖尿病、糖耐量异常引起的相关周围神经病，以及尿毒症周围神经病、甲状腺疾病相关性周围神经病、维生素缺乏或过量等引起的周围神经病。

（2）外伤和压迫性疾病：如嵌压性周围神经病、急慢性外伤性周围神经病。

（3）免疫介导性疾病：如吉兰-巴雷综合征、淀粉样变性多发性神经病、血管炎性周围神经病、副蛋白血症性周围神经病、结节病性周围神经病。

（4）感染性疾病：如人类免疫缺陷病毒相关周围神经病、Lyme病性周围神经病、麻风性周围神经病。

（5）药物或其他理化因素：如呋喃唑酮、拉米夫定等药物或酒精、砷、铊等的中毒。

（6）肿瘤相关性周围神经病：肿瘤直接浸润或远隔效应导致。

此外还有隐源性痛性周围神经病，也称特发性痛性感觉性神经病[1]。

痛性周围神经病的治疗包括对因治疗和对症治疗，其中对症治疗主要包括药物治疗、物理治疗、介入治疗、外科手术、心理治疗、中医中药治疗。而药物治疗所用药物包括抗惊厥药、抗抑郁药、镇静药和局部用利多卡因等。介入治疗以神经阻滞、微创治疗为主。

2. PRP治疗痛性周围神经病的临床研究

PRP对痛性周围神经病的治疗主要表现在嵌压性周围神经病中的应用，以及少数在糖尿病性周围神经病和麻风性周围神经病中的尝试。

PRP在嵌压性周围神经病的治疗中，以对腕管综合征的治疗为代表。腕管综合征是最常见的周围神经卡压性疾病，典型的症状是正中神经支配区的手指麻木、刺痛、疼痛或有烧灼感，或夜间感觉异常，还可有腕部肌腱发炎。腕管综合征的治疗包括药物治疗、夜间夹板固定、物理治疗、局部类固醇注射等。

2017年，Wu等进行了一项前瞻性随机对照单盲试验，将60例单侧轻中度腕管综合征患者随机分成PRP组和对照组，PRP组在超声引导下注射3mL PRP，对照组给予夜间夹板固定，采用VAS评分作为主要观察指标，

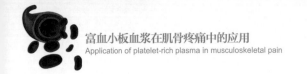

次要观察指标是波士顿腕管综合征问卷（Boston carpal tunnel syndrome questionnaire，BCTQ）、正中神经横截面积、正中神经电生理指标和手指肌力，在治疗前和治疗后1个月、3个月、6个月分别进行评估。结果显示，治疗6个月后PRP组的VAS评分、BCTQ评分、正中神经横截面积均较对照组显著减低，这提示PRP可以显著缓解腕管综合征患者的疼痛[2]。2018年，Michael-Alexander开展了一项随机对照临床研究，探讨单次注射PRP可否改善轻中度腕管综合征患者的临床症状。他们将50例轻度至中度的腕管综合征患者分为PRP组和对照组（注射生理盐水），利用快速DASH问卷在治疗前和治疗后4周、12周进行评估。结果显示，根据快速DASH问卷，PRP组成功率为76.9%，对照组成功率为33.3%，提示超声引导下单次注射PRP治疗腕管综合征的疗效肯定[3]。2019年，Shen等进行了一项前瞻性随机单盲试验，纳入52例单侧中度腕管综合征患者，分为PRP组和5%葡萄糖组，在注射前和注射后1个月、3个月、6个月进行BCTQ评分、正中神经横截面积和正中神经电生理指标的评估。结果显示，PRP组相较于对照组在随访3个月时BCTQ评分显著降低，随访6个月时正中神经远端运动潜伏期显著缩短，6个月时正中神经横截面积显著减少[4]。2019年，Senna等开展了一项随机对照研究，将98例轻中度特发性的腕管综合征患者分为PRP注射组和类固醇注射组，在治疗前和治疗后1个月、3个月评估VAS评分、BCTQ评分、正中神经感觉和运动功能的电生理表现，并用超声检测正中神经的形态学改变。结果显示，PRP注射组患者的临床症状、正中神经电生理和正中神经横截面积在治疗后1个月、3个月时有明显改善，并且在3个月的随访期间，PRP注射组在临床表现、腕肘段正中神经运动传导速度、正中神经感觉潜伏期和正中神经感觉传导方面较类固醇注射组都有明显改善，提示PRP可有效治疗轻中度腕管综合征，并在改善疼痛、功能及正中神经感觉和运动功能的电生理指标上优于类固醇[5]。

2019年，Chang等比较了PRP联合体外冲击波治疗中度腕管综合征与单独应用PRP治疗的疗效差异。他们将40例中度腕管综合征患者分为PRP组和PRP联合体外冲击波组，以基线状态和注射后1个月、3个月、6个月时的BCTQ评分、电生理检查、正中神经横截面积的变化来评估两种方法的疗效。结果显示，PRP联合体外冲击波组相较于PRP组没有明显差异[6]。2020年，Trull-Ahuir等评估了PRP在腕关节韧带松解术后辅助治疗轻度至重度腕管综合征的效果。他们将50例轻度至重度腕管综合征患者分为腕关节韧带松解术+PRP组和腕关节韧带松解术+贫血小板血浆（PPP）组，观察指标包括基线时和治疗后6周的握力、Wong-Baker Faces量表、BCTQ评分、南安普敦伤口评估量表。结果显示，两组患者术后疼痛、症状严重程度和功能均有改善，且只有腕关节韧带松解术+PRP组在6周随访过程中恢复了术前握力水平[7]。以上研究提示，PRP在治疗轻度、中度和重度腕管综合征时均有较好的疗效，在改善疼痛、功能、神经电生理指标方面均有效果，可与腕关节松解术、物理治疗等配合应用。

在麻风性周围神经病的治疗方面，2014年Anjayani等进行了一项随机双盲对照临床试验，他们纳入了60例麻风性周围神经病患者，试验组注射1mL PRP，对照组注射1mL PPP，通过比较治疗前和治疗2周后两点辨别试验结果和VAS评分来判断皮肤感觉敏感度的改变情况。结果显示，试验组VAS评分和两点辨别试验结果较对照组均出现明显改变，提示PRP可促进麻风性周围神经病皮肤敏感性的改变[8]。

在糖尿病性周围神经病的治疗方面，2020年Hassanien等通过一项随机前瞻性试验来探讨注射PRP治疗糖尿病性周围神经病的临床疗效。该试验共纳入60例Ⅱ型糖尿病合并糖尿病性周围神经病的患者，随机分为PRP+药物治疗组和药物治疗组，在治疗前和治疗后1个月、3个月、6个月分别对患者进行VAS评分和改良多伦多临床神经病变评分（modified Toronto

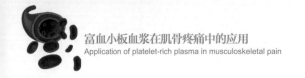
clinical neuropathy score，mTCNS）。结果显示，PRP+药物治疗组VAS评分和mTCNS评分较药物治疗组有明显改善，提示注射PRP是减轻糖尿病性周围神经病疼痛、麻木和增强周围神经功能的有效方法[9]。

3. PRP治疗痛性周围神经病的基础研究

研究显示，PRP可以促进周围神经损伤后的再生[10]。PRP含有多种生长因子，其中一些被认为可促进神经再生，例如胰岛素样生长因子–Ⅰ（IGF–Ⅰ）、血小板源性生长因子（PDGF）、转化生长因子–β（TGF–β）、碱性成纤维细胞生长因子（bFGF）、血管内皮生长因子（VEGF）。

IGF–Ⅰ受体主要表达于轴突、神经末梢、施万细胞、运动神经元胞体，可以参与激活下游两条信号通路，包括PI–3K和MAPK。PI–3K可活化在神经元存活中起重要作用的蛋白激酶B/Akt，而MAPK的活化也可使神经突起生长，促进细胞存活。总体来说，IGF–Ⅰ作为运动、感觉和交感神经元的神经营养因子，可促进生长锥运动、神经突起生长，并防止细胞凋亡。TGF–β2和TGF–β3在施万细胞的增殖分化调节中起核心作用，体外研究发现将慢性失神经干细胞与TGF–β共同孵育可以恢复体内的生长支持表型。bFGF可由受损轴突、施万细胞、内皮细胞、成纤维细胞、巨噬细胞合成和释放，明显诱导Ras/MAPK的激活，从而促进神经突起的生长。研究表明，在过度表达bFGF的小鼠中，再生有髓轴突的数量增加了一倍。VEGF作为一种有效的血管生长因子，可刺激内皮细胞的增殖和迁移，此外VEGF和内皮细胞跨膜受体FLK–1结合，可激活MAPK途径和PI–3K/Akt途径，促进细胞增殖并介导抗凋亡作用。研究还表明，VEGF可作为一种神经营养因子，促进神经突起生长和施万细胞增殖[10-11]。

2008年，Sariguney等将40只Wistar大鼠动物分为五组，其中A组（$n=$4）仅从坐骨切迹至分叉处解剖出右坐骨神经，其余组则切断坐骨神经并用以下方法修复：B组（$n=8$）用2根缝合线，C组（$n=8$）用6根缝合线，

D组（$n=10$）用2根缝合线和PRP，E组（$n=10$）用6根缝合线和PRP。将D组和E组分别与B组和C组进行比较，结果发现加用PRP治疗的大鼠肌电图潜伏期缩短，组织学检查发现髓鞘层增厚[12]，这提示PRP有助于坐骨神经的再髓鞘化。2009年，Ding等制作了24只雄性SD大鼠的双侧神经挤压动物模型，然后应用PRP治疗海绵体损伤部位，结果显示PRP对海绵体功能的恢复和海绵体神经的再生具有积极作用[13]。2019年，Zhu等制作了50只家兔挤压伤模型，然后比较正常对照组、模型组、超短波治疗组、PRP治疗组、PRP+超短波治疗组家兔的神经功能、神经电生理、再生神经的组织学和形态学，以及靶肌肉的恢复情况。结果显示：PRP+超短波治疗组轴突再生早，复合肌肉动作电位出现阳性早；在干预后第12周，组织学评估显示PRP+超短波治疗组和正常对照组中S-100蛋白的表达相似。此外，形态学评估显示，与超短波治疗组和PRP治疗组相比，PRP+超短波治疗组有髓神经纤维密度和直径以及髓鞘厚度均显著增加。靶肌肉的形态计量学显示，PRP+超短波治疗组的肌肉体积百分比降低最少。超声检查显示，挤压伤后12周，靶肌肉的硬度和灌注参数改善最好。因此，在挤压伤模型中，超声引导下连续注射PRP联合小剂量超短波辐射对促进轴突功能恢复和减少靶肌肉萎缩具有协同作用[14]。

以上研究提示，PRP对周围神经的再生轴突再髓鞘化过程具有促进作用。

（许珍）

参考文献

[1] 中华医学会神经病学分会肌电图与临床神经电生理学组，中华医学会神经病学分会神经肌肉病学组．痛性周围神经病的诊断和治疗共识[J]．中华神经科杂志，2012，45（11）：824-827．

[2] WU Y T, HO T Y, CHOU Y C, et al. Six-month efficacy of platelet-rich plasma for carpal tunnel syndrome：a prospective randomized，single-blind controlled trial[J]．Sci

Rep, 2017, 7（1）: 94.

[3] MALAHIAS M A, NIKOLAOU V S, JOHNSON E O, et al. Platelet-rich plasma ultrasound-guided injection in the treatment of carpal tunnel syndrome: a placebo-controlled clinical study[J]. J Tissue Eng Regen Med, 2018, 12（1）: e1480-e1488.

[4] SHEN Y P, LI T Y, CHOU Y C, et al. Comparison of perineural platelet-rich plasma and dextrose injections for moderate carpal tunnel syndrome: a prospective randomized, single-blind, head-to-head comparative trial[J]. J Tissue Eng Regen Med, 2019, 13（11）: 2009-2017.

[5] SENNA M K, SHAAT R M, ALI A. Platelet-rich plasma in treatment of patients with idiopathic carpal tunnel syndrome[J]. Clin Rheumatol, 2019, 38（6）: 3643-3654.

[6] CHANG C Y, CHEN L C, CHOU Y C, et al. The Effectiveness of platelet-rich plasma and radial extracorporeal shock wave compared with platelet-rich plasma in the treatment of moderate carpal tunnel syndrome[J]. Pain Med, 2020, 21（8）: 1668-1675.

[7] TRULL-AHUIR C, SALA D, CHISMOL-ABAD J, et al. Efficacy of platelet-rich plasma as an adjuvant to surgical carpal ligament release: a prospective, randomized controlled clinical trial[J]. Sci Rep, 2020, 10（1）: 2085.

[8] ANJAYANI S, WIROHADIDJOJO Y W, ADAM A M, et al. Sensory improvement of leprosy peripheral neuropathy in patients treated with perineural injection of platelet-rich plasma[J]. Int J Dermatol, 2014, 53（1）: 109-113.

[9] HASSANIEN M, ELAWAMY A, KAMEL E Z, et al. Perineural platelet-rich plasma for diabetic neuropathic pain, could it make a difference? [J]. Pain Med, 2020, 21（4）: 757-765.

[10] YU W J, WANG J, YIN J. Platelet-rich plasma: a promising product for treatment of peripheral nerve regeneration after nerve injury[J]. Int J Neurosci, 2011, 121（4）: 176-180.

[11] SÁNCHEZ M, ANITUA E, DELGADO D, et al. Platelet-rich plasma, a source of autologous growth factors and biomimetic scaffold for peripheral nerve regeneration[J]. Expert Opin Biol Ther, 2017, 17（2）: 197-212.

[12] SARIGUNEY Y, YAVUZER R, ELMAS C, et al. Effect of platelet-rich plasma on peripheral nerve regeneration[J]. J Reconstr Microsurg, 2008, 24（3）: 159-167.

[13] DING X G, LI S W, ZHENG X M, et al. The effect of platelet-rich plasma on cavernous nerve regeneration in a rat model[J]. Asian J Androl, 2009, 11（2）: 215-221.

[14] ZHU Y Q, JIN Z, FANG J, et al. Platelet-rich plasma combined with low-dose ultrashort wave therapy accelerates peripheral nerve regeneration[J]. Tissue Eng Part A, 2019, 26（3-4）: 178-192.

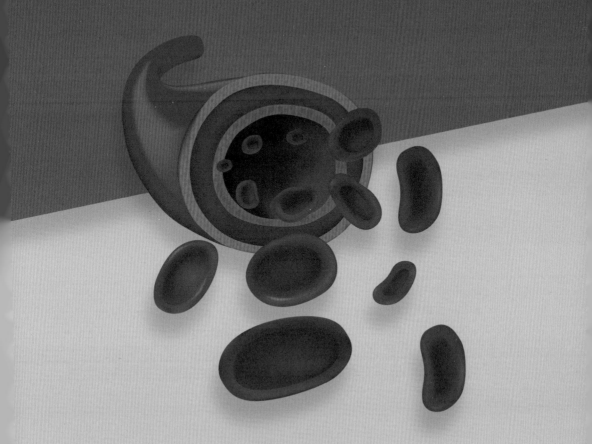

第六章

富血小板血浆治疗技术的
质量控制

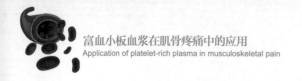
第一节 疼痛性疾病的诊断原则

国际疼痛研究学会对疼痛的定义是"与实际的或者潜在的组织损伤，或者与关于这种损伤的描述有关的一种令人不愉快的感觉和情感体验"。疼痛性疾病是以疼痛为主要症状，病因与病理机制相对明确或不明的一大类慢性疾病的总称，其中主要是慢性疼痛[1-2]。疾病的正确诊断是有效治疗的基础，尤其应注意鉴别诊断，避免误诊和漏诊。疼痛性疾病的诊断应基于病因学、病理生理学的深层次机制，需充分考虑到疼痛部位、性质、程度以及疼痛对患者生理功能和社会参与的影响[3-4]。同时，慢性疼痛患者通常伴随着焦虑、抑郁症状，因此患者心理状态和行为认知变化也是影响病情进展的关键因素[5-6]。

一、疼痛性疾病的诊断

疼痛性疾病的诊断主要依靠病史采集（主诉、现病史和既往史等）、全面的体格检查及疼痛相关的特异性体格检查、实验室检查、影像学检查、神经电生理检查和心理学检查等。

1. 病史采集

（1）一般资料：包括性别、年龄、职业、民族、婚育状况等，临床典型的疼痛病症可能与上述因素有关。

（2）诱因：指诱发疼痛的明显及潜在病因，如感染、外伤、过劳、疲劳等。

（3）疼痛特征：包括疼痛部位、性质、持续时间、伴随症状及加重或缓解因素。在疼痛性质方面，有几种疼痛较为典型，如神经病理性疼痛多表现为电击样痛、烧灼样痛和刺痛等，内脏痛多表现为钝痛、绞痛和胀痛等。

（4）既往史、个人史及家族史：应注意外伤史、手术史、食物药物过敏史、用药史以及与本次发病有关的既往诊疗经历，以此作为安全有效治疗的前提。

2. 体格检查

体格检查是指通过视诊、触诊、叩诊、听诊等获取客观评估信息的方法，包括全身检查和一般检查，最好按照头面部、上肢、胸腹、腰背、下肢的顺序进行检查。对于疼痛患者，也推荐按体位顺序检查，目的是减少因体位变动加重疼痛，提高诊疗效率（神经系统检查应置于全身检查和一般检查之中）。重点检查应针对疼痛部位本身，从皮肤开始，进行触觉、痛觉、温度觉等感觉检查，逐渐向深层结构（筋膜、肌肉、肌腱、韧带、骨关节）等展开检查。但应注意，虽然对于多数疼痛性疾病来说，疼痛部位即为病变所在，但有些疼痛远离病变部位，反映了支配该区域的神经病变或该神经走行经过区域的病变，同样要作为诊断的重要考量[7-8]。

3. 实验室检查

合理地进行实验室检查对于评估疼痛性疾病具有重要的价值，同时也是规避漏诊或误诊的重要途径。疼痛性疾病相关的实验室检查包括血液检查、红细胞沉降率（ESR）、C-反应蛋白（CRP）检查、抗链球菌溶血素O试验（抗O试验）及尿酸含量测定等[9]。

4. 影像学检查

影像学检查可作为疼痛疾病诊断和探究病理生理改变的重要依据，目前临床常用的影像学检查方法包括X线、CT、MRI、发射型计算机断层成像（ECT）、超声、骨扫描、正电子发射体层成像（PET）等[10-11]。

（1）X线：X线检查的特点为空间分辨率高但密度分辨率不足，适用于骨和含气组织显像，对于判断骨折及脱位等情况具有优势。

（2）CT：CT具有很高的空间分辨率，成像速度较快，有助于清晰显示骨组织和软组织钙化，但其对比度较差。如注射造影剂，能显示半月板、腕管及椎间盘，即造影剂强化可进一步提高组织密度和分辨率。

（3）MRI：①MRI具有多参数的成像模式，是一种高对比度检查方法，可使组织影像更加清晰，显示软组织的对比度高于CT，可使关节软骨、肌肉、韧带、椎间盘等组织直接成像；②无骨伪影干扰；③在患者体位不变的情况下，可通过变换层面选择梯度磁场，行横、矢、冠或斜位断层扫描，从而使得在三维空间上观察人体成为现实；③通过磁场来进行扫描成像，是一种无辐射、较为安全的检查方法。

（4）ECT：ECT近年来发展较快，临床诊断价值较大。随着医用放射性核素和核医学仪器的迅速发展，人体内很多组织器官如心、脑、骨骼和骨髓等均可使用放射性核素行ECT检查。ECT不仅可显示脏器或病变组织的形态结构，还可以提供脏器或病变组织的功能和代谢信息。

（5）超声：超声检查具有无创、实时性、安全和短期内可重复等优点，因此其在疼痛性疾病评估中的作用日益得到重视。超声可进一步划分为A、B、M、D等型，但B型超声（B超）能够实时显像，且切面图像与人体解剖相似，因此其在临床上的应用最为广泛。例如，在骨骼肌肉疼痛的诊断方面，B超不但可观察组织结构，而且可在检查中实时观察肌肉、肌腱的运动情况，因此可更直观地展示病变对功能的影响。如今，超声引导下的疼痛微创治疗已逐渐成为康复医学科、疼痛科等的特色技术，可弥补X线、CT引导技术的部分缺陷，正获得越来越多临床工作者的重视和青睐。超声引导下富血小板血浆（PRP）注射技术正是基于超声成像，逐渐发展形成的一套相对完善的诊断、治疗体系，目前已成为疼痛性疾病诊疗的重要方法。

此外，影像学检查还包括PET、红外热成像等。但应注意不要过度依赖影像学检查，需结合患者病史、体格检查等资料进行针对性的综合判断。

5. 神经电生理学检查

肌电图、神经传导测定、诱发电位检查是诊断神经肌肉疾病的基本方法，有助于提供可靠的神经系统功能的信息，对于神经、肌肉损伤引起的疼痛性疾病具有重要诊断价值[12-13]。

综上所述，完整的临床诊断应当涵盖病因、病理生理、解剖部位的情况，同时对疾病进行分期和分型，以便进行治疗并判断预后。根据疼痛部位、疼痛性质、疼痛程度及特点，寻找疼痛病因和疼痛机制，综合体格检查、实验室检查及影像学检查可为临床诊断提供依据。

二、疼痛性疾病治疗的整体原则

通常情况下，疼痛性疾病的病因复杂，临床表现各异，且患者对疼痛的耐受程度及治疗反应差异较大，很难界定统一的治疗标准，应注意治疗的个性化和灵活性。尽管如此，为了保证医疗质量和医疗安全，仍需重视疼痛性疾病治疗的整体原则。

1. 重视诊断，先诊断后治疗

对于疼痛性疾病，应重视诊断和鉴别诊断，避免原发疾病被症状掩盖，做到"有的放矢"。如采取诊断性治疗，必须目的明确，很多情况下患者疼痛难忍时常需及时止痛、缓解症状，但这种措施绝不是最终目的，需在症状缓解后进一步完善诊断，避免"头痛医头、脚痛医脚"。应重视首诊获得的各项检查结果和治疗效果评价，对复诊患者应核实诊断正确

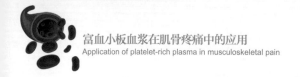
性，必要时应纠正诊断并完善治疗方案。

2. 选择综合治疗手段和安全、有效的原则

判定某种药物或某项治疗的疗效，不应以短期效果来判定，必须以远期预后为终点做疗效评价。疼痛性疾病的治疗要注意合理用药，例如：对于癌性疼痛，应采用WHO三阶梯药物治疗，以"口服为主，主动按时给药、按阶梯给药、个体化给药"为原则；对于非癌性疼痛，应用镇痛药物时要坚持足疗程，不宜频繁换药或同类药物重叠使用。在治疗方案的选择上，应"先简后繁，先无创后有创"，即以简单、无创、安全地达到治疗目的为原则。此外，疼痛性疾病患者常合并多种疾病以及精神心理障碍（焦虑、抑郁等），因此应根据不同患者的特点，身心兼顾，标本兼治，采用多元化的治疗手段以提高疗效。

3. 注意节约医疗资源，尽量减轻医疗负担

在"以患者为中心"的前提下，选择各种疗法和药物时应依据获益、风险和经济负担择优而定，充分且合理地利用医疗资源。

以超声引导下应用PRP注射技术治疗骨骼肌肉疼痛为例，接诊医生应根据疼痛性疾病的诊治原则，进行充分的病史采集、体格检查，结合实验室检查和影像学检查结果，在准确诊断的基础上实施PRP注射治疗。对于拟接受PRP注射的患者需进行认真筛查，注意避免该项治疗的绝对禁忌证和相对禁忌证（依据国际细胞学会的《富血小板血浆应用指南》）。

PRP注射治疗的适应证：①骨性关节炎；②慢性筋膜炎（背部/足底筋膜炎）；③肌腱病（Achilles肌腱病）、慢性肌腱炎（网球肘、肱二头肌长头肌腱炎）；④软组织损伤（肩袖损伤，膝/踝关节韧带、肌肉/肌腱拉伤）；⑤骨折愈合不良、骨髓炎（作为辅助治疗手段）；⑥股骨头坏死；⑦椎间盘退变、腰椎间盘突出伴慢性疼痛；⑧神经病理疼痛，如带状疱疹后神经痛、偏头痛、烧伤瘢痕疼痛等；⑨伤口愈合不良、糖尿病足、

压疮。

PRP注射治疗的绝对禁忌证：①血小板功能障碍综合征；②严重血小板减少；③血流动力学不稳定；④败血症；⑤手术部位局部感染；⑥患者有明显精神心理异常、认知障碍或其他躯体疾病，以致影响治疗效果观察。

PRP注射治疗的相对禁忌证：①非甾体抗炎药（NSAID）停药未超过48h；②1个月内患处曾注射过皮质类固醇；③2周内全身应用过皮质类固醇；④吸烟；⑤近期有发热或其他疾病；⑥癌症，特别是恶性骨肿瘤或造血系统癌症；⑦血红蛋白<10g/dL；⑧血小板<10^5/μL。

（栾烁　马超）

参考文献

[1] WILLIAMS A C C, CRAIG K D. Updating the definition of pain[J]. Pain, 2016, 157
（11）：2420-2423.

[2] BOUHASSIRA D. Neuropathic pain: definition, assessment and epidemiology[J]. Rev
Neurol（Paris）, 2019, 175（1-2）：16-25.

[3] BARON R, BINDER A, WASNER G. Neuropathic pain: diagnosis,
pathophysiological mechanisms, and treatment[J]. Lancet Neurol, 2010, 9（8）：
807-819.

[4] VARDEH D, MANNION R J, WOOLF C J. Toward a mechanism-based approach to
pain diagnosis[J]. J Pain, 2016, 17（9 Suppl）：T50-T69.

[5] MICHAELIDES A, ZIS P. Depression, anxiety and acute pain: links and management
challenges[J]. Postgrad Med, 2019, 131（7）：438-444.

[6] GUREJE O. Comorbidity of pain and anxiety disorders[J]. Curr Psychiatry Rep, 2008,
10（4）：318-322.

[7] LALANI I, ARGOFF C E. History and physical examination of the pain
patient[M]//DUBIN A. Practical management of pain: Fifth Edition. Elsevier, 2014:
151-161.

[8] HERR K. Pain assessment strategies in older patients[J]. J Pain, 2011, 12（3 Suppl
1）：S3-S13.

[9] RANNOU F, OUANES W, BOUTRON I, et al. High-sensitivity C-reactive protein
in chronic low back pain with vertebral end-plate Modic signal changes[J]. Arthritis

Rheum, 2007, 57（7）: 1311-1315.

[10] SERBAN O, POROJAN M, DEAC M, et al. Pain in bilateral knee osteoarthritis-correlations between clinical examination, radiological, and ultrasonographical findings[J]. Med Ultrason, 2016, 18（3）: 318-325.

[11] BEATTIE P F, DOWDA M, FEUERSTEIN M. Differentiating sensory and affective-sensory pain descriptions in patients undergoing magnetic resonance imaging for persistent low back pain[J]. Pain, 2004, 110（1-2）: 189-196.

[12] CANDOTTI C T, LOSS J F, PRESSI A M, et al. Electromyography for assessment of pain in low back muscles[J]. Phys Ther, 2008, 88（9）: 1061-1067.

[13] GARCIA-LARREA L, HAGIWARA K. Electrophysiology in diagnosis and management of neuropathic pain[J]. Rev Neurol（Paris）, 2019, 175（1-2）: 26-37.

第二节　富血小板血浆临床应用与制备方法

一、富血小板血浆临床应用实施条件

富血小板血浆（PRP）临床应用需要满足一定的要求和实施条件，具体如下。

1. 医院要求

具有血制品制备实验室的二级以上医院。

2. 制作科室资质要求

通过医院医务科新技术临床应用审批并备案。

3. 制备室基本要求

（1）布局合理，符合功能流程，洁污分开，分为污染区、清洁区、无菌区。

（2）操作室内部设施、温控、湿控要求应当符合环境卫生学管理和医院感染控制的基本要求，需配备紫外线灯和空气消毒机。

（3）地面、墙面、天花板等应光滑、无孔隙、防潮、耐清洁消毒。

（4）操作室内设采血区、PRP制备区和注射区。

（5）采血区应设有治疗车及采血所需物品，PRP制备区应配备超净台和离心机，注射区应配备超声机1台、注射用床1张、治疗车1台。

（6）准备药物、细胞治疗或做前期准备时，应有专门的地点，有足够的空间，且设计合理，能最大限度降低空气中微生物污染的风险。

（7）操作室内应设置洗手池和一次性擦手纸。

（8）操作室内应配备锐器箱、医用废弃物箱和垃圾箱各1个。

（9）用于临床项目的设施应保持干净、整洁、有序。

4．设备及耗材要求

（1）设备：①PRP制备用离心机；②血制品制备超净工作台；③标签打印系统；④超声机1台（用于引导注射）。

（2）耗材：①实验室制备PRP所需的所有耗材（图6-1）均应符合国家3类耗材的管理规定。②使用符合国家标准的PRP制备套装产品（国产或进口成品）。

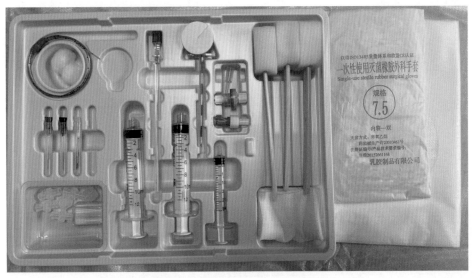

图6-1 实验室制备PRP所需耗材

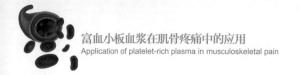
5. 人员管理

（1）科室应成立医院感染管理小组，由科主任、护士长、监控医生、监控护士组成，督促落实各项医院感染预防与控制措施。

（2）项目负责人应是在司法管辖权临床执业范围内经认证和注册的职业医师，并且受过疾病治疗的专业培训，在担任临床项目主管之前应先接受专业培训，但在疾病治疗领域有10年以上经验的除外。

（3）项目主管应该有两年直接参与相关疾病住院治疗和门诊诊疗管理的经验，负责行政和临床操作管理，监督相关标准和法律法规的执行，监督临床项目参与成员的工作情况。

（4）PRP制备医生需是获得司法管辖权临床执业范围内经认证和注册的执业医师，并且已经接受PRP制备的专业技术培训。

（5）采血人员应是经过正规培训，且在疾病治疗领域有丰富的患者管理经验的护士。采血过程中一旦发生紧急事件，应迅速通知临床医生。

（6）应有专人负责患者满意度调查、不良事件的登记备案以及治疗后疗效的随访。

（7）临床PRP治疗项目中应有有资质或经过培训的咨询专家或专家团队，能够处理患者需要的关键医疗护理事务。

二、临床医用自体富血小板血浆制备流程规范

1. 静脉采血流程

（1）准备采血用物，包括载有抗凝剂的无菌注射器、采血针头、无菌棉签、止血带、安尔碘皮肤消毒剂等。

（2）护士核对医嘱、采血执行单及条码上的姓名、床号、住院号、治疗项目等。

（3）护士进行自我介绍，对患者进行反核对，并解释抽血目的，评估患者局部采血皮肤及血管的情况。

（4）采血时按无菌操作原则穿刺肘正中静脉或前臂内侧静脉或手背静脉，见回血后抽取静脉血，将血液缓缓吸入无菌注射器中，禁止内推血液，采血后及时颠倒混匀，动作要轻缓。

（5）采血完毕后，再次核对患者姓名、床号和住院号，将用过的器材放在规定的回收箱内，并及时将采好的血交给制备PRP的医生。

（6）对患者进行宣教，穿刺部位的压迫力度、时间以不出血为宜，禁止按摩。

2. 二次离心法制备PRP流程

（1）消毒：用75%的酒精擦拭无菌超净台台面，放入备用耗材（无菌预充式导管、无菌离心管套件、5mL注射器、试管架、无菌镊子、无菌纱布、无菌注射针头、无菌锐器盒、无菌废弃物盒）；打开超净台紫外线灯和房间紫外线灯，消毒至少20min；关闭紫外线灯，打开超净台日光灯并持续吹风，待用。

（2）全血样品转移：操作者常规手消毒后，戴清洁手套，用75%的酒精擦拭载有血液样品的注射器外壁，置于超净台台面，按无菌操作要求依次取出无菌预充式导管和导管盖子，预充式导管和导管盖子均口朝上放置，将血液标本由注射器经导管口注入导管内，导管盖子盖紧，置于试管架上，操作中避免接触导管口和盖子接口端。

（3）离心全血样品：保持离心机底座稳定，预充式导管口朝下放置，对称放入配平管后离心，离心力400g，离心时间10min。

（4）排出红细胞：离心完毕后（图6-2），常规手消毒，垂直取出预充式导管，用75%的酒精纱布擦拭后，垂直于地面置于超净台试管架上待用，忌倾斜或翻转预充式导管。取无菌离心管，拧下离心管盖子，将离心管置于试管架上备用；打开无菌注射针头外包装备用。在导管始终保持垂直的状态下，将载有血液样品的导管盖子拧下，盖子口保持无菌朝上置于台面，取无菌注射针头旋转固定于导管口，将预充式导管的推杆旋转拧紧至导管活塞，取下注射针针帽，将针头垂直悬于离心管口，忌触碰离心管壁，缓慢轻推活塞，保留血浆成分，将底层暗红色成分推至离心管中，后将针帽盖好，拧下注射针头，丢弃至无菌锐器盒中；将导管盖子拧紧至预充式导管口，置于试管架上。

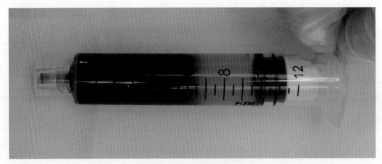

图6-2　第一次离心后

（5）离心血浆样品：保持离心机底座稳定，预充式导管口朝下放置，对称放置配平管后离心，离心力700g，离心时间10min。

（6）提取PRP：离心完毕后，常规手消毒，垂直取出预充式导管，用75%的酒精纱布擦拭后，垂直于地面置于超净台试管架上待用，忌倾斜或翻转预充式导管。取无菌离心管，拧下离心管盖子，将离心管置于试管架上备用；打开无菌注射针头和无菌注射器外包装备用。在导管始终保持垂直的状态下，将载有血浆样品的预充式导管盖子拧下，盖子口保持无菌朝上置于台面上，取无菌注射针头旋转固定于导管口，将预充式导管的推杆旋转拧紧至导管活塞，取下注射针针帽，将针头垂直悬于离心管口，忌触碰离心管壁，缓慢轻推活塞，保留1～2mm血细胞层及上层血浆成分，将中下层PRP注入无菌注射器中备用，后将导管针头的针帽盖好，拧下注射针头，丢弃至无菌锐器盒中；将载有PRP的无菌注射器装好针头备用。见图6-3至图6-5。

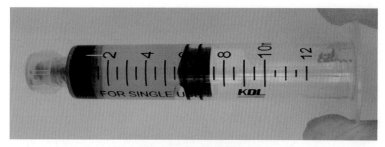

图6-3　第二次离心后

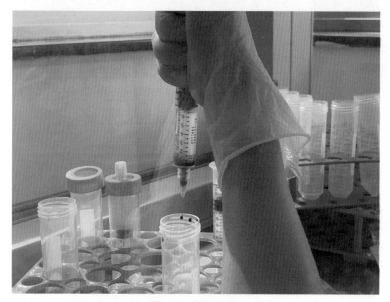

图6-4　提取PRP

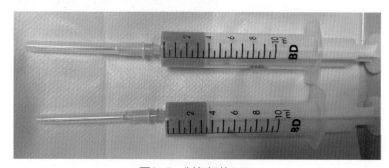

图6-5　制备好的PRP

（7）PRP制备后整理：恢复超净台、离心机整洁，补充待用耗材，用75%的酒精擦拭超净台台面，紫外线消毒。

三、质量管理规范

制备好的PRP需每月定期进行浓度检测，登记在册，以确保符合临床应用标准。见图6-6、图6-7。

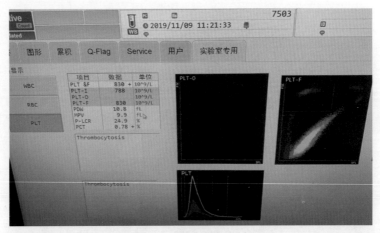

图6-6　PRP检测（1）

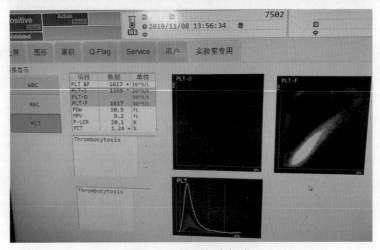

图6-7　PRP检测（2）

科室开展PRP注射治疗需有相应的质量管理体系。

（1）完整的质量管理体系包括临床试验、样本采集和制备单位的质量管理。

（2）开展PRP制备、超声引导下注射均应在医院医务科备案。

（3）质量管理方案包括制备和注射每个关键步骤的标准操作规程、完整的管控文件、每个患者的评估和治疗记录、相关医护人员定期进行继续教育等。

（4）开展相关临床试验需通过医院临床伦理委员会审批，参与的患者签署知情同意书。研究过程中，医院伦理委员会应定期对研究进行监察访问，以保证研究方案的所有内容都得到严格遵守且研究资料填写正确。研究人员必须经过统一培训，记录方式与判断标准应统一。整个临床试验过程均应严格按照规范进行PRP制备和超声引导注射等操作。研究者应按病例报告表的填写要求，如实、详细、认真记录病例报告表中各项内容，以确保病例报告表内容完整、真实、可靠。临床试验中所有观察结果和发现都应加以核实，以保证数据的可靠性，确保临床试验中各项结论来源于原始数据。在临床试验和数据处理阶段均应有专人负责数据管理。

（栾烁　伍少玲）

第三节　疗　效　评　价

疼痛患者经过PRP治疗后，需定期进行疗效评价。临床上对疼痛性疾病进行疗效评价，主要是了解治疗后疼痛的部位、强度、性质、发作情况及伴随症状等的变化，以明确现有治疗的效果。目前临床上对于疼痛的疗效评价既依靠患者自身的主观评定也包括客观测量的评定。

一、疗效评价方法

1. 单维评定方法

在疼痛治疗过程中，不仅要了解患者有无疼痛，还要了解患者疼痛强度的变化[1]。

（1）语言分级评分法（verbal rating scale，VRS）：将描绘疼痛强度的词汇通过测量尺的图形或数值表达，使描绘疼痛强度的梯度词汇更容易为患者所理解。

（2）视觉模拟评分法（visual analog scale，VAS）：是一种简单、有效、常用的测量方法。方法是画一条水平粗直线，通常为10cm，在线两端分别附注表示不同疼痛强度的词语，如一端为"无痛"，另一端为"最剧烈的疼痛"，患者根据自己所感受的疼痛程度，在直线上的某点做一记号，以表示疼痛的强度及心理上的冲击，从起点至记号处的距离长度（cm）就是疼痛的评分值。让患者及时评价不同时间点疼痛的绝对值，如PRP治疗前后对比疼痛的变化可以得到恰当的疗效评价[2]。

（3）数字分级评分法（numerical rating scale，NRS）：此方法要求患者用0到10这11个点来描述疼痛的强度。0表示无疼痛，疼痛较强时增加点数，10表示最剧烈的疼痛。此方法容易被患者理解和接受，可以口述也可以记录，结果较为可靠。

2. 疼痛问卷表

疼痛问卷表（pain questionnaires）是根据疼痛的生理感受、情感因素和认识成分等多方面因素设计而成的，因此能较准确地评价疼痛的强度与性质，常用的有麦吉尔疼痛问卷（McGill pain questionnaire，MPQ）、简化麦吉尔疼痛问卷（short-form of McGill pain questionnaire，SF-MPQ）、简明疼痛问卷表（brief pain qusetionnaire，BPQ）等[3-4]。

3. 痛阈测定

利用机械、温度、电流等物理刺激或药物刺激，使被试者确认刺激强度逐步增加到疼痛产生的一点即是痛阈[5]。如果将刺激的强度继续增加至患者无法忍耐，则此时的刺激强度为耐痛阈。

4. 功能评定

指评价患者疼痛部位的功能障碍情况（如Harris髋关节评分[6]、WOMAC量表[7]等）和基本的日常生活活动功能（如家务活动能力评价，包括坐、站、走、躺等在内的活动评价以及业余爱好情况评价等）。

5. 生物力学评定

包括柔韧性、耐力（活动时间测试、平板或功率自行车测试）、肌肉力量（重复举一物体的次数等）的评价。

6. 心理和行为测定

由于疼痛对人体的生理和心理都会造成一定的影响，所以疼痛患者经常表现出一些行为改变，如面部表情[8]、躯体姿势、行为和肌紧张度等。通过观察记录这些变化，可为临床疼痛评价提供一些较客观的辅助依据[9]。

7. 影像学评估

可以根据具体情况选用超声、X线、CT或MRI来评估PRP注射效果。

8. 生理、生化测定

疼痛常可引发机体各项生理指标的变化，如慢性疼痛患者皮质醇升高，血浆及脑脊液中的β–内啡肽降低，急性疼痛患者β–内啡肽升高。因此疼痛评价还可以通过生理测定法或生化测定法来实现，也可以根据心率、血压、呼吸、肺活量、脑电图等的变化对疼痛进行评定。

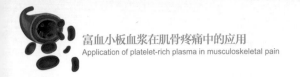
二、疗效评价制度

以PRP治疗为例，完善、及时的疗效评价是技术质量控制的关键环节。对于疼痛性疾病患者，应完善随访制度和随访流程。

（1）建立出院患者随访信息登记制度。建立患者随访档案，详细记录姓名、年龄、单位、住址、联系电话、诊断、住院治疗情况、随访情况等，由患者住院期间的主管医生及护士负责填写，档案由专人负责管理。

（2）随访方式包括门诊随访、电话随访、邮件随访、上门随诊、再次入院治疗等，随访的内容包括了解患者出院后的疼痛变化和恢复情况，指导患者进行日常康复，并收集是否有再次接受PRP治疗的指征及治疗时机等信息。

（3）随访时间应根据患者病情而定，一般患者出院1个月内应随访至少1次，此后根据临床需要定期随访。

（4）负责随访的第一责任人为主管医生，应根据随访情况决定是否与上级医生、科主任一起随访，并总结治疗经验。

（5）科主任或PRP项目负责人应对出院患者随访情况每月至少检查1次，定期总结、督导。

具体来讲，根据《富血小板血浆应用指南》的推荐，应注意完善PRP治疗后随访：①一般在术后/注射后2～6周对患者进行重新评估，具体包括充分观察疼痛部位、功能状态、注射部位等的情况，并讨论应重点关注的问题和未来的治疗方向。②应使用有效的疗效评估方法记录患者反应。③并发症、患者反应和所有其他相关数据应输入跟踪系统。④再次注射的考量应以患者为中心，并根据功能评估的结果做出临床决策。一般在身体各部位的具体注射次数难有定论，应进行个性化考量。

（栾烁）

参考文献

[1]　WILLIAMSON A, HOGGART B. Pain: a review of three commonly used pain rating scales[J]. J Clin Nurs, 2005, 14（7）: 798-804.

[2]　TODD K H, FUNK J P. The minimum clinically important difference in physician-assigned visual analog pain scores[J]. Acad Emerg Med, 1996, 3（2）: 142-146.

[3]　HAWKER G A, MIAN S, KENDZERSKA T, et al. Measures of adult pain: visual analog scale for pain（VAS Pain）, numeric rating scale for pain（NRS Pain）, McGill pain questionnaire（MPQ）, short-form McGill pain questionnaire（SF-MPQ）, chronic pain grade scale（CPGS）, short form-36 bodily pain scale（SF-36 BPS）, and measure of intermittent and constant osteoarthritis pain（ICOAP）[J]. Arthritis Care Res（Hoboken）, 2011, 63（Suppl 11）: S240-S252.

[4]　MAIN C J. Pain assessment in context: a state of the science review of the McGill pain questionnaire 40 years on[J]. Pain, 2016, 157（7）: 1387-1399.

[5]　GRANGES G, LITTLEJOHN G. Pressure pain threshold in pain-free subjects, in patients with chronic regional pain syndromes, and in patients with fibromyalgia syndrome[J]. Arthritis Rheum, 1993, 36（5）: 642-646.

[6]　HARRIS W H. Traumatic arthritis of the hip after dislocation and acetabular fractures: treatment by mold arthroplasty. An end-result study using a new method of result evaluation[J]. J Bone Joint Surg Am, 1969, 51（4）: 737-755.

[7]　MCCONNELL S, KOLOPACK P, DAVIS A M. The Western Ontario and McMaster Universities Osteoarthritis Index（WOMAC）: a review of its utility and measurement properties[J]. Arthritis Rheum, 2001, 45（5）: 453-461.

[8]　SCHIAVENATO M. Facial expression and pain assessment in the pediatric patient: the primal face of pain[J]. J Spec Pediatr Nurs, 2008, 13（2）: 89-97.

[9]　GORCZYCA R, FILIP R, WALCZAK E. Psychological aspects of pain[J]. Ann Agric Environ Med, 2013（1）: 23-27.

第四节　应用富血小板血浆可能存在的风险与处置预案

　　尽管PRP由自体全血经离心制备而成，目前普遍认为其不具免疫原性及感染性疾病传播风险，但并非所有的PRP治疗都能达到临床疗效标准，甚至可能发生严重不良事件[1]。本节主要介绍PRP治疗的相关风险。PRP治疗的相关风险与干细胞治疗部分类似，涉及医用材料、PRP类型、PRP的获取和制备、医护人员操作水平和注射部位等方面，大致可分为内在因素、外在因素和临床因素[2]。

　　（1）与特定细胞类型固有特性相关的危险因素（内在因素）：目前部分学者认为富白细胞血小板血浆（LR-PRP）中的高浓度白细胞在损伤部位可释放白细胞介素-6、白细胞介素-8、肿瘤坏死因子-α等多种炎症因子，介导炎症反应和氧化应激，可导致注射后患者疼痛加剧，有时伴局部肿胀和关节活动范围减小，但此类反应多具有自限性，一般在注射后2~3天可自行消退。

　　（2）与医用材料相关的风险（外在因素）：不规范的采血、离心、制备及储存可能损害PRP质量，未使用抗凝剂或抗凝剂保存不当、过期等可引起血液在采血管内触发凝血反应；使用Ⅲ类医用耗材以外的采血管、注射器等，可能导致血制品与容器内壁的涂层发生反应而出现不良反应。血小板浓度不达标会出现疼痛等临床症状无改善的情况。有研究表明，高于基线2.5倍左右的PRP对软骨细胞再生、新生血管形成等有积极作用，低于此浓度的PRP往往无法达到治疗效果，而一旦浓度过高，将对细胞的生长代谢产生抑制作用，对组织修复产生负面影响。

　　（3）非特有的临床相关危险因素（临床因素）：使用不合格、过期的医用材料或在制备过程、皮肤清洁和器械消毒过程、注射操作过程等多个节点中发生污染可造成感染。一旦发生关节感染，将引发严重的不良后果，甚至可能导致残疾和死亡。

显然，上述风险都应该得到重视。尽管大多数学者认为，相比于干细胞治疗，PRP相对安全性较高，但基于风险的多样性及不良反应的严重性，仍要求每一位医护人员在实施PRP治疗时先对患者、环境和自身进行全方位的精准评估和全程严格质量把控，个体化、精准化评估和标准化质量把控有助于提高PRP在临床应用中的安全性和有效性。

对于临床中存在的相关风险应以预防为主，首先，科室应对医护人员进行系统化培训和考核，确保所有操作人员的业务能力达标；医院和科室应完善和落实相关制度，对环境及设备消毒、PRP制备和操作流程等采取规范化管理及专人负责制等，避免发生血制品污染；在选择医用材料时，应选择有资质的厂家和PRP专用医疗器械及一次性使用耗材。治疗前应与患者及家属积极沟通和疏导，以提高患者对相关知识的理解和依从性；对于轻微的自限性不良反应如轻微注射部位疼痛加剧和关节肿胀等，可予以冰敷、制动、口服非甾体类药物或止痛药物；一旦出现感染，必须立即完善相关检验检查，根据感染类别及病情轻重程度使用针对性抗生素，出现全身感染症状者应及时进行全身抗感染治疗，必要时行脓肿切开引流、清创、关节腔灌洗治疗或手术治疗[3]。

（王少玲）

参考文献

[1] KAWASE T, OKUDA K. Comprehensive quality control of the regenerative therapy using platelet concentrates: the current situation and prospects in Japan[J]. Biomed Res Int, 2018（7）: 1-10.

[2] HERBERTS C A, KWA M S, HERMSEN H P. Risk factors in the development of stem cell therapy[J]. J Transl Med, 2011, 22（9）: 1-14.

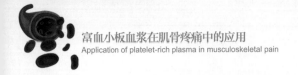

[3] STEVENS D L, BISNO A L, CHAMBERS H F, et al. Practice guidelines for the diagnosis and management of skin and soft tissue infections: 2014 update by the Infectious Diseases Society of America[J]. Clin Infect Dis, 2014, 59（2）: e10-e52.

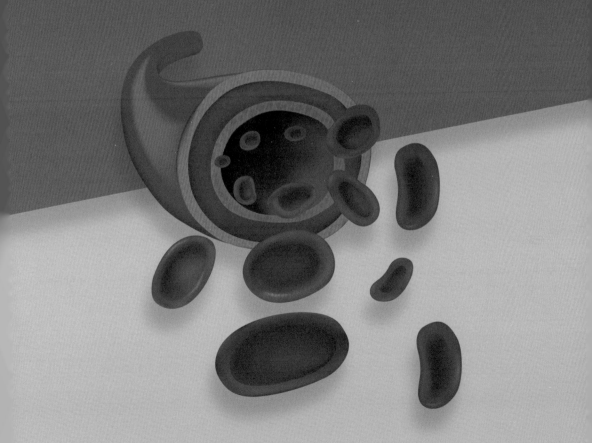

第七章

富血小板血浆研究展望

第一节　再生医学与富血小板血浆

富血小板血浆（PRP）在临床上来源广泛，制备方便，可以促进肌腱、韧带、软骨和骨组织再生，因此骨科、运动医学、口腔科和许多其他医学科室均已开展PRP的临床应用。

1. PRP复合支架在骨缺损修复中的应用

PRP在骨组织工程领域得到广泛应用，已作为细胞载体和/或成骨和成血管的生长因子来源。El Backly等[1]报道，羟基磷灰石–β–磷酸三钙支架与PRP结合具有促进兔颅骨缺损骨修复的作用。作者提出PRP可通过提供组织再生的关键生长因子来影响局部组织微环境，从而增强祖细胞募集、胶原蛋白和骨基质的沉积，并在支架和骨骼之间建立连接。Oryan等[2]研究报道，羟基磷灰石和β–磷酸三钙联合壳聚糖/明胶/富血小板凝胶可促进大鼠桡骨缺损模型骨愈合。Alidadi等[3]研究报道，明胶支架内嵌血小板凝胶可促进大鼠临界大小桡骨缺损骨愈合。Shibata等[4]报道，PRP和可生物降解的明胶水凝胶可增强兔胸骨缺损骨的修复。其研究结果表明，局部应用可降解的明胶水凝胶可控制PRP持续释放多种生长因子，对术后早期胸骨愈合有明显的促进作用。

骨组织再生工程还将PRP与细胞结合使用，其中PRP既可作为细胞载体，又可作为自体生长因子的供体来源。Yu等[5]报道，自体PRP可以作为骨诱导因子，改善由骨髓间充质干细胞（BMSCs）和β–磷酸三钙制成的组织工程骨的骨再生能力，促进兔桡骨缺损骨修复。Liao等[6]使用生物相容性热凝胶水凝胶、透明质酸–g–壳聚糖–g–聚（N–异丙基丙烯酰胺）（HA–CPN）作为三维有机凝胶基质，用于捕获兔脂肪来源的干细胞

（rASCs），将双相磷酸钙（BCP）陶瓷微粒作为矿化骨基质嵌入凝胶基质中，使PRP的骨诱导性能进一步强化。其研究结果显示，通过将PRP和BCP结合为HA-CPN的骨诱导和骨传导因子，成功地证明了热凝胶复合水凝胶支架可以促进rASCs的骨生成，可用于骨组织工程。Nakano等[7]报道，用添加PRP的明胶海绵包裹去分化的大鼠脂肪间充质干细胞有促进兔颅骨缺损骨修复的作用。

2. PRP在骨软骨、软骨缺损修复中的应用

PRP在组织工程中的应用不仅限于骨组织，已有实验证实了PRP在骨软骨和软骨修复中的作用。大多数研究都将PRP作为软骨细胞或祖细胞的载体[8]。Beigi等[9]研究报道，活化的PRP可促进三维海藻酸支架包裹的脂肪干细胞的软骨分化，促进兔膝关节软骨缺损修复。Barlian等[10]研究报道，添加抗坏血酸和PRP的胶原蛋白/丝素蛋白混合支架可促进人脐带间充质干细胞的软骨分化。Rosadi等[11]研究报道，PRP可诱导人脂肪源性干细胞在丝素支架上的软骨分化。

3. PRP在口腔科的应用

一份临床报告表明，PRP联合Bio-oss人工骨粉促进牙种植体周围骨缺损修复的效果显著，PRP能够加快和提升牙种植体周围骨缺损的修复速度和修复质量，使种植修复的疗效得以长期保持，值得在临床中推广应用[12]。

4. PRP在软组织修复中的应用

PRP活化后会形成柔软的水凝胶，成为软组织修复的最佳材料。PRP已被用于脂肪和皮肤损伤修复，并用作黏合剂来闭合伤口。Notodihardjo等[13]报道，PRP结合可生物降解的明胶水凝胶可促进血管生成和小鼠创面愈合。Spanò等[14]报道，由PRP、冷沉淀、凝血酶和葡萄糖酸钙混合产生的膜样物质可作为生物活性黏合剂，促进慢性溃疡小鼠模型的伤口修复。Myung等[15]研究报道，PRP可通过增强脐带间充质干细胞的血管生成

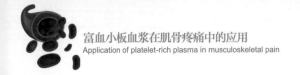
因子的分泌来提高其治疗大鼠皮肤创伤模型的修复效果。

5. 总结

以上研究报道表明，PRP已在各种再生医学中得到广泛应用，如作为自体水凝胶细胞载体，或者用作促进细胞黏附、血管生成或组织再生的生长因子来源。对于后者，一些研究提出如何在更长的时间内维持生长因子的释放尤其重要，例如应用明胶结合的纤维蛋白水凝胶包裹活化PRP来缓释生长因子。但是大多数研究并未探究PRP的作用方式。此外，PRP一般会作为材料的一部分用于与细胞和生物材料的复合，但此类研究无法明确具体成分的作用。这些不足说明在再生医学中PRP的作用特点、作用大小仍然不明确。作为生长因子的自体递送载体，PRP具有发展成为再生疗法固有部分的潜力。为了明确在临床环境中应用PRP的安全性和可预测性，将来进行系统且深入的研究至关重要。

（汪衍雪）

参考文献

[1] EL BACKLY R M, ZAKY S H, CANCIANI B, et al. Platelet rich plasma enhances osteoconductive properties of a hydroxyapatite-β-tricalcium phosphate scaffold（Skelite™）for late healing of critical size rabbit calvarial defects[J]. Journal of Cranio-Maxillofacial Surgery, 2014, 42（5）: e70-e79.

[2] ORYAN A, ALIDADI S, BIGHAM-SADEGH A, et al. Chitosan/gelatin/platelet gel enriched by a combination of hydroxyapatite and beta-tricalcium phosphate in healing of a radial bone defect model in rat[J]. International Journal of Biological Macromolecules, 2017, 101: 630-637.

[3] ALIDADI S, ORYAN A, BIGHAM-SADEGH A, et al. Role of platelet gel embedded within gelatin scaffold on healing of experimentally induced critical-sized radial bone defects in rats[J]. International orthopaedics, 2017, 41（4）: 805-812.

[4] SHIBATA M, TAKAGI G, KUDO M, et al. Enhanced sternal healing through platelet-rich plasma and biodegradable gelatin hydrogel[J]. Tissue Engineering Part A, 2018, 24（17-18）: 1406-1412.

[5] YU T B, PAN H Z, HU Y L, et al. Autologous platelet-rich plasma induces bone

formation of tissue-engineered bone with bone marrow mesenchymal stem cells on beta-tricalcium phosphate ceramics[J]. Journal of Orthopaedic Surgery and Research, 2017, 12（1）: 1-10.

[6] LIAO H T, TSAI M J, BRAHMAYYA M, et al. Bone regeneration using adipose-derived stem cells in injectable thermo-gelling hydrogel scaffold containing platelet-rich plasma and biphasic calcium phosphate[J]. International Journal of Molecular Sciences, 2018, 19（9）: 2537.

[7] NAKANO K, KUBO H, NAKAJIMA M, et al. Bone regeneration using rat-derived dedifferentiated fat cells combined with activated platelet-rich plasma[J]. Materials, 2020, 13（22）: 5097.

[8] Xie X T, Wang Y, Zhao C J, et al. Comparative evaluation of MSCs from bone marrow and adipose tissue seeded in PRP-derived scaffold for cartilage regeneration[J]. Biomaterials, 2012, 33（29）: 7008-7018.

[9] BEIGI M, ATEFI A, GHANAEI H, et al. Activated platelet-rich plasma improves cartilage regeneration using adipose stem cells encapsulated in a 3D alginate scaffold[J]. Journal of Tissue Engineering and Regenerative Medicine, 2018, 12（6）: 1327-1338.

[10] BARLIAN A, JUDAWISASTRA H, RIDWAN A, et al. Chondrogenic differentiation of Wharton's Jelly mesenchymal stem cells on silk spidroin-fibroin mix scaffold supplemented with L-ascorbic acid and platelet rich plasma[J]. Scientific Reports, 2020, 10（1）: 1-18.

[11] ROSADI I, KARINA K, ROSLIANA I, et al. In vitro study of cartilage tissue engineering using human adipose-derived stem cells induced by platelet-rich plasma and cultured on silk fibroin scaffold[J]. Stem Cell Research & Therapy, 2019, 10（1）: 369.

[12] 吴晓虹, 刘伟东. 富血小板血浆联合Bio-oss人工骨粉在牙种植体周围骨缺损修复中的应用效果观察[J]. 中国基层医药, 2019, 26（13）: 1611-1615.

[13] NOTODIHARDJO P V, MORIMOTO N, KAKUDO N, et al. Gelatin hydrogel impregnated with platelet-rich plasma releasate promotes angiogenesis and wound healing in murine model[J]. Journal of Artificial Organs, 2015, 18（1）: 64-71.

[14] SPANÒ R, MURAGLIA A, TODESCHI M R, et al. Platelet-rich plasma-based bioactive membrane as a new advanced wound care tool[J]. Journal of Tissue Engineering and Regenerative Medicine, 2018, 12（1）: e82-e96.

[15] MYUNG H, JANG H, MYUNG J K, et al. Platelet-rich plasma improves the therapeutic efficacy of mesenchymal stem cells by enhancing their secretion of angiogenic factors in a combined radiation and wound injury model[J]. Experimental dermatology, 2020, 29（2）: 158-167.

第二节　细胞医学与富血小板血浆

目前大量研究在探索应用富血小板血浆（PRP）取代胎牛血清用于间充质干细胞（MSCs）的体外扩增，以避免胎牛血清在临床应用中可能引发的免疫排斥反应。PRP可在干细胞的增殖、分化、迁移和免疫调节功能方面起重要作用。

1. 富血小板血浆对干细胞增殖的影响

国内研究学者从人骨髓血中分离获得BMSCs，分别加入到2%、5%、10%、20%的PRP培养液中培养，以10%的胎牛血清（fetal bovine serum，FBS）组作为对照组。结果显示，5%～10%的PRP组与对照组在细胞培养过程中均促进了BMSCs的增殖，其中，10%的PRP组细胞扩增数量最大，表明PRP在适宜浓度下可以促进BMSCs的生长[1]。林颢等[2]研究发现，脐带血PRP对人脐带间充质干细胞的生长有促进作用，且浓度为750pg/mL以上的PRP作用显著。Lai等[3]研究发现，1%的PRP可以显著促进人脂肪间充质干细胞的扩增。Zhang等[4]以不同浓度PRP对人子宫内膜干细胞进行培养，发现10%的PRP促进细胞扩增的效果最强，并且优于10%的FBS组。研究表明，与胎牛血清相比，PRP可延迟干细胞衰老表型的出现，使染色体稳定的时间更长[5]。

2. 富血小板血浆对干细胞分化的影响

间充质干细胞可以在不同诱导条件下分化为多种中胚层来源的细胞类型，包括软骨细胞、成骨细胞等[6]。研究显示，PRP可增强脂肪间充质干细胞和骨髓间充质干细胞的软骨分化和细胞外软骨基质合成[7]。张晔等的研究结果显示，1%的PRP可增强人骨髓间充质干细胞成骨分化[8]。Gersch

等[9]的研究显示，10%的PRP可促进人脂肪间充质干细胞的自发成骨分化。这些结果表明，PRP可以保持干细胞的特性，并且不妨碍其向骨、软骨的分化。

3. 富血小板血浆对细胞迁移与黏附的影响

细胞迁移可以反映细胞的运动与修复能力，鲜有文献探讨PRP诱导MSCs迁移的潜力，PRP能否增强前体细胞的迁移并成功黏附定植是提高骨再生能力的关键[7]。研究显示，脐带血来源PRP、成人PRP和成人PPP在促进细胞迁移方面都比胎牛血清更有效[10]。Gersch等[9]的研究显示，激活的PRP可改善脂肪间充质干细胞的黏附及其随后的增殖。Wang等[11]研究发现，PRP不仅可促进子宫内膜间充质干细胞的增殖和迁移能力，还可增强其黏附能力。

4. 富血小板血浆对干细胞免疫反应调节的影响

MSCs可以通过抑制T淋巴细胞的增殖来调节免疫应答[12]。MSCs也可以抑制其他特异性免疫细胞的增殖和功能，包括B淋巴细胞、NK细胞和树突状细胞。此外，MSCs可改变免疫细胞的细胞因子分泌谱，产生抗炎表型[13]。PRP可通过增强MSCs抑制T淋巴细胞增殖和激活的作用来保持其免疫特权潜能[13]。值得注意的是，超高浓度的血小板（10倍）可削弱MSCs对T淋巴细胞和NK细胞的抑制作用，并刺激炎症因子IL-6、IL-8和T细胞激活性低分泌因子（RANTES）的分泌[14]。上述结果表明，在添加PRP的培养基中培养MSCs可防止潜在的动物病原体的传播和异种免疫反应。

从整体上概括，PRP可刺激间充质干细胞增殖，保留间充质干细胞的多能性，且不干扰任何谱系分化，还可增强细胞迁移与黏附，保留间充质干细胞的免疫潜能，并可能延迟衰老表型的出现。但是目前将精确的分子和生物机制联系起来的相关报道尚少，许多知识的空白需要进一步的实验来填补。

（汪衍雪）

参考文献

[1] 谭金娣，陈福扬，史欣，等．富血小板血浆对干细胞增殖及分化作用的研究进展 [J]．口腔医学，2017，37（8）：743-745．

[2] 林颢，李鹏，孙杰聪，等．富血小板血浆对人脐带间充质干细胞增殖及成骨分化的影响[J]．广东医学，2016，37（9）：1274-1277．

[3] LAI F, KAKUDO N, MORIMOTO N, et al. Preparing activated platelet-rich plasma for culturing human adipose-derived stem cells[J]. Journal of Visualized Experiments, 2020（159）：32421005.

[4] ZHANG S W, LI P P, YUAN Z W, et al. Effects of platelet-rich plasma on the activity of human menstrual blood-derived stromal cells in vitro[J]. Stem cell research & therapy, 2018, 9（1）：48.

[5] CRESPO-DIAZ R, BEHFAR A, BUTLER G W, et al. Platelet lysate consisting of a natural repair proteome supports human mesenchymal stem cell proliferation and chromosomal stability[J]. Cell Transplant, 2011, 20（6）：797-811.

[6] QIAN Y, HAN Q X, CHEN W, et al. Platelet-rich plasma derived growth factors contribute to stem cell differentiation in musculoskeletal regeneration[J]. Frontiers in chemistry, 2017, 5：89.

[7] RUBIO-AZPEITIA E, ANDIA I. Partnership between platelet-rich plasma and mesenchymal stem cells: in vitro experience[J]. Muscles Ligaments Tendons J, 2014, 4（1）：52-62.

[8] 张晔，曾炳芳，张长青，等．富血小板血浆对体外培养骨髓间充质干细胞增殖及成骨活性的作用[J]．中国修复重建外科杂志，2005（2）：109-113．

[9] GERSCH R P, GLAHN J, TECCE M G, et al. Platelet rich plasma augments adipose-derived stem cell growth and differentiation[J]. Aesthet Surg J, 2017, 37（6）：723-729.

[10] MURPHY M B, BLASHKI D, BUCHANAN R M, et al. Adult and umbilical cord blood-derived platelet-rich plasma for mesenchymal stem cell proliferation, chemotaxis, and cryo-preservation[J]. Biomaterials, 2012, 33（21）：5308-5316.

[11] WANG X H, LIU L, MOU S M, et al. Investigation of platelet-rich plasma in increasing proliferation and migration of endometrial mesenchymal stem cells and improving pregnancy outcome of patients with thin endometrium[J]. Journal of Cellular Biochemistry, 2019, 120（5）：7403-7411.

[12] JONSDOTTIR-BUCH S M, SIGURGRIMSDOTTIR H, LIEDER R, et al. Expired and pathogen-inactivated platelet concentrates support differentiation and immunomodulation of mesenchymal stromal cells in culture[J]. Cell transplantation, 2015, 24（8）：1545-1554.

[13] FLEMMING A, SCHALLMOSER K, STRUNK D, et al. Immunomodulative efficacy of bone marrow-derived mesenchymal stem cells cultured in human platelet lysate[J]. Journal of Clinical Immunology, 2011, 31（6）: 1143-1156.

[14] ABDELRAZIK H, SPAGGIARI G M, CHIOSSONE L, et al. Mesenchymal stem cells expanded in human platelet lysate display a decreased inhibitory capacity on T- and NK-cell proliferation and function[J]. European Journal of Immunology, 2011, 41（11）: 3281-3290.

第三节　干细胞治疗与富血小板血浆治疗

干细胞治疗和富血小板血浆（PRP）治疗是再生医学中的两个重要方面[1]。骨髓间充质干细胞（BMSCs）、脐带间充质干细胞（hUC-MSCs）、脂肪间充质干细胞（ASCs）等干细胞可以成功地应用于组织再生领域。从全血中分离出来的天然产物PRP可以分泌多种生长因子（GF）来调节生理活动。这些GF可以刺激不同的干细胞增殖和分化，并保持干细胞的特性[2]。因此，在再生医学中，尤其是在骨骼、软骨和肌腱的修复中，两种治疗方法的组合受到广泛的期待。

1. 富血小板血浆联合干细胞治疗疾病的临床研究

哈承志等[3]研究报道，膝关节腔内PRP与hUC-MSCs联合注射治疗200例轻中度膝关节骨关节炎患者，疗效优于单纯注射PRP或hUC-MSCs，且优于注射玻璃酸钠。治疗后1个月、3个月、6个月、12个月，联合注射组VAS评分与美国膝关节协会（AKS）评分改善最明显；治疗后3周，关节液中炎症因子IL-1β、TNF-α、前列腺E_2（PGE_2）、MMP-13及软骨寡聚基质蛋白降低最明显；治疗后6个月，MRI显示联合注射组退化的软骨修复最明显。

Mayoly等[4]报道，脂肪微粒联合PRP注射治疗3例K-L分级为Ⅳ级的腕关节炎患者，在治疗后1年，VAS评分、DASH评分和PRWE功能评分均明显改善。Bastos等[5]研究报道，对膝关节炎患者进行膝关节腔内自体PRP与自体BMSCs联合注射，疗效优于单纯注射BMSCs，也优于注射糖皮质激素。治疗后1个月、2个月、3个月、6个月、9个月和12个月，联合注射组膝关节损伤和骨关节炎结果评分与关节活动度改善最明显；治疗后12个月，关节液中炎症因子IL-10降低最明显。

Lamo-Espinosa等[6]进行了多中心临床研究，采用自体LP-PRP与自体BMSCs联合注射治疗60例膝关节炎患者，在注射后3个月、6个月、12个月随访，联合注射组患者VAS、WOMAC评分都优于单纯PRP注射组；在注射后12个月行X线和MRI评估时发现，膝关节间隙和关节损伤程度改变不明显。

2. 富血小板血浆联合干细胞治疗疾病的基础研究

张波等[7]研究PRP与同种异体BMSCs联合治疗兔股骨头坏死时发现，各治疗组都能改善股骨头骨细胞增殖、减少骨陷窝空缺率，其中联合组治疗效果最佳。王位等[8]体外实验研究发现：20%的PRP裂解液在体外可显著促进hUC-MSCs的增殖、成肌腱分化；PRP联合hUC-MSCs促进大鼠受损跟腱愈合的作用最为显著；在促进大鼠跟腱愈合方面，单独应用hUC-MSCs较单独应用PRP效果更好，而PRP可以增强hUC-MSCs促进大鼠受损跟腱愈合的能力。解光越等[9]研究发现，LR-PRP和兔滑膜干细胞均可促进兔膝关节软骨损伤修复，联合治疗组较单独治疗组效果好。Vural等[10]报道，采用VEGF过表达的ASCs联合PRP治疗大鼠原发性卵巢功能不全，结果联合治疗组大鼠卵泡计数和卵巢功能较单纯ASCs治疗组和单纯PRP治疗组改善明显。Myung等[11]研究发现，在大鼠辐射后伤口延迟愈合模型中，PRP联合hUC-MSCs治疗伤口愈合最快，作者提出PRP是通过增强hUC-MSCs血管生成因子的分泌来提高其治疗效果的。

3. 结语

细胞治疗有巨大的临床应用潜力。然而，细胞移植后面临着复杂而恶劣的环境，局部缺氧、氧化应激和炎症可能导致细胞大规模丧失或死亡，进而影响细胞治疗效果。PRP可以增强干细胞的干性特性。以上一些研究资料显示，PRP联合干细胞的治疗效果往往优于单纯干细胞治疗或单纯PRP治疗，这种联合治疗在各个学科代表了一种有前途有希望的方法。但治疗的相关分子机制研究尚处于待完善阶段，并且在临床研究中对细胞移植的风险评估尤其重要，因为临床疗效和安全性取决于对各种因素、培养条件和质量风险管理的控制。

（汪衍雪）

参考文献

[1] QIAN Y, HAN Q X, CHEN W, et al. Platelet-rich plasma derived growth factors contribute to stem cell differentiation in musculoskeletal regeneration[J]. Frontiers in chemistry, 2017, 5：89.

[2] TOBITA M, TAJIMA S, MIZUNO H. Adipose tissue-derived mesenchymal stem cells and platelet-rich plasma：stem cell transplantation methods that enhance stemness[J]. Stem cell research & therapy, 2015, 6（206）：215.

[3] 哈承志，李伟，任少达，等. 富血小板血浆联合间充质干细胞治疗膝骨关节炎的疗效[J]. 中华关节外科杂志（电子版），2018, 12（5）：644-652.

[4] MAYOLY A, INIESTA A, CURVALE C, et al. Development of autologous platelet-rich plasma mixed-microfat as an advanced therapy medicinal product for intra-articular injection of radio-carpal osteoarthritis：from validation data to preliminary clinical results[J]. International Journal of Molecular Sciences, 2019, 20（5）：1111.

[5] BASTOS R, MATHIAS M, ANDRADE R, et al. Intra-articular injection of culture-expanded mesenchymal stem cells with or without addition of platelet-rich plasma is effective in decreasing pain and symptoms in knee osteoarthritis：a controlled, double-blind clinical trial[J]. Knee surgery, sports traumatology, arthroscopy：official journal of the ESSKA, 2020, 28（6）：1989-1999.

[6] LAMO-ESPINOSA J M, BLANCO J F, SANCHEZ M, et al. Phase II multicenter randomized controlled clinical trial on the efficacy of intra-articular injection of autologous bone marrow mesenchymal stem cells with platelet rich plasma for the treatment of knee

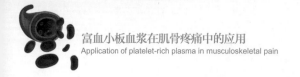

osteoarthritis[J]. J Transl Med，2020，18（1）：356.

[7] 张波，韦冰丹，甘坤宁，等. 富血小板血浆联合骨髓间充质干细胞对兔股骨头坏死BMP-2/Smads通路的影响[J]. 中国骨质疏松杂志，2016，22（2）：131-134.

[8] 王位，付宇翀，周梅，等. 人脐带间充质干细胞联合富含血小板血浆促进大鼠跟腱损伤的修复[J]. 第三军医大学学报，2017，39（2）：185-191.

[9] 解光越，陈阳，张志勇，等. 富白细胞血小板血浆联合兔滑膜干细胞促进膝关节软骨损伤修复的研究[J]. 中华实验外科杂志，2017，34（10）：1718-1720.

[10] VURAL B，DURUKSU G，VURAL F，et al. Effects of VEGF（+）mesenchymal stem cells and platelet-rich plasma on inbred rat ovarian functions in cyclophosphamide-induced premature ovarian insufficiency model[J]. Stem Cell Rev Rep，2019，15（4）：558-573.

[11] MYUNG H，JANG H，MYUNG J K，et al. Platelet-rich plasma improves the therapeutic efficacy of mesenchymal stem cells by enhancing their secretion of angiogenic factors in a combined radiation and wound injury model[J]. Experimental Dermatology，2020，29（2）：158-167.

第四节　富血小板血浆研究展望

富血小板血浆（PRP）具有抑制炎性反应、促进组织修复、控制感染和构建生物支架的潜能，目前在临床上普遍应用于骨科、口腔科、皮肤科、疼痛科、康复科、整形外科等。

一、PRP在临床上的应用

目前，PRP在临床上的应用主要包括以下方面。

1. 促进关节软骨的修复

PRP激活后可释放多种生长因子，有促进软骨修复的功能。其中被人们广泛认同的有血管生长因子、转化生长因子及胰岛素样生长因子。近年来，大量临床研究已证实，PRP治疗关节软骨退行性疾病是安全、有效的，其中以治疗膝骨关节炎为主。

PRP制备简单，价格便宜，可能成为未来治疗关节骨病的新手段。血管生成因子（VGF）的局部应用被证明对局部血管生长、骨形成细胞聚集和骨化有利，可以促进骨修复；TGF-β1能促进骨细胞的增殖；胰岛素样生长因子（IGF）可提升软骨细胞外基质的合成，应用于非老龄人群或关节炎患者，还有控制软骨基质分解代谢的作用。血小板源性生长因子（PDGF）能够促使细胞进行合成与代谢，降低IL-1β活性，减少软骨细胞凋亡，导致这一变化的诱因可能是抗炎效应[1-3]。

中山大学孙逸仙纪念医院康复医学科于2020年发表了一项临床回顾研究，分析了超声引导下PRP注射对不同严重程度KOA的疗效及疗效差异，受试者依据K-L分级标准分为0、Ⅰ、Ⅱ、Ⅲ、Ⅳ级组，各组患者均接受4次PRP关节腔注射治疗，注射间隔为1周。结果显示：Ⅰ、Ⅱ、Ⅲ级组患者注射PRP后VAS评分和WOMAC评分均随时间明显改善（$P < 0.001$）；各组治疗后3个月、6个月分别与治疗前相比，VAS评分、WOMAC评分均改善明显（$P < 0.05$）。该结果提示超声引导下关节腔注射PRP可有效缓解轻、中度KOA疼痛，改善患者功能障碍[4]。

2. 肌腱损伤的修复

PRP是自体来源的富含高浓度血小板的血浆，含有丰富的生长因子，如VEFG、TGF-β、PDGF、IGF和EGF等，这些生长因子能诱导细胞信号传导，从而刺激组织血管生成、肌腱细胞增殖和分化以及新基质形成，对肌腱细胞的胶原蛋白合成、内源性生长因子的产生有积极作用。除生长因子以外，PRP包含的其他成分如白细胞介素、趋化因子、蛋白酶、蛋白酶抑制剂、鞘脂、血栓素、5-羟色胺等，可在肌腱损伤的早期阶段发挥抗炎作用[5-6]，目前已应用于肱骨外上髁炎、跟腱损伤、慢性跟腱炎、肩袖损伤等常见肌腱损伤变性的治疗，表现出一定的临床疗效。

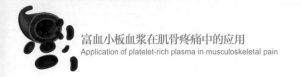
中山大学孙逸仙纪念医院康复医学科予多名中老年肩袖损伤患者超声引导下冈上肌腱撕裂处PRP注射，每10天1次，连续3次，并给予康复治疗，结果注射后2周患者肩痛、关节活动度明显改善。

3. 骨缺损的修复

应用PRP修复骨组织在体外细胞实验和动物模型中均展现出较好的愈合效果，但是在临床应用中疗效不一。细胞因子的介入能刺激骨微环境的再生能力，促进骨折修复。临床研究表明，在骨折内固定术中或术后联合应用PRP，可明显促进骨痂生长和骨折的愈合[7]。

中山大学孙逸仙纪念医院康复医学科对1例43岁距骨骨折内固定术后1年多的男性患者予超声引导下骨不连处PRP注射，每2周1次，连续8次，结合运动训练，半年后复查CT，可见距骨内固定后骨不连处有明显骨痂生长，患者步行时疼痛改善。

2020年，中山大学孙逸仙纪念医院康复医学科报道了1例超声引导下髋关节腔PRP注射改善青少年ARCO Ⅳ期ONFH的临床个案：患者为16岁女性，MRI示双侧股骨头塌陷并双侧髋关节间隙狭窄、关节腔大量积液。经PRP注射（4.5mL/侧，治疗频率1次/周，连续5次）并配合常规康复治疗，9个月后随访，患者VAS评分从7分改善至3分，双髋ROM改善，Harris髋关节评分和WOMAC评分均有明显改善，且能耐受长时间站立及短距离步行，复查MRI结果示双侧塌陷较前改善，积液明显减少，骨坏死体积减小，双侧关节间隙较前增大[8]。

4. 难愈性伤口修复

PRP促进慢性难愈性创面修复的主要机制：①血小板经活化后释放多种功效强大的生长因子；②PRP中含有大量白细胞，例如中性粒细胞、单核细胞和淋巴细胞，此类细胞以多种方式参与到抗感染过程中；③PRP中有3种血液黏附因子，即纤维蛋白、纤维连接蛋白和玻连蛋白。纤维蛋白可以在局部形成组织修复过程中必需的三维结构，以包裹血小板和白细胞，避免其流失，使细胞在修复过程有爬行支撑[9-11]。

中山大学孙逸仙纪念医院康复医学科应用PRP凝胶治疗多例外伤后难愈性创面，可观察到创面无感染、愈合速度较前快。

5. 口腔科、皮肤科、整形美容科等的应用

PRP在口腔种植骨再生中的应用效果明显，能显著减少骨吸收率，临床治疗效果更确切，同时治疗过程也比较安全可靠。PRP在皮肤科中也得到广泛的应用，涉及治疗脱发、皮肤年轻化、瘢痕修复、创面愈合等多个领域。而对于面部皱纹、皮肤光损伤等，开展局部使用PRP、皮肤注射PRP或者两种方式相结合的方案进行治疗，部分患者数周就会有面容的改变。

二、PRP的应用优势和存在问题

临床应用PRP具有许多独特的优势，如PRP由患者自体外周血制备，没有免疫原性，同时含有大量的生长因子，其制备过程相对精简，也可应用产品化的套装快速制备，制成的PRP性质稳定。

PRP在临床上应用的有效性仍有一定的争议。PRP中的成分和活性蛋白多而复杂，其各自如何发挥作用和/或协同作用的机制仍然不完全清楚，其相互激活的调节信号和活性蛋白释放的序列与时间都是未解开的谜团。

PRP中的血小板含量是多少才有最好的临床效果，目前还没有统一的标准，有研究提出血小板浓度应为基线血小板浓度的4～8倍[12]。相关资料显示，4～5倍的血小板浓度能有效促使骨组织及软组织的修复，而超过此浓度并不能体现出更佳的治疗效果。

三、结语

PRP富含多种生长因子，这些生长因子相互协调，能促进患者软骨、肌腱、韧带等组织的修复和再生，促进骨骼生长，加速创面愈合。PRP治疗作为一项新技术，其适应证的选择、制备和注射的过程、注射后的康复训练等各个环节均很重要。作为自体血液的浓缩部分，PRP可以改善和加速组织的愈合，与同种异体移植物比较，不会发生血源性传染性疾病的传播及免疫性反应。但是，目前大部分PRP治疗缺乏大规模的多中心、前瞻性、随机对照研究，对于PRP的合适治疗浓度范围没有统一的标准，制备装置和方法不一致，缺乏标准化的PRP制备技术，注射剂量和次数等均存在较大差异。未来对PRP治疗的研究应集中解决以上问题，增加长期临床效果的前瞻性研究。另外，PRP联合干细胞治疗也是一个趋势，配合超声引导下注射技术、精准靶点注入技术等，有希望使PRP治疗成为成熟的常规治疗，为肌骨疼痛疾病的治疗提供新方向。

（伍少玲）

参考文献

[1] PATEL S, DHILLON M S, AGGARWAL S, et al. Treatment with platelet-rich plasma is more effective than placebo for knee osteoarthritis: a prospective, double-blind, randomized trial[J]. Am J Sports Med, 2013, 41（2）: 356-364.

[2] CERZA F, CARNI S, CARCANGIU A, et al. Comparison between hyalumnic acid and platelet-rich plasma, intra-articular infiltration in the treatmen to fgonanhrosis[J]. Am J Sports Med, 2012, 40（12）: 2822-2827.

[3] ANDIA I, MAFFULLI N. Platelet-rich plasma for managing pain and inflammation in osteoarthritis[J]. Nat Rev Rheumatol, 2013, 9（12）: 721-730.

[4] 栾烁，栗晓，林彩娜，等. 超声引导下关节腔注射富血小板血浆治疗膝骨性关节炎疗效的回顾性研究[J]. 华西医学，2020，35（5）: 568-573.

[5] DOCHEVA D, MULLER S A, MAJEWSKI M, et al. Biologics for tendon repair[J].

Adv Drug Deliv Rev, 2015, 84: 222-239.

[6] RAJABI H, SHEIKHANI SHAHIN H, NOROUZIAN M, et al. The healing effects of aquatic activities and allogenic injection of platelet-rich plasma (PRP) on injuries of Achilles tendon in experimental rat[J]. World J Plast Surg, 2015, 4 (1): 66-73.

[7] CHELLINI F, TANI A, VALLONE L, et al. Platelet-rich plasma prevents in vitro transforming growth factor-beta1-induced fibroblast to myofibroblast transition: involvement of vascular endothelial growth factor (VEGF) -A/VEGF receptor-1-mediated signaling (dagger) [J]. Cells, 2018, 7 (9): 142.

[8] LUAN S, LIU C C, LIN C N, et al. Platelet-rich plasma for the treatment of adolescent late-stage femoral head necrosis: a case report[J]. Regen Med, 2020, 15 (9): 2067-2073.

[9] RAMOS-TORRECILLAS J, GARCIA-MARTFNEZ O, DE LUNA-BERTOS E, et al. Effectiveness of platelet-rich plasma and hyaluronic acid for the treatment and care of pressure ulcers[J]. Biol Res Nurs, 2015, 17 (2): 152-158.

[10] OSTVAR O, SHADVAR S, YAHAGHI E, et al. Effect of platelet-rich plasma on the healing of cutaneous defects exposed to acute to chronic wounds: a clinico-histopathologie study in rabbits[J/OL]. Diagn Pathol, 2015, 10 (1): 85[2020-02-01]. https://www.Onacademic.com/detail/journal-1000039955105110-383a.html. DOI: 10.1186/s13000-015-0327-8.

[11] GENTILE P, GARCOVICH S. Systematic review-the potential implications of different platelet-rich plasma (PRP) concentrations in regenerative medicine for tissue repair[J]. Int J Mol Sci, 2020, 21 (16): 5702.

[12] MAZZOCCA A D, MCCARTHY M B, CHOWANIEC D M, et al. The positive effects of different Platelet-Rich plasma methods on human muscle, bone, and tendon cells[J]. Am J Sports Med, 2012, 40 (8): 1742-1749.

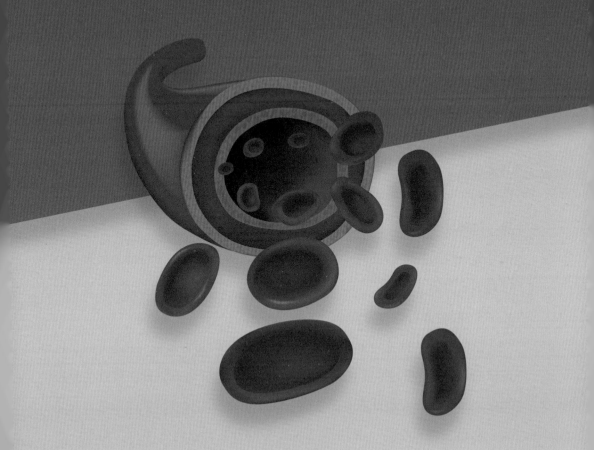

第八章

超声引导下富血小板血浆注射技术

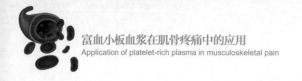
第一节　概　　述

一、超声仪的基本结构

1. 超声仪的组成

超声仪主要由探头、计算机信号处理系统、图像存储和显示系统组成。探头的主要功能是通过陶瓷晶体的正负压电效应发射和接收超声波。计算机信号处理系统的主要功能是对接收到的模拟信号或数字信号进行放大、滤波等后处理。图像存储和显示系统的主要功能是传输、存储已经处理好的图像信息并通过显示器加以显示。

2. 超声成像原理

超声波进入人体后，遇到人体组织不同的界面时，会产生反射、散射及多普勒（Doppler）信号等，形成回波，携带信息的回波被接收、放大和处理后，以不同的形式显示在显示器上，即为声像图，声像图属于断层图像。超声成像过程：探头发射超声波进入人体→产生反射、散射及Doppler信号等→探头接收回波→将声信号转变为电信号→主机进行信号处理→显示器显示图像。

3. 彩色多普勒血流成像的作用

彩色多普勒血流成像（彩超）包括二维灰阶切面显像（B超）和彩色显像两部分。B型超声仪是使用最广泛的超声仪，可提供超声检查的基础图像。高质量的彩超要求有满意的二维灰阶切面图像和清晰的彩色血流显像。彩超主要对脏器、肿块及外周血管的分布、走向、多少、粗细、形态及血流速度等多项参数加以显示，在注射药物时还可以显示药物扩散方向。

4. 超声仪的使用步骤

（1）开机。按超声仪的电源开关即可开机。

（2）选择探头。根据靶目标的深浅选择合适的探头。

（3）输入患者资料。按患者信息输入键输入患者的一般信息。

（4）选择超声模式。根据检查需要，分别选择二维灰阶模式、彩色血流显示模式或多普勒频谱模式等。利用彩色多普勒效应可以帮助鉴别血管并显示注射药物时药物的扩散方向。

（5）调节深度。根据靶目标的深浅调节深度，选择适宜的深度可更好地显示靶目标。适宜的深度是指将靶目标置于声图像的正中或使深度比靶目标深1cm。

（6）调节增益。调节近场、远场或总增益可使靶目标显示清晰。超声波在穿过组织时会发生衰减，调节增益补偿衰减，能使组织结构回声较均匀。

（7）调节焦点。选择适宜的焦点数，并调节聚焦深度，以使聚焦深度与靶目标深度一致。

（8）存储图像。先按冻结键冻结所需图像，然后回放图像至最满意时再按储存键储存静态图像，也可实时储存动态图像。图像可存于超声工作站或超声仪主机内。

（9）体标、测量和标记。按体标键选择合适的体标。按测量键测量图像内任意两点的距离。按箭头键图像内会出现箭头，将箭头移动到靶目标处即可进行标记，也可以用文字进行标记。

5. 临床科室使用超声引导穿刺或注射的特点

（1）图像清晰。特别是二维灰阶切面图像分辨率好。

（2）操作简单。可根据临床需要加载实用的新技术。

（3）携带方便，易在床旁操作。

（4）能实时储存静态图像和动态图像。

建议超声仪配备线阵高频探头和凸阵低频探头，有条件者可以再配一个专用穿刺探头。

二、超声探头的选择

（1）探头是超声仪的基本部件，探头中的关键部件是具有压电效应的晶片，它是超声换能器，其作用是对电能和声能进行互相转换。探头既是超声波的发出装置，也是超声波的接收装置。

（2）根据探头内晶片的排列方式，可将探头分为线阵探头、相控阵探头、凸阵探头等。根据探头发出的超声波频率，可将探头分为低频探头与高频探头。高频探头频率高、波长短、分辨率高、穿透力差，低频探头频率低、波长长、分辨率低、穿透力好。

（3）探头的选择主要取决于靶目标的深度。靶目标较表浅时，选择高频线阵探头，分辨率高，图像显示更清楚；靶目标较深时，选择低频凸阵探头，分辨率低，但可增加可视范围，有利于寻找靶目标。对于表浅的靶目标（深度＜4cm），可选 7～14MHz的探头；对于深度在 4～6cm的靶目标，可用 5～7MHz的探头；对于深度＞6cm的靶目标，可选 3～5MHz的探头。

三、不同组织的超声成像特点

根据声像图的灰度不同，可将回声强弱区分为强回声、高回声、等回声、低回声、无回声。灰度越明亮，表示回声越强。回声的高低强弱一般以所检查组织器官的正常回声为标准或将病变部位回声与周围正常组织器官回声进行比较后确定。

掌握肌肉骨骼系统各组织结构的正常声像图表现，是对该组织结构进行准确定位及判断有无病变的重要基础。肌肉骨骼系统各组织结构的正常声像图表现如下。

（1）皮肤及皮下组织：皮肤的表皮与真皮在声像图上不易区分，均呈带状高回声。皮下组织浅层为脂肪组织，呈低回声；深层为筋膜组织，呈带状高回声；脂肪组织内的疏松结缔组织呈线状高回声。

（2）肌肉：肌肉由肌纤维组成。肌肉纵切面声像图中，肌束呈低回声，肌束膜与肌束平行，呈线状高回声，肌外膜、肌间隔呈较肌束膜厚的线状高回声。肌肉横切面声像图多表现为圆形或类圆形，其中肌束呈点状低回声，肌束膜、肌外膜和肌间隔表现为点状或线状高回声，相互交错呈筛网状。

（3）肌腱：肌腱起着连接肌肉与骨骼的作用。肌腱纵切面声像图的回声高于肌肉，呈条索状，由多个相互平行的线状高回声构成，有腱鞘的肌腱在肌腱周围可见线状低回声。肌腱横断面声像图为圆形或扁平状，呈细小点状高回声结构。

（4）韧带：韧带连接相邻两骨，主要存在于关节周围，有稳固关节的作用。韧带由致密纤维结缔组织构成，声像图表现为带状高回声，两端连于骨。

（5）滑囊：滑囊是由结缔组织和滑膜形成的潜在封闭腔隙，多位于肌腱、韧带、肌肉与骨接触而又相互滑动处。滑囊的声像图中，囊壁为线状高回声，囊腔呈线状低回声。

（6）筋膜：筋膜分为浅筋膜和深筋膜，浅筋膜由疏松结缔组织构

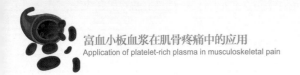

成，深筋膜由胶原纤维构成。筋膜在声像图上表现为厚薄不等的线状或带状高回声。

（7）神经：神经由聚集成束的神经纤维构成，外面由结缔组织包绕。声像图上正常神经回声高于肌肉，低于肌腱。其纵切面呈长纤维状高回声与低回声相间，横断面呈椭圆形高回声，内有点状低回声，呈筛网状结构。

（8）关节：关节由骨端关节面、关节囊和关节腔组成。关节面表面为关节软骨。声像图上关节软骨表现为较薄、厚度一致、光滑连续的低回声结构；骨端骨皮质位于软骨深面，呈薄而光滑的线状强回声，后方有声影；滑膜不易显示；关节腔内液体无回声；关节内韧带呈均匀的带状低回声。

四、超声各向异性伪像的鉴别

伪像是由超声波本身的物理特性（如方向性、反射与折射、穿透力等）、仪器性能和检查操作等多种因素造成的非人体本身的真实图像。

超声的声像图是断层图像，涉及声学、医学及电子学等基础知识，并不是简单的解剖断面图像的重建。对于非影像专业的临床医生来说，如果没有经过系统的超声医学基础知识的学习，在实际应用超声过程中可能对伪像特别是肌骨超声经常出现的各向异性伪像认识不足，从而造成误诊。

各向异性是指由于声束不能同时保持与韧带、肌腱、肌肉等呈垂直方向，导致同一韧带、肌腱、肌肉等在声像图上的回声强弱不同，回声不均。可以通过侧动探头，改变扫查方向，调整声束入射角观察回声的变化来鉴别各向异性伪像。

五、超声扫查技术

1. 探头的使用

根据穿刺的部位和深度选择合适的高频线阵探头或低频凸阵探头。握持探头的姿势要恰当，避免以不恰当的方式过紧地握取探头，这样不便于灵活调整探头方向。正确的握持方式应以拇指、食指和中指握住探头底部，小指和无名指作为支点放在患者身体上，这样既可稳定探头，也可灵活控制探头方向和力度。检查时应避免对探头过度施压，以免导致图像变形或表浅结构显示不清。

2. 选择合适频率

探头发射的超声波频率越高，获取的图像的分辨率越高，但是超声波频率增高会降低其穿透力，影响对较深部组织结构的观察，因而在进行浅表部位注射时应选用高频探头，进行深部组织注射时应选用低频探头。

3. 耦合剂的使用

可选用无菌耦合剂或将探头做无菌处理，以防止注射部位感染。

4. 选择合适深度

根据靶目标的深度选择合适的图像深度，使所需观察的结构占据屏幕的大部分区域。深度过大会导致图像太小，既不利于观察细节也浪费了屏幕空间；深度过小则有可能导致靶目标位于图像底部，使其与周围组织结构之间的关系不能充分显示或缺乏对比，导致所能获得的信息不足。

5. 选择适当的焦点区

图像的焦点区是声束聚焦的位置，该水平的图像显示最清晰，因而应将焦点位置设置在靶目标水平。焦点区设置过浅会导致深部结构图像清晰度下降，而焦点区设置过深会降低浅层结构图像的清晰度。另外，焦点区

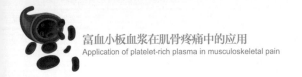
数量一般设置为1～2个，不宜过多，否则会降低图像的帧频。

6. 调节增益

增益可增加或减少图像的亮度或灰阶。一般情况下，增益调节至所观察的组织结构具有适当的亮度即可。增益过高会导致图像过亮，影响对图像细节的观察；增益过低会导致图像过暗，结构显示不清。

7. 时间增益补偿

超声波在介质中传播时，其能量会随着传播距离的增加而衰减，因而被探头接收的反射回来的超声信号也会逐渐减少，导致图像远场结构清晰度下降。为了解决上述问题，可调节某一区域的时间增益补偿（time gain compensate，TGC）按键增大增益。向右移动按键，相应区域的图像变亮；向左移动按键，相应区域的图像则变暗。常规扫查时，初始状态下通常将所有按键保持在中线位置，当需要增加或降低某一特定区域图像的增益时，才移动相应的按键。

六、平面内/外进针的技术特点

参考穿刺针相对于探头的方向，可将进针方式分为平面内进针和平面外进针。平面内进针时，穿刺针平行于探头，因而整个进针路径和针尖都可以显示；平面外进针时，穿刺针垂直于探头，难以显示进针路径，仅可显示注射针的横截面，表现为一个点状强回声。由于平面内进针可在同一个平面内同时显示进针路径、针尖、靶目标的位置关系，所以操作更加安全，可有效避免损伤其他重要结构，同时可根据具体位置实时调节进针方向和角度。相比之下，平面外进针由于难以显示整个进针路径和针尖，仅可显示进针路径的某个位置，因而有时难以把控穿刺的角度，并且易误伤其他结构；但是当靶目标位置特别表浅并接近进针点时，可以选择平面外注射。穿刺时也可以平面内进针为主，结合平面外进针以观察针尖，避免容积效应。见图8-1A、图8-1B、图8-2A、图8-2B。

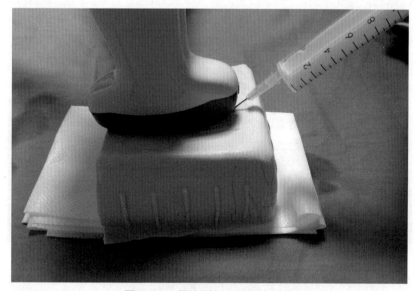

图8-1A　超声引导下平面内进针

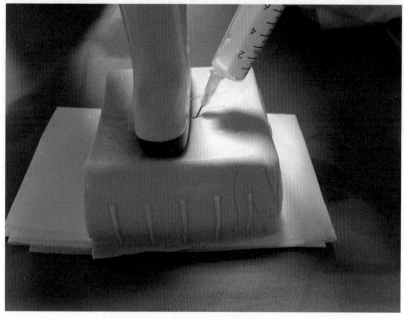

图8-1B　超声引导下平面外进针

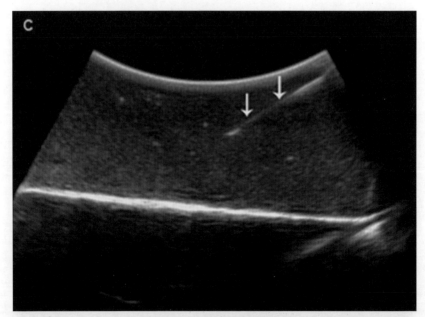

图8-2A 平面内进针声像图

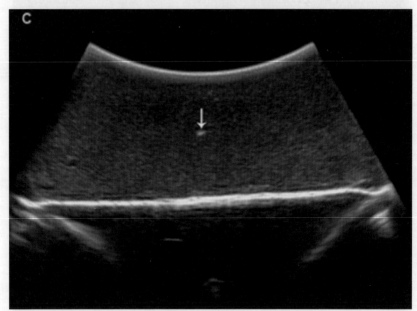

图8-2B 平面外进针声像图

七、如何使进针路径清楚显影

当超声探头发射的声束与观察的靶目标相垂直时，探头接收的反射声波最多，成像最清晰；声束方向与靶目标之间的倾斜角度越大（即入射角越大），探头接收的回波信号就越少，就会导致伪像出现，图像的清晰度就会降低。基于该原理，在穿刺时需尽量让声束方向与穿刺针接近垂直。

为了能清晰显示穿刺针，应预先对需注射的病变区域进行超声扫查，通过调节图像的深度、焦点位置、探头频率、增益水平等参数来优化图像，并且需先行设计穿刺路径，测量到达靶目标的穿刺距离及靶目标的深度。进针路径应安全、易于操作，同时尽可能让注射针与声束的方向接近垂直，以减少注射针的各向异性伪像。目前有些超声仪器配备了穿刺针增强技术，或者声束偏转功能以增强对穿刺针的显示，以下几个操作方法有助于增强对进针路径及针尖的显示。

（1）当靶目标的位置较深时，进针路径与声束方向往往会接近平行，针尖难以显示，可以选择距离靶目标稍远的位置进针，以减小进针路径和皮肤之间的角度，从而使进针路径与声束的方向接近垂直以更好地显示针头。

（2）当靶目标位置非常表浅时，可在探头的进针一端堆聚无菌耦合剂形成一个斜坡，或使用无菌耦合垫，这样注射针在接触皮肤之前也可清晰地显示出来。

（3）肩关节、腕关节、膝关节、踝关节等相关结构病变需进行注射治疗时，如纵切面进针路径过于倾斜而出现各向异性，可尝试采用横切面进针，避开血管、神经等结构，根据穿刺靶目标的深度，利用关节的自然弧度在相应体表的稍低位置进针，这样可使进针路径更垂直于声束。

八、注射过程中的操作技术

1. 注射前准备

详细的病史采集、全面的体格检查和明确的诊断是注射治疗前必须完成的，用以确定患者是否适合进行注射治疗。还需要确定病灶部位，选择好注射药物，同时准备好发生过敏反应或并发症时的急救措施。

（1）注射室准备：注射室应具备足够的工作空间以利于进行超声引导下的注射操作，需设置患者观察区、医疗物品准备区、无菌医疗用品放置区、污染医疗用品储存区、患者等候区以及医务人员专用洗手池。此外，注射室还应具备可调节高度和角度的治疗床、良好的通风系统、可调节无影灯、医用气体管道系统、急救用品以及急救呼叫系统等。

（2）超声仪准备：需准备好合格、适用的超声仪。

（3）患者知情同意和准备：术者应遵循规范化流程，对患者做好解释工作，取得患者的信任和合作，解除患者紧张及焦虑的情绪。务必使患者明确可能发生的不良反应，如注射过程中或注射后可能出现注射部位疼痛、感染、肌腱断裂、注射部位色素沉着以及严重过敏反应等。在详细了解以上情况后，患者应签署知情同意书。

（4）PRP制备：按照本书第二章第三节介绍的方法在严格无菌操作下制备PRP。

（5）器具准备：根据注射部位和目的，选择不同型号的无菌注射器和注射针头，此外，还需准备Ⅱ型或Ⅲ型安尔碘皮肤消毒液、敷贴、无菌棉签、无菌手套和无菌铺巾等。

（6）注射体位和部位：注射时患者一般取卧位，位置要舒适，也可采用其他体位。注射部位应该充分暴露并严格消毒，必要时用标记笔标出相应的注射部位。应选择相对安全的注射部位，尽量避开血管和神经。

（7）注射剂量和容量：药液需通过生理盐水稀释以增加容量。当注射足够容量的药液充分浸润发炎的关节和滑囊内面时，药液的张力可起到牵拉、松解粘连的作用。不同部位的关节注射容量不同，如膝关节、肩关节、髋关节需3～5mL，手关节和腕关节等小关节通常需1～2mL，手指或足趾关节可注射0.5mL。

2. 无菌技术

超声引导下的注射治疗过程必须严格遵从无菌原则。临床上用的Ⅱ型或Ⅲ型安尔碘消毒液可以用于注射部位皮肤消毒；严格的手卫生是预防和控制感染的重要措施，注射时无菌手套、无菌帽、口罩也是必不可少的用品；超声探头以及探头连线可以用消毒铺巾覆盖，必要时可以使用无菌的探头帽。

3. 超声引导下的PRP注射

详见本章第二至第四节。

4. 注射后的处理

注射完成后注射局部的皮肤消毒后应用无菌敷料覆盖，患者需留观至少半小时，如无不适可离开。实施注射治疗的医生需做好相关的工作记录，并向患者说明注射后可能出现的各种反应。对于疼痛缓解一段时间后复发或者疼痛加重的患者，可以嘱其用冰袋冷敷或者口服一般止痛药物，1周后返院复诊。在注射治疗后，患者应积极采取以下方式促进恢复：

（1）必要时制动：视损伤部位而定，例如膝关节注射后减少长时间步行有利于功能恢复，而腕关节治疗后制动可能会加重病情，肌腱和滑囊劳损时在不加剧疼痛的情况下可保持日常活动。

（2）康复锻炼：在不加剧疼痛的情况下，应尽量保持日常活动，而在症状缓解以后需要进行行之有效的运动疗法，如适应性功能锻炼、强化

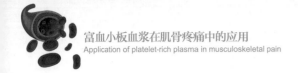

性功能锻炼和辅助器械锻炼。

（3）预防复发：应保持人体正常姿势，消除不良的活动和体位。

（伍少玲　马超）

第二节　超声引导下的上肢注射技术

本节主要介绍上肢疼痛疾患中临床疗效较肯定的超声引导下PRP注射技术。

一、超声引导下冈上肌腱损伤的PRP注射

患者取坐位，患侧上肢叉腰，高频超声探头纵向置于肩峰和肱骨大结节间，可清楚显示冈上肌腱损伤处（局部回声不均匀）。常规消毒，采用平面外进针方式，将穿刺针刺入至肌腱损伤处，如回抽无血，则注入自体PRP 1~3mL，拔针、按压局部后常规贴无菌敷贴。见图8-3A、图8-3B。

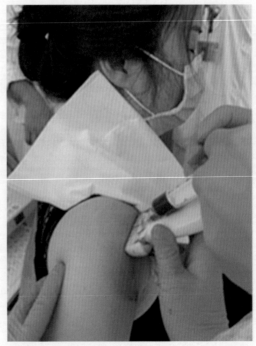

图8-3A　超声引导下冈上肌腱损伤的PRP注射

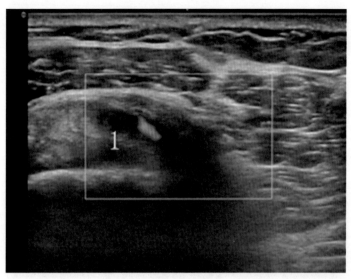

1：冈上肌腱

图8-3B　超声引导下冈上肌腱损伤的PRP注射声像图（彩色多普勒超声显示PRP注入）

二、超声引导下肩峰下-三角肌下滑囊的PRP注射

　　患者取仰卧位或坐位，超声探头置于肩峰与肱骨大结节之间，可清楚显示肩峰下及三角肌下和冈上肌腱之间、低回声的滑囊。常规消毒，从探头的外侧端以平面内进针方式，由外侧向内侧缓慢进针，当观察到针尖进入滑囊后回抽，如无血，则缓慢注入PRP 3mL，见图8-4A。注射过程应无明

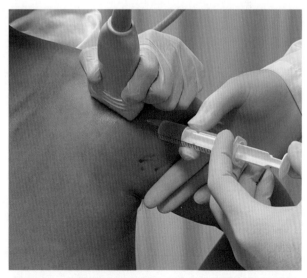

图8-4A　超声引导下肩峰下-三角肌下滑囊的PRP注射

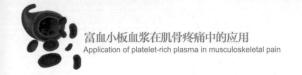
显阻力，超声可实时观察到PRP在滑囊内均匀散开，见图8-4B。注射完毕后拔针、按压局部，贴上无菌敷贴。

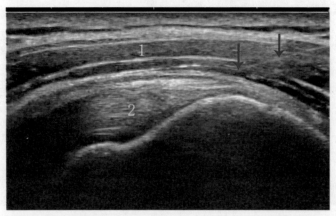

1：三角肌；2：冈上肌腱；红色箭头示进针路径

图8-4B　超声引导下肩峰下-三角肌下滑囊的PRP注射声像图

三、超声引导下肩关节腔（盂肱关节腔）的PRP注射

患者取侧卧位，患肩在上，上肢呈前屈、内旋位撑于治疗床上，斜冠状位放置探头于肩胛冈中下方，平行于冈下肌腱纤维。探头沿肩胛冈向外扫描至肱骨头时，可于肩胛冈与肱骨头夹角处清楚地显示肱骨头、关节盂、后盂唇的边缘。采用平面外进针方式，将穿刺针缓慢刺入，当观察到针尖进入关节腔后回抽，如无血，则缓慢注射PRP 3～5mL；注射过程应无明显阻力，确保药物在关节腔内均匀散开，可应用彩色多普勒超声实时观察PRP的弥散；注射完毕后，拔针、按压局部，贴上无菌敷贴。见图8-5A、图8-5B。

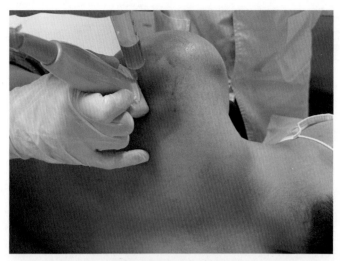

图8-5A　超声引导下盂肱关节腔的PRP注射

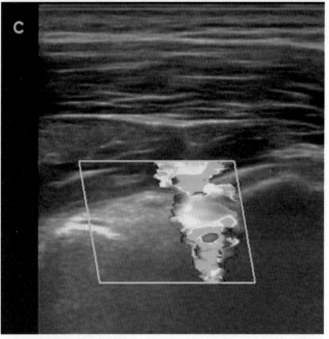

图8-5B　超声引导下盂肱关节腔的PRP注射（彩色多普勒超声显示PRP的弥散）

四、超声引导下肱骨外上髁的PRP注射

患者取坐位或仰卧位，屈肘90°，前臂平放于治疗台上；选择高频线阵探头，将探头置于肱骨外上髁纵切显示伸肌总腱长轴；声像图可见患侧伸肌总腱较健侧增厚，回声不均匀。超声显示肱骨外上髁、伸肌总腱、肱桡关节和桡骨头，采用平面内进针方式，注射针以一定角度刺入，将PRP1～2mL注入总伸肌腱附着处；注射完毕后拔针、按压局部，贴上无菌敷贴。见图8-6A、图8-6B。

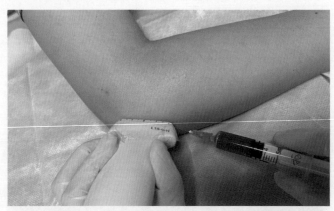

图8-6A　超声引导下肱骨外上髁的PRP注射

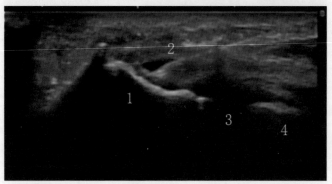

1：肱骨外上髁；2：伸肌总腱；3：肱桡关节；4：桡骨头

图8-6B　超声引导下肱骨外上髁的PRP注射声像图

五、超声引导下腕关节腔（桡腕关节腔）的PRP注射

患者取坐位或仰卧位，手腕置于桌面或床面，掌心朝下；选择高频线阵探头，将探头置于关节长轴切面，显示桡骨、舟骨之间低回声的关节腔，可见关节间隙增大、骨皮质不规则等表现，有时可见骨侵蚀和关节腔积液。采用平面外进针方式，穿刺针缓慢渐入，穿刺至关节间隙，局部注入PRP 0.5～1mL，超声可实时观察到药液在关节腔内弥散；注射完毕后拔针、按压局部，贴上无菌敷贴。见图8-7A、图8-7B。

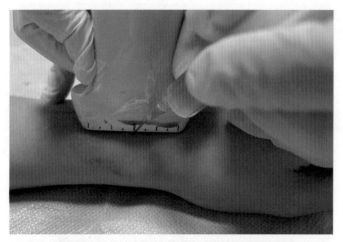

图8-7A　超声引导下桡腕关节腔的PRP注射

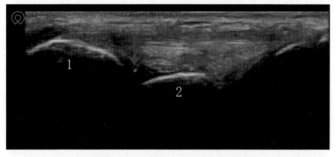

1：桡骨；2：舟骨；红色箭头示针尖

图8-7B　超声引导下桡腕关节腔的PRP注射声像图

六、超声引导下腕管综合征的PRP注射

患者取坐位或仰卧位，手腕部置于桌面或床面，掌心朝上；将高频线阵探头横向置于腕部短轴切面，声像图可清晰显示腕横韧带及深面筛网状正中神经、腕管肌腱，应用彩色多普勒显示腕部桡动脉和尺动脉，以确定进针点和进针路径；选择离正中神经较远的尺侧或桡侧进针，一般以正中神经和尺动脉之间为进针点；采用平面内进针方式，穿刺针缓慢渐入，分别穿刺至正中神经的浅面和深面，以水分离的方式将PRP 3mL缓慢注入，包绕正中神经；注射完毕后拔针、按压局部，贴上无菌敷贴。见图8-8A、图8-8B。

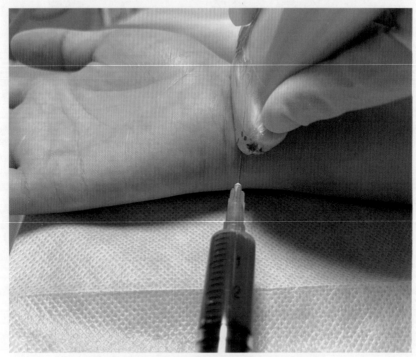

图8-8A　超声引导下腕管综合征的PRP注射

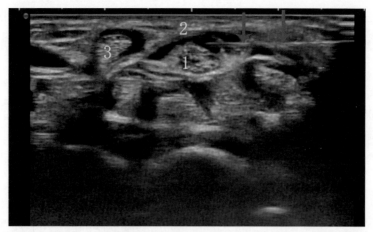

1：正中神经；2：腕横韧带；3：桡侧腕屈肌腱；红色箭头示进针路径

图8-8B　超声引导下腕管综合征的PRP注射声像图

（马超　伍少玲）

第三节　超声引导下的下肢注射技术

本节主要介绍下肢疼痛疾患中临床疗效较肯定的超声引导下PRP注射技术。

一、超声引导下髋关节腔的PRP注射

患者取仰卧位，髋关节置于中立位，触诊腹股沟区，标记股动脉、股静脉的体表位置；使超声探头长轴与股骨头和股骨颈平行，置于髋关节上方，显示股骨头、髋臼和髋关节腔；确定注射靶点，应用彩色多普勒观察毗邻血管情况，确定进针点和进针路径；常规消毒后，采用平面外进针方式将注射针缓慢刺入，实时调整针尖方向至针尖进入髋关节腔，回抽无积

液或血液后注入PRP 4～5mL，注射过程应无明显阻力，彩色多普勒超声实时观察PRP的弥散情况；注射完毕后拔针、按压局部，贴上无菌敷贴。见图8-9A、图8-9B。

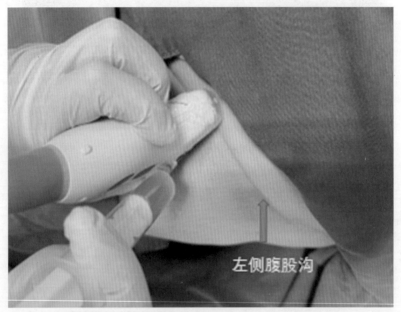

图8-9A　超声引导下髋关节腔的PRP注射

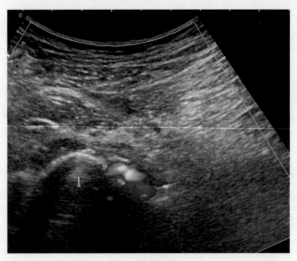

1：股骨头

图8-9B　超声引导下髋关节腔的PRP注射声像图（彩色多普勒超声显示PRP注入）

二、超声引导下膝部的PRP注射

1. 超声引导下膝关节腔的PRP注射

为减少对膝关节软骨的损伤及不必要的穿刺损伤，髌上囊已成为膝关节腔注射中安全、有效的常规首选部位。患者取平卧位，患侧下肢置中立位，避免髋外旋；膝下垫薄枕，保持患膝屈20°～30°。注射前，用高频线阵探头纵向对髌骨上方2～3cm范围内进行扫查。对于髌上囊有积液的患者，选择积液厚度最深处作为拟进针点；对于无明显积液的患者，通过患者主动屈膝或在操作者协助下屈膝来确认髌上囊间隙，在局部皮肤上标注拟进针点。常规消毒注射区域皮肤，将探头长轴垂直于股骨长轴走行方向放置，调整探头待滑囊及股骨皮质均清晰显示后，采用平面内进针方式将注射针刺入皮肤，注意调整探头和注射针的位置，待屏幕上清晰显示注射针针尖位置处于髌上囊内时，注入PRP 4～5mL，如有积液可将积液抽完后进行注射，注射过程应无明显阻力。彩色多普勒超声可实时观察到PRP在滑囊内均匀散开。注射完成后，拔出注射针，消毒并覆盖敷料。见图8-10A、图8-10B。

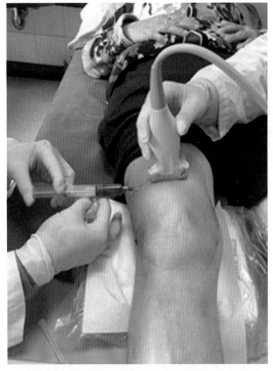

图8-10A 超声引导下膝关节腔的PRP注射

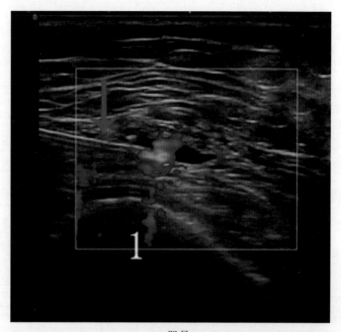

1：股骨

图8-10B　超声引导下膝关节腔的PRP注射声像图
（彩色多普勒超声显示PRP注入）

2. 超声引导下膝周肌腱/韧带的PRP注射

膝骨关节炎患者膝周肌腱或韧带常存在痛点，如鹅足腱、髂胫束附着点、膝侧副韧带等，可同时给予PRP注射。

患者取平卧位，患侧下肢置中立位，膝下垫薄枕，保持患膝屈20°～30°，触诊、标记痛点位置；常规消毒注射区域皮肤，可根据个人注射经验，采用平面内或平面外进针方式将注射针刺入皮肤至靶点，局部注射PRP 1mL，超声可实时观察到PRP在膝周肌腱/韧带均匀散开；注射完成后，拔出注射针，消毒并覆盖敷料。见图8-11A、图8-11B。

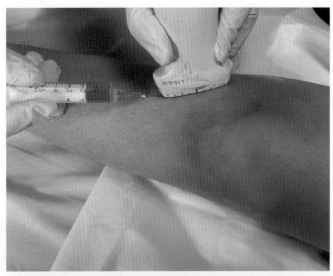

图8-11A　超声引导下鹅足腱平面内的PRP注射

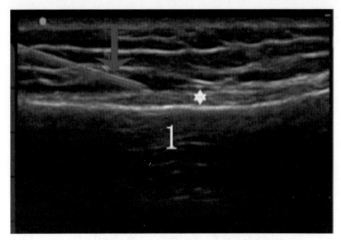

1：胫骨；红色箭头示进针路径；星号处为鹅足腱

图8-11B　超声引导下鹅足腱平面内的PRP注射声像图

三、超声引导下跟腱/跟腱旁组织的PRP注射

对于跟腱撕裂或慢性跟腱病，可在跟腱局部注射PRP 1mL；对于跟腱滑囊炎，可将PRP 1～1.5mL注射到跟骨后滑囊。

患者取俯卧位，脚悬于床尾，采用高频探头显示跟腱病变较明显区域，常规消毒注射区域皮肤，可根据个人经验，将探头横向置于跟腱病变处，采用平面内进针方式将注射针缓慢刺入至靶点，局部注入PRP，见图8-12A、图8-12B。也可将探头纵向

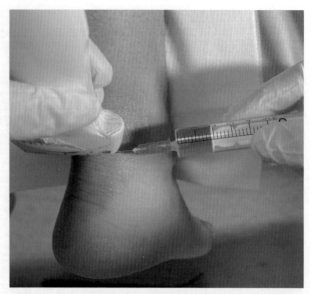

图8-12A　超声引导下跟腱短轴-平面内的PRP注射

置于跟腱病变处，采用平面外进针方式将注射针缓慢刺入至靶点，局部注入PRP，见图8-13A、图8-13B。超声可实时观察到PRP在跟腱/跟腱旁组织中均匀散开。注射完成后，拔出注射针，消毒并覆盖敷料。

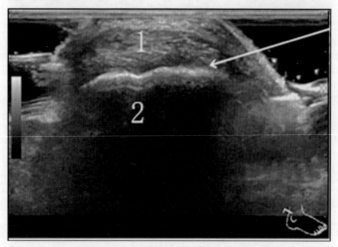

1：跟腱；2：跟骨；箭头示模拟进针路径

图8-12B　超声引导下跟腱短轴-平面内的PRP注射声像图

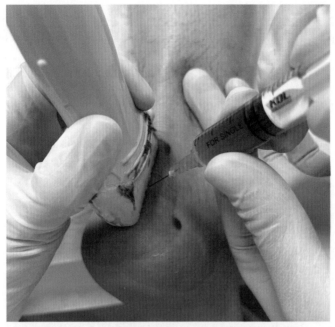

图8-13A　超声引导下跟腱长轴-平面外的PRP注射

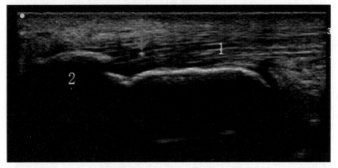

1：跟腱；2：跟骨；红色箭头示针尖

图8-13B　超声引导下跟腱长轴-平面外的PRP注射声像图

四、超声引导下跖筋膜的PRP注射

患者取俯卧位，脚悬于床尾（或屈膝），将高频探头（10～15MHz）纵向置于足底跟骨上，显示病变跖筋膜区域，声像图可见跟骨附着处局部跖筋膜增厚。常规消毒注射区域皮肤，可根据个人经验，将探头纵向置于跖筋膜病变处，采用平面外进针方式，将注射针从足底皮肤缓慢刺入至靶点（跖筋膜与跟骨附着处之间），局部注入PRP。也可将探头横向置于跖筋膜病变处，采用平面内进针方式，将注射针从足内侧缓慢刺入至靶点，局部注入PRP，见图8-14A、图8-14B。超声可实时观察到PRP在跖筋膜中均匀散开。注射完成后，拔出注射针，消毒并覆盖敷料。

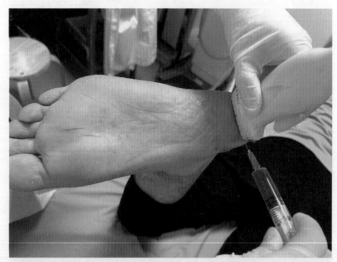

图8-14A　超声引导下跖筋膜短轴-平面内的PRP注射

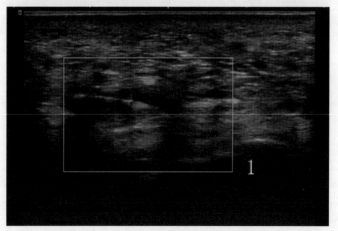

1：跟骨

图8-14B　超声引导下跖筋膜短轴-平面内的PRP注射声像图
（彩色多普勒超声显示PRP注入）

五、超声引导下骨不连的PRP注射

患者取平卧位，采用高频探头纵向沿胫骨/距骨扫查，仔细寻找骨不连处；常规消毒注射区域皮肤，采用平面外进针方式，将注射针从患处皮肤缓慢刺入至靶点，局部注入PRP 1～2mL。超声可实时观察到PRP在骨不连处均匀散开。注射完成后，拔出注射针，消毒并覆盖敷料。胫骨骨折术后骨不连的PRP注射见图8-15A至图8-15D，距骨骨折术后骨不连的PRP注射见图8-16A、图8-16B。

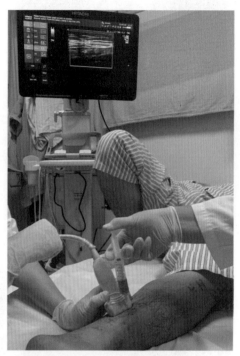

图8-15A 胫骨骨折术后骨不连的PRP注射

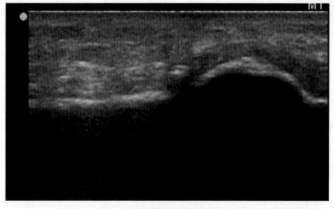

红色箭头示针尖

图8-15B 胫骨骨折术后骨不连的PRP注射声像图

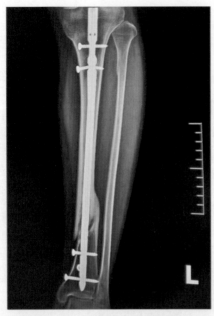

图8-15C　胫骨骨折术后X线片

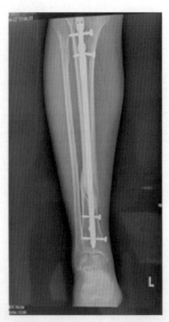

图8-15D　PRP注射1个月后的X线片

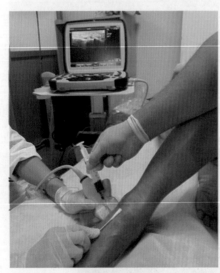

图8-16A　距骨骨折术后骨不连的PRP
　　　　　注射

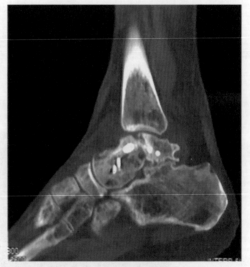

图8-16B　距骨骨折术后CT片

（伍少玲　马超）

第四节　超声引导下腰部注射技术

本节主要介绍超声引导下腰神经根的PRP注射。

患者取俯卧位，腹部垫薄枕以减少腰椎前凸，先触诊进行腰椎定位和标记；常规皮肤消毒，将低频（3～5MHz）凸阵探头纵向置于后正中线，显示腰椎棘突长轴，然后逐渐向侧方移动至腰椎关节突关节长轴，显示腰椎关节突关节长轴特征性高回声"驼峰征"线，其骨性结构为上、下关节突；确定注射靶点，应用彩色多普勒超声观察毗邻血管情况，确定进针点和进针路径；采用平面外注射方式，从垂直于探头长轴压迹的中间位置进针，按拟定路径进入，接近靶点时需缓慢进入，直至针尖到达靶点位置；回抽无血液和脑脊液后，注入少量生理盐水以观察弥散情况，或应用彩色多普勒超声确定针尖位置是否接近腰动脉，最后注入自体PRP 3～4mL。注射完毕后拔针，消毒，常规贴无菌敷贴。见图8-17A、图8-17B。

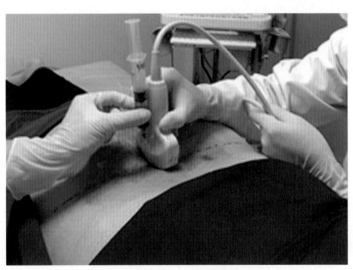

图8-17A　超声引导下腰神经根的PRP注射

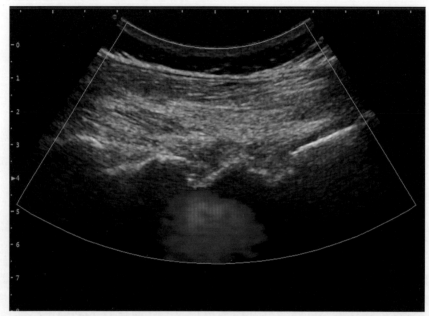

图8-17B　超声引导下腰神经根的PRP注射声像图（彩色多普勒超声显示PRP弥散）

（马超　伍少玲）

附 录

作者团队研究成果展示

　　本附录所载文章均为作者团队近几年的研究成果，讲述了PRP注射治疗部分肌骨疼痛相关疾病的临床效果，特影印于书后，以供读者参考。

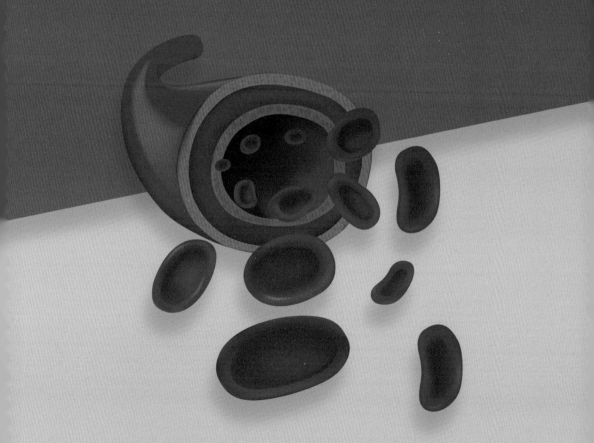

Case Report

For reprint orders, please contact: reprints@futuremedicine.com

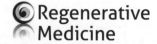

Regenerative Medicine

Platelet-rich plasma for the treatment of adolescent late-stage femoral head necrosis: a case report

Shuo Luan[1], Cuicui Liu[1], Caina Lin[1], Chao Ma*,[1] & Shaoling Wu**,[1]

[1]Department of Rehabilitation Medicine, Sun Yat-sen Memorial Hospital, No.107 Yanjiang West Road, Guangzhou 510120, China
*Author for correspondence: ma_chao99@126.com
**Author for correspondence: wushaolinggz@126.com

Osteonecrosis of femoral head (ONFH) is a disabling and intractable disease. Previous studies reported the increasing failure rates of total hip arthroplasty in younger patients, thus there should be special considerations for the adolescents. In this paper, we present a case of an adolescent female with late-stage glucocorticoid-induced ONFH (according to the Association Research Circulation Osseous classification system, Association Research Circulation Osseous IV). The patient received five consecutive ultrasound-guided intra-articular injections of platelet-rich plasma, and the therapeutic effects were assessed by visual analog scale, joint range of motion, Western Ontario and McMaster Universities Osteoarthritis Index, Harris Hip Score and magnetic resonance imaging. At 9-month follow-up, clinical and radiological reassessments demonstrated favorable outcomes. This case highlights the therapeutic potential of platelet-rich plasma injections for the late-stage ONFH, especially for adolescent patients.

First draft submitted: 26 April 2020; Accepted for publication: 22 October 2020; Published online: 26 November 2020

Keywords: ARCO stage IV • glucocorticoid-induced osteonecrosis of the femoral head • platelet-rich plasma • regenerative medicine • ultrasound-guided injection

Background

Osteonecrosis of femoral head (ONFH) is a devastating chronic disease, which is affecting millions of people worldwide. Multiple causes and risk factors are associated with the nontraumatic ONFH, including glucocorticoid use, alcohol abuse, HIV infection and Gaucher's disease. [1]. Glucocorticoid-induced ONFH accounts for about 25–50% of nontraumatic ONFH cases [2]. Current treatment options for ONFH consist of both nonsurgical treatments (e.g., pharmacotherapy, physical therapies and assistant devices) and surgical treatments (e.g., bone grafting, core decompression and total hip arthroplasty [THA]) [3,4]. In general, physical therapy and analgesic medication might help to relieve pain at the early-stage of ONFH. However, for late-stage patients with collapsed lesions on weight-bearing joint surfaces, it is likely that the patient will need to undergo hip arthroplasty eventually.

In recent years, platelet-rich plasma (PRP) has been widely used as an adjuvant biological therapy in many musculoskeletal diseases, including bone nonunion, tendinopathy injury and degenerative osteoarthritis [5–7]. Although the exact mechanism causing the favorable outcomes is yet to be elucidated, PRP has been demonstrated to hold therapeutic potential for ONFH in both animal experiments and preliminary clinical studies [8,9].

Case presentation

Herein, we present a 16-year-old adolescent female who was referred to our rehabilitation department in January 2019 with chief complaints of progressive bilateral hip pain and stiffness for the preceding 5 months. She was diagnosed with pituicytoma and underwent the microsurgical removal of the pituicytoma at the Guangdong Hospital of Traditional Chinese Medicine (Guangdong Province, China) in January 2018. It should be noted, prior to the onset of symptoms, the patient previously attended school and was able to undergo regular physical activity as normal, and her past medical history was unremarkable. Following surgery, she received hydrocortisone replacement treatment (10 mg am and 5 mg pm, a daily dose of 15 mg) for 8 months due to postoperative hypopituitarism.

Future Medicine

10.2217/rme-2020-0057 © 2020 Future Medicine Ltd   *Regen. Med.* (Epub ahead of print)   ISSN 1746-0751

Case Report   Luan, Liu, Lin, Ma & Wu

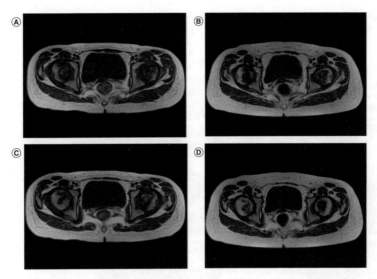

Figure 1.   Comparisons of horizontal T1-weighted images of bilateral femoral heads pretreatment and at 9-month follow-up. Decreased necrotic lesions were detected at the 9-month follow-up **(B & D)** compared with the pretreatment **(A & C)**.

Table 1. Comparisons of outcome measurements (visual analog scale, Western Ontario and McMaster Universities Osteoarthritis Index and Harris Hip Score): pretreatment, during platelet-rich plasma treatment and 9-month follow-up.

	Pretreatment	Post the 1st injection	Post the 3rd injection	Post the 5th injection	9 month follow-up
VAS	7	5	3	3	3
WOMAC	59	49	26	17	15
Pain subscale	9	7	4	3	3
Stiffness subscale	6	4	2	0	0
Physical function subscale	44	38	20	14	12
HHS	29.05	30.1	51.35	59.65	63.65
Pain subscale	10	10	20	20	20
Function subscale	12	13	24	32	36
Motion subscale	3.05	3.1	3.35	3.65	3.65
Deformity subscale	4	4	4	4	4

HHS: Harris Hip Score; VAS: Visual analog scale; WOMAC: Western Ontario and McMaster Universities Osteoarthritis Index.

However, the patient began to develop progressive hip pain by the fifth month, with the symptoms exacerbated after standing or walking for long periods.

The patient visited the orthopedics clinic of Sun Yat-sen Memorial Hospital (Guangzhou, China) in May 2018 and x-ray examination indicated bilateral osteonecrosis. She took analgesic medication and acupuncture for pain relief until she revisited the rehabilitation clinic at Sun Yat-sen Memorial Hospital due to severe pain in January 2019. MRI was ordered and the collapsed femoral heads with joint-space narrowing and joint effusion were observed (Association Research Circulation Osseous [ARCO] classification IV, **Figure** 1A & C; **Figure** 2A, C, E & G) [10]. Upon admission, the patient exhibited tenderness over bilateral femoral heads without fever, rubor, or skin lesions. She reported severe pain (visual analog scale 7/10) (**Table** 1). Physical examination showed significantly

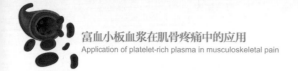

Platelet-rich plasma for the treatment of adolescent late-stage femoral head necrosis: a case report   Case Report

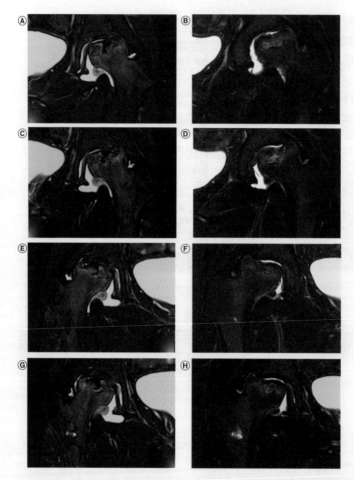

Figure 2.   Comparisons of coronal fat-suppressed T2-weighted images of bilateral femoral heads pretreatment and 9-month follow-up. Pretreatment scans indicated extensive collapses and narrowed joint space **(A, C, E & G).** At 9 months after treatment, the images demonstrated reduced collapse and less joint effusion. The mixed signal intensities indicated the probable bone reconstruction **(B, D, F & H).**

decreasing ranges of motion (ROM) and muscle weakness of the bilateral hips **(Table 2)**. The Harris Hip Score was 29 (pain subscale: 10; function subscale: 12; motion subscale: 3.05; deformity subscale: 4). Western Ontario and McMaster Universities Osteoarthritis Index score was 59 (pain subscale: 9; stiffness subscale: 6; physical function subscale: 44) **(Table 1)**. The patient exhibited no neurologic signs or meningeal signs.

The patient and her guardians refused to undergo any form of surgical treatment and decided to try a minimally invasive alternative. The written informed consent outlining the risks and benefits of intra-articular PRP injections

Table 2. Comparisons of outcome measurements (range of motion and muscle strengths): pretreatment, during platelet-rich plasma treatment and 9-month follow-up.

Range of motion	Pretreatment		Post the 1st injection		Post the 3rd injection		Post the 5th injection		9 month follow-up	
	Left	Right	Left	Right	Left	Right	Left	Right	Left	Right
Flexion	33°	35°	37°	37°	47°	43°	55°	52°	55°	53°
Extension	14°	14°	16°	16°	18°	17°	28°	25°	25°	25°
Abduction	15°	15°	16°	16°	20°	22°	33°	32°	30°	30°
Adduction	15°	15°	18°	18°	30°	30°	32°	32°	30°	30°
Internal rotation	17°	16°	18°	18°	23°	25°	25°	27°	26°	30°
External rotation	25°	25°	25°	25°	28°	28°	32°	30°	30°	30°
Muscle strength	**Left**	**Right**	**Left**	**Right**	**Left**	**Right**	**Left**	**Right**	**Left**	**Right**
Flexor	2+	2+	2+	2+	3	2+	3	3-	3	3
Extensor	3-	3-	3-	3-	3-	3-	3-	3-	3-	3-
Abductor	2+	2+	2+	2+	3-	2+	3-	3-	3-	3-
Adductor	2+	2+	2+	2+	3	3	3	3	3	3
Internal rotator	(–)	(–)	(–)	(–)	2+	2+	3-	3-	3-	3-
External rotator	(–)	(–)	(–)	(–)	2+	2+	3-	3-	3-	3-

(–): Unable to operate the assessment due to severe pain inhibition.

was obtained before treatment. The study protocol was approved by the Ethics Committee of Sun Yat-sen Memorial Hospital, Sun Yat-sen University.

A total of 36 ml of blood sample was drawn from the antecubital vein into 10-ml syringes containing 1 ml 3.8% (w/v) sodium citrate. The blood samples were centrifuged for 10 min at 1600 r.p.m. at room temperature (23°C) to separate the red blood cells from the buffy coat (containing platelets and white blood cells) and plasma. The supernatant buffy coat and the upper plasma layer were then harvested and transferred into new centrifuge tubes without disturbing the red blood cell layer. Then, the samples were centrifuged again for 10 min at 3200 r.p.m. at room temperature. The lower fraction of the plasma was collected, which contained approximately 10 ml of concentrated PRP. A sample of 1 ml PRP was sent to the laboratory for quantitative analysis of platelet and leukocyte counts. All procedures were performed under sterile conditions.

Sonographic examinations and ultrasound-guided injections were performed by a qualified doctor using SON-IMAGE HS1 PLUS with a low-frequency convex array. After sterile preparation and general local anesthesia (1% lidocaine, 2ml), the injection was performed using a 9-gauge needle. A total of 4.5 ml PRP was injected into each hip joint and the anterosuperior, parasagittal approach allowed for the even distribution of PRP on the cartilage of femoral head and acetabulum (**Figure 3**). The patient underwent five consecutive intra-articular PRP injections with a 1-week interval. Regular rehabilitation programs were usually restarted on the second day after each injection. Physical exercises based on her age (ROM exercise, muscle strengthening and load-bearing control) were supervised by an experienced physical therapist. By the third month after treatment, the follow-up was performed via phone. The patient adhered to family training and could tolerate longer walks with prolonged pain relief (visual analog scale [VAS], 3/10).

On January 4th, 2020, the patient revisited our clinic setting for clinical and MRI assessments. She presented with moderate pain (VAS, 3/10), an increased Harris Hip Score of 64 (pain subscale: 20; function subscale: 36; motion subscale: 3.65; deformity subscale: 4), and a decreased Western Ontario and McMaster Universities Osteoarthritis Index score of 15 (pain subscale: 3; stiffness subscale: 0; physical function subscale: 12) (**Table 1**). The evaluations also showed functional improvements in hip flexor and adductor strength (3/5) and ROM of multiple directions (**Table 2**). She could tolerate prolonged sitting and longer walks without assistive devices. The MRI showed improved coronal and horizontal images of bilateral femoral heads with decreased necrotic volume, filled lacunae in the osseous matrix and widened joint space (**Figure** 1B & D; **Figure** 2B, D, F & H).

Discussion

This case highlighted the dilemma of treating adolescent ONFH. For the first time, we presented a case of adolescent late-stage ONFH that was effectively treated with multiple intra-articular hip injections of PRP. We propose that PRP might play a positive role in promoting osteonecrosis healing and functional recovery.

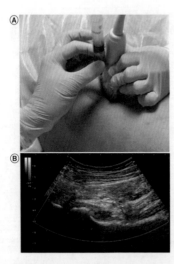

Figure 3. **Ultrasound-guided intra-articular injections of platelet-rich plasma. (A)** Low-frequency convex array was aligned with the long axis of the femoral head and the PRP was injected by anterosuperior, parasagittal approach. **(B)** Direct visualization of the PRP injected into the hip joint.
PRP: Platelet-rich plasma.

In general, ONFH patients should be given an accurate diagnosis and appropriate treatment at a very early stage. Unfortunately, many factors lead to delayed diagnosis and inadequate therapy. Recent years have seen considerable developments in THA and other surgical procedures, however, there should be some special considerations for adolescent treatment options [11,12]. First, there is little doubt that the ultimate goal of ONFH management is to preserve hip function and postpone the occurrence of mechanical failure [13,14]. In the present case, this female could be considered too young for hip replacements. Adolescents usually stay active, which leads to extra stress on hips and earlier wear-out of artificial hips. It was reported that 60% of implants were estimated to last about 25 years, which indicated that young patients are very likely to require revision surgeries at some point [15]. This helps to explain why the adolescents and their guardians are often reluctant to accept THA, besides the multiple surgical risks. Moreover, bone tissues might be regenerated by local progenitor cells and the epiphyseal plate under the beneficial stimulus of PRP. The optimum treatment of adolescent ONFH should be focused on hip preserving strategies and providing a more appropriate environment for further restorations.

As one of the most commonly used biologic therapies, intra-articular PRP injection seems to hold promise for musculoskeletal regenerative medicine. PRP consists of different kinds of growth factors, such as PDGF, VEGF, IGF-1 and TGF, which helps to provide the optimal environment for osteoblast activities, cartilage repair and revascularization [16,17]. Tao *et al.* once reported that PRP exosomes could prevent cell apoptosis and promote angiogenesis, thus maintaining osteogenic differentiation and osteogenesis in a rat model of ONFH [8]. Ultrasound-guided PRP injections have many advantages, including being minimally invasive, real-time visualization and the ability to identify and characterize target regions [18,19]. Considering the above, it appears reasonable to recommend autologous PRP as a possible alternative for all stages of ONFH, especially for younger patients in need of preserving hip functions. Pak *et al.* previously reported the complete resolution of an early-stage femoral head avascular necrosis (ARCO I) case treated with mixtures of adipose tissue-derived stem cells and PRP via intra-articular injection [9].

Few studies have been published that focus on the application of PRP in the late-stages of ONFH (ARCO III, IV). Thus far, most published studies support that the prognosis for ONFH is generally worse if the patient is symptomatic with large volumes of collapse. In the present case, we performed both clinical and imaging evaluations, including the Harris Hip Score and MRI, in line with recommendations in the Chinese Guideline for the Diagnosis and Treatment of ONFH in adults [13,14]. In her first visit, the patient presented with severe pain (visual analog scale 7/10), serious functional impairment and bilateral femoral head collapse changes in MRI. Generally, the most used protocol for this type of degenerative injury includes 2–3 injections, however, we agreed

10.2217/rme-2020-0057

to perform two treatment courses combined with rehabilitation during her one-month hospitalization based on the patient's wishes and the severity of her hip condition.

The improvements in strength and HHS may not be considered high enough for the patient to resume full normal daily activity, however, the therapeutic efficacy evaluated by clinical and MRI evaluations demonstrated notable improvements. Specifically, there was a marked improvement in her sitting posture (from 'unable to sit in any chair' to 'sitting comfortably in an ordinary chair for 1 hour') and gait (from 'severe limp' to 'slight limp'). The patient could also walk with tolerated pain by 9 months follow-up, which is necessary for her schooling and social activities. The PRP treatment failed to achieve complete pain relief or reverse the collapse, however, this case highlights that age is another key factor for ONFH treatment options [13]. The patient may have to undergo THA at some point in the future, however, surgery before adulthood may not have been suitable timing.

The current case study does however have several limitations that should be acknowledged. First, the therapeutic mechanisms of PRP could not be verified directly in this case, even though the reduced symptoms, decreased necrosis volume and effusion absorption were observed. A longer follow-up of the current case, including clinical and MRI evaluations, is still necessary. Also, modified specific assessment tools, such as International Hip Outcome Tool (SC-iHOT-33) and Hip Outcome Score, should be given full consideration for young patients [20]. More prospective evidence, especially randomized controlled trials with longer follow-up and larger numbers of cases will be needed in the future.

Conclusion

Glucocorticoid-induced ONFH is a disabling disease and adolescent ONFH management requires additional concerns for hip joint preservation and restoration. In this paper, we presented a case of an adolescent late-stage glucocorticoid-induced ONFH (ARCO stage IV) treated with PRP. Ultrasound-guided intra-articular injections of PRP may hold promise for ONFH of all stages, especially for adolescent patients.

Translational perspective

Femoral head necrosis is characterized by decreased osteogenic activity and increased osteocyte apoptosis. Autologous PRP containing growth factors as well as highly concentrated platelets has attracted the attention of many researchers in regenerative and restorative medicine in recent years. Due to severe morphological changes and mechanical problems of the affected hip joints, the therapeutic effect of PRP for late-stage femoral head necrosis has rarely been studied in previous literature. We hope this case study may help to offer a new perspective for the integrated management of adolescent femoral head necrosis. Moreover, further research is needed into the mechanism by which PRP treatment affects unmatured bone tissues and bone marrow mesenchymal cells of adolescent patients. Besides the ultrasound-guided injections, PRP usage combined with bone tissue engineering also deserves more attention for future translational research and applications.

Summary points

- Glucocorticoid-induced osteonecrosis of femoral head (ONFH) is an important health problem worldwide, which may have a detrimental effect on the overall quality of life of ONFH patients.
- This case concerned the dilemma of treating adolescent ONFH, since lifetime risk of revision of total hip arthroplasty increased and conventional conservative management could be challenging in treating late-stage ONFH of younger patients.
- In this case, the repetitive ultrasound-guided intra-articular injections of platelet-rich plasma were effective in treating an adolescent ONFH (Association Research Circulation Osseous stage IV). Favorable outcomes were obtained with clinical and radiological reassessments at 9-month follow-up.
- Ultrasound-guided platelet-rich plasma injections may hold promise for ONFH of all stages, especially for adolescent patients. Therapeutic mechanisms of joint restoration and protection are needed for future exploration.

Financial & competing interests disclosure

This study was funded by National Natural Science Foundation of China (81671088, 81771201 and 81972152) and Sun Yat-Sen Clinical Research Cultivating Program (SYS-C-201704, SYS-C-202002). The authors have no other relevant financial involvement or financial conflict with the subject matter or materials mentioned in the manuscript apart from the above disclosed. The authors declare no conflict of interest.

No writing assistance was utilized in the production of this manuscript.

Platelet-rich plasma for the treatment of adolescent late-stage femoral head necrosis: a case report   Case Report

Ethical conduct of research

The authors state that they have obtained verbal and written informed consent from the patient for the inclusion of their medical and treatment history within this case report.

References

1. Arbab D, Konig DP. Atraumatic femoral head necrosis in adults. *Dtsch. Arztebl. Int.* 113(3), 31–38 (2016).

2. Yoon BH, Jones LC, Chen CH *et al.* Etiologic classification criteria of ARCO on femoral head osteonecrosis part 1: glucocorticoid-associated osteonecrosis. *J. Arthroplasty* 34(1), 163–168 e161 (2019).

3. Cao HJ, Guan HF, Lai YX, Qin L, Wang XL. Review of various treatment options and potential therapies for osteonecrosis of the femoral head. *J. Orthop. Transl.* 4, 57–70 (2016).

4. Mont MA, Cherian JJ, Sierra RJ, Jones LC, Lieberman JR. Nontraumatic osteonecrosis of the femoral head: where do we stand today? *J. Bone Joint Surg. Am.* 97a(19), 1604–1627 (2015).

5. Engebretsen L, Steffen K, Alsousou J *et al.* IOC consensus paper on the use of platelet-rich plasma in sports medicine. *Brit. J. Sport. Med.* 44(15), 1072–1081 (2010).

6. Fice MP, Miller JC, Christian R *et al.* The role of platelet-rich plasma in cartilage pathology: an updated systematic review of the basic science evidence. *Arthroscopy* 35(3), 961–976 e963 (2019).

7. Andia I, Maffulli N. Platelet-rich plasma for managing pain and inflammation in osteoarthritis. *Nat. Rev. Rheumatol.* 9(12), 721–730 (2013).

8. Tao SC, Yuan T, Rui BY, Zhu ZZ, Guo SC, Zhang CQ. Exosomes derived from human platelet-rich plasma prevent apoptosis induced by glucocorticoid-associated endoplasmic reticulum stress in rat osteonecrosis of the femoral head via the Akt/Bad/Bcl-2 signal pathway. *Theranostics* 7(3), 733–750 (2017).

9. Pak J, Lee JH, Jeon JH, Lee SH. Complete resolution of avascular necrosis of the human femoral head treated with adipose tissue-derived stem cells and platelet-rich plasma. *J. Int. Med. Res.* 42(6), 1353–1362 (2014).

10. Yoon BH, Mont MA, Koo KH *et al.* The 2019 revised version of association research circulation osseous staging system of osteonecrosis of the femoral head. *J. Arthroplasty* 35(4), 933–940 (2020).

11. Luo ZY, Wang D, Huang ZY, Wang HY, Zhou ZK. Knee and hip replacements and the risk of revision. *Lancet* 394(10200), e30 (2019).

12. Schreurs BW, Hannink G. Total joint arthroplasty in younger patients: heading for trouble? *Lancet* 389(10077), 1374–1375 (2017).

13. Zhao D, Zhang F, Wang B *et al.* Guidelines for clinical diagnosis and treatment of osteonecrosis of the femoral head in adults (2019 version). *J. Orthop. Transl.* 21, 100–110 (2020).

14. Microsurgery Department of the Orthopedics Branch of the Chinese Medical Doctor Association *et al.* Chinese guideline for the diagnosis and treatment of osteonecrosis of the femoral head in adults. *Orthop.Surg.* 9(1), 3–12 (2017).

15. Evans JT, Evans JP, Walker RW, Blom AW, Whitehouse MR, Sayers A. How long does a hip replacement last? A systematic review and meta-analysis of case series and national registry reports with more than 15 years of follow-up. *Lancet* 393(10172), 647–654 (2019).

16. Oryan A, Alidadi S, Moshiri A. Platelet-rich plasma for bone healing and regeneration. *Expert Opin. Biol. Ther.* 16(2), 213–232 (2016).

17. Guadilla J, Fiz N, Andia I, Sanchez M. Arthroscopic management and platelet-rich plasma therapy for avascular necrosis of the hip. *Knee Surg. Sports Traumatol. Arthrosc.* 20(2), 393–398 (2012).

18. Zhang S, Wang F, Ke S *et al.* The effectiveness of ultrasound-guided steroid injection combined with miniscalpel-needle release in the treatment of carpal tunnel syndrome vs. steroid injection alone: a randomized controlled study. *Biomed. Res. Int.* 2019, 9498656 (2019).

19. Wan Q, Yang H, Li X *et al.* Ultrasound-guided versus fluoroscopy-guided deep cervical plexus block for the treatment of cervicogenic headache. *Biomed. Res. Int.* 2017, 4654803 (2017).

20. Li DH, Wang W, Li X *et al.* Development of a valid simplified Chinese version of the International Hip Outcome Tool (SC-iHOT-33) in young patients having total hip arthroplasty. *Osteoarthr. Cartilage* 25(1), 94–98 (2017).

Journal of Pain Research

Dovepress
open access to scientific and medical research

Open Access Full Text Article

ORIGINAL RESEARCH

Comparisons of Ultrasound-Guided Platelet-Rich Plasma Intra-Articular Injection and Extracorporeal Shock Wave Therapy in Treating ARCO I–III Symptomatic Non-Traumatic Femoral Head Necrosis: A Randomized Controlled Clinical Trial

Shuo Luan*, Shaoling Wang*, Caina Lin, Shengnuo Fan, Cuicui Liu, Chao Ma [ID], Shaoling Wu [ID]

Department of Rehabilitation Medicine, Sun Yat-sen Memorial Hospital, Sun Yat-sen University, Guangzhou, 510120, Guangdong, People's Republic of China

*These authors contributed equally to this work

Correspondence: Shaoling Wu; Chao Ma, Email wushl@mail.sysu.edu.cn; machao@mail.sysu.edu.cn

Background and Objective: Osteonecrosis of the femoral head (ONFH) is a devastating disease, and there is some evidence that extracorporeal shock wave therapy (ESWT) and intra-articular platelet-rich plasma (PRP) injection might alleviate pain and improve joint function in individuals with ONFH. The objective of this study was to compare the effectiveness and safety of PRP and ESWT in symptomatic ONFH patients.

Methods: A total of 60 patients aged 40–79 with unilateral ONFH at Association Research Circulation Osseous (ARCO) stages I, II, and III were randomly assigned to the PRP (N=30) or the ESWT group (N=30). Four treatment sessions were provided in both groups. Assessments were performed at baseline, and 1-, 3-, 6-, and 12-month. Primary outcomes were measured by the visual analogue scale (VAS), and pressure pain thresholds (PPTs). Secondary outcomes were assessed by Western Ontario and McMaster Universities Osteoarthritis Index (WOMAC), Harris Hip Score (HHS), and magnetic resonance imaging (MRI). The linear mixed-model analysis was used to evaluate the differences between groups and within groups and the "group by time" interaction effects.

Results: There were significant differences between groups in terms of changes over time for VAS, PPTs, WOMAC, and HHS since 3-month and maintained up to 12-month (P<0.05, except for PPTs at 12-month). The simple main effects showed that the patients in PRP group had greater improvements in VAS (mean difference = −0.82, 95% CI [−1.39, −0.25], P=0.005), WOMAC (mean difference = −4.19, 95% CI [−7.00, −1.37], P=0.004), and HHS (mean difference = 5.28, 95% CI [1.94, 8.62], P=0.002). No related adverse events were reported.

Conclusion: This study supported the effectiveness and safety of both the PRP injection and ESWT in treating ONFH patients. For symptomatic patients with ONFH, intra-articular PRP injection appeared superior to ESWT in pain relief and functional improvement.

Keywords: necrosis of the femoral head, platelet-rich plasma, ultrasound-guided intra-articular injection, extracorporeal shock wave therapy

Introduction

Osteonecrosis of the femoral head (ONFH) may lead to progressive pain, hip joint dysfunction, and severely decreased life quality, affecting more and more patients worldwide. The aetiologies of ONFH are multifactorial and complicated, including both traumatic and non-traumatic (corticosteroid use, alcohol consumption, smoking, and genetic) causes.[1–3]

Received: 5 November 2021
Accepted: 18 January 2022
Published: 5 February 2022

341

© 2022 Luan et al. This work is published and licensed by Dove Medical Press Limited. The full terms of this license are available at https://www.dovepress.com/terms.php and incorporate the Creative Commons Attribution — Non Commercial (unported, v3.0) License (http://creativecommons.org/licenses/by-nc/3.0/). By accessing the work you hereby accept the Terms. Non-commercial uses of the work are permitted without any further permission from Dove Medical Press Limited, provided the work is properly attributed. For permission for commercial use of this work, please see paragraphs 4.2 and 5 of our Terms (https://www.dovepress.com/terms.php).

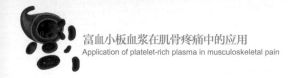
Histopathological changes of ONFH are usually characterized by osteocytes death and empty lacunae in the osseous matrix, which further develops into low bone mass, and subchondral trabecular collapse.[4] Among the various diagnostic imaging examinations, MRI remains the most important diagnostic method with relatively high sensitivity and specificity, especially for patients with early-stage ONFH. The latest version of the Association Research Circulation Osseous (ARCO) classification system was revised in 2019, which has been proposed as one of the most popular classification systems for ONFH worldwide.[5] In particular, not all avascular bone necrosis shares the same causes. For example, the possible correlation between the tyrosine kinase inhibitors, immunosuppressants, monoclonal antibodies, rapamycin inhibitors, and selective estrogen receptor modulators, and osteonecrosis of the jaws should be highlighted.[6]

Up to now, there are still no unified guidelines or recommendations for ONFH treatment, especially for patients accompanied by varying levels of pain symptoms. It is well accepted that patients with ARCO stage I and II were at early stages, with ARCO stage III and IV disease at late stages.[7] For patients with early-stage ONFH, joint-preserving procedures are recommended, including both the non-surgical options (drugs, extracorporeal shock wave, and biologic treatment) and surgical options (core decompression, vascularized bone graft, and so on).[8–10] Core decompression (CD) helps reduce the pressure in the femoral head, opens up the hardening zone, and further enhances the new bone regeneration.[11] Total hip arthroplasty (THA) remains the most widespread and the only definitive procedure for end-stage ONFH patients.[12] However, ONFH occurs predominantly in younger patients who are generally physically active and inclined to preserve the structural integrity of their joints. Thus, there is an urgent demand for developing safe and effective joint-preserving treatments.[13] Extracorporeal shock wave therapy (ESWT) is a non-invasive and safe treatment proven effective in treating ONFH.[14] It was proposed that ESWT helped to promote the revascularization and regeneration process of ONFH.[15,16] Pilot clinical studies also confirmed the analgesic and therapeutic effects of ESWT in treating ONFH.

Relatively, the platelet-rich plasma (PRP) intra-articular injection has not been fully discussed for ONFH management. While the use of PRP gel in association with core decompression as a surgical treatment has been much discussed and tried by various authors.[17] Over the past few decades, PRP has emerged as a popular biologic treatment for many musculoskeletal diseases, including knee osteoarthritis, delayed or non-unions, osteonecrosis of the jaws, and tendon injuries.[18–21] It is well-accepted that PRP has the potential to promote the healing process due to the autologous blood growth factors (GFs) released from α-granules within platelets.[22,23] In 2017, Tao et al reported that the exosomes derived from human PRP via the tail vein injection could relieve apoptosis, promote angiogenesis and osteogenic differentiation in a rat model of ONFH.[24] Recently, researchers have been paying more attention to the analgesic effects of PRP. Several clinical studies have demonstrated that PRP helped relieve pain symptoms in chronic diseases, including osteoarthritis and osteonecrosis, but the potential mechanisms are not fully understood. Even though the intra-articular PRP injection for hip osteoarthritis has revealed satisfactory treatment outcomes, little evidence on its effectiveness and safety in ONFH management existed.[18,25] In 2020, our team reported that the intra-articular PRP injections improved pain symptoms and imaging findings of a late-stage ONFH (ARCO stage IV) patient.[26] Despite the promising in vitro and in vivo results, it is still necessary to confirm the therapeutic effects of PRP through clinical randomized controlled trials.

The objective of this study was to compare the therapeutic effects of ultrasound-guided intra-articular PRP injections and extracorporeal shock wave therapy (ESWT) in symptomatic unilateral ONFH patients at ARCO I–III stages. Considering the various etiologies, the present study focused on the non-traumatic ONFH.

Materials and Methods
Study Design
This was a randomized, single-blind, parallel-group study with a 12-month follow-up. We aimed to evaluate the effectiveness and safety of intra-articular injection of PRP for treating ONFH compared to ESWT.

Participants and Study Procedure
The participants were recruited from the Department of Rehabilitation Medicine of Sun Yat-sen Memorial Hospital, Sun Yat-sen University from June 2019 to December 2019. This study was approved by the Medical Ethics Committee of Sun

Dovepress

Yat-sen Memorial Hospital (2019-KY-086). The study protocol was registered at the Chinese Clinical Trial Registry (ID: ChiCTR1900023601).

Patients who met the following criteria were included: 1) between 40 and 80 years old, 2) diagnosed with non-traumatic ONFH for over 3 months; 3) ONFH identified by X-ray/MRI, accompanied with clinical symptoms and signs; 4) Visual Analogue Scale (VAS) ≥ 4; 5) ARCO stages I, II and III; 6) resistant to non-morphine or failed to respond to previous physical therapies. Exclusion criteria included 1) hip surgery history; 2) combined with infection, joint tumors, or tuberculosis; 3) blood coagulation disorders, or a history of drug abuse or oral anticoagulation; 4) abnormal psychological, cognitive disorders; 5) not suitable for injection because of local infection; 6) received the intra-articular injections in the past 3 months; 7) pregnancy.

At the baseline evaluation, all eligible participants' demographic characteristics, medical history, and laboratory tests (blood biochemistry and blood cell analysis) were collected. Detailed physical and radiological examinations including the primary outcomes (Visual Analogue Scale and pressure pain thresholds) and secondary outcomes (Western Ontario and McMaster Universities Osteoarthritis Index, Harris Hip Score, and MRI) were evaluated before randomized allocation by a trained physician. The MRI scannings were used to assess the ARCO stages. All patients gave written informed consent to participate in the study.

The enrolled patients were randomly assigned at 1:1 ratio into the PRP group (N=30) or ESWT group (N=30). The randomization was conducted using the Website tool (https://www.random.org/). No other analgesic drugs or physical therapies were administered to the patients in both groups during the treatment and 12-month follow-up period. The baseline and follow-up outcome assessors and data administrators were blinded to the allocation, but the patients and treatment providers were not blinded because of the nature of this trial design.

Interventions

Extracorporeal Shock Wave Treatment

The ESWT was applied using Gymna Shockmaster 500 and the femoral artery was confirmed with ultrasound Doppler beforehand to avoid potential injuries. Patients were treated with the affected hip in mild adduction and internal rotation. The ESWT procedures were performed without anesthesia and the clean coupling gel was used at the interface to decrease the loss of energy between the probe and skin. Before treatment, the physician reviewed the MRI scannings to ensure that the impulses were focused around the necrotic tissue of the femoral head. Four selected spots were located on the hardened layer around the lesion based on patients' MRI scannings, and a dose of 1000 impulses at an energy flux density (EFD) of 0.50 mJ/mm^2 was applied at each point in one single session, for about 15 minutes. Patients received consecutive four weekly sessions of treatment in the entire cycle. After each session, patients were instructed to walk with crutches (partial weight-bearing). The ESWT procedure was replicable and performed by the same operator. The study nurse recorded adverse reactions, including persistent unbearable pain and swelling.

Ultrasound-Guided Intra-Articular Platelet-Rich Plasma Injection

The PRP preparation procedures were performed under sterile conditions. A total of 18 mL of whole-blood sample was drawn from the antecubital vein into 10-mL syringes containing 1 mL 3.8% (w/v) sodium citrate. The autologous PRP was prepared in a two-step centrifugation process and the harvest and transfer methods were the same as our previously described protocol.[26] At room temperature (23°C), the blood samples were centrifuged for 10 min at 1600 revolutions per minute (r.p.m.). The supernatant buffy coat and plasma were transferred into the other tubes. Then, the samples were centrifuged at 3200 r.p.m for another 10 min and the lower layer plasma was obtained as concentrated PRP. A small sample of PRP (0.5mL) was usually sent to the laboratory for quantitative analysis of platelet and leukocyte counts.

Similar to the injection protocol introduced in our previous study, the PRP injections were performed with patients in the supine position.[26] All the injections were performed using SONIMAGE HS1 PLUS. Preliminary sonographic examinations including the ultrasound Doppler of the affected hip were performed to identify the vascular and nerve structures. Before injection, the intra-articular fluid would be evacuated if presented. We usually chose 20–22G needles for injections according to patients' individualized body sizes. With the low-frequency convex array (C5-2, 2–5MHz) probe aligned along the long axis of the femoral neck, the needle was advanced into the anterior joint recess at the

https://doi.org/10.2147/JPR.S347961

DovePress

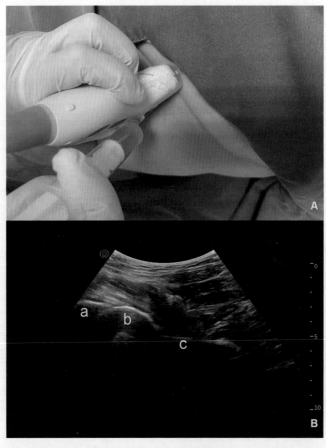

Figure 1 Ultrasound-guided PRP injection for ONFH. The low-frequency convex array probe was aligned with the long axis of the affected femoral head (**A**) and the needle was advanced using anterior longitudinal approach (**B**). (a) acetabulum; (b) femoral head; (c) femoral neck.

femoral head-neck junction. PRP diffusion could be visualized under sonographic guidance. The tolerable hip joint motion of the affected side was assisted by a physician assistant to ensure the PRP distribution on the ball-and-socket synovial joint. All patients in the PRP group received four weekly injections at a one-week interval (see Figure 1). All adverse reactions and complications, including persistent joint swelling, infections, allergies, and severe posttreatment pain were recorded by the study nurse in written form.

Assessment Outcomes

The primary outcomes included the VAS and PPTs, and the secondary outcomes included the WOMAC, HHS, and MRI scannings. The clinical outcome assessments were scheduled at baseline before randomization and at 1, 3, 6, and 12

Dovepress　　　　　　　　　　　　　　　　　　　　　　　　　　　　　　　

months post-treatment. In particular, the MRI was evaluated at baseline and 12-month follow-up. The assessors were blinded to the type of treatment administered.

Visual Analogue Scale (VAS)

Visual Analogue Scale (VAS) provides a simple way to subjectively evaluate pain intensity, which has been widely used in clinical practice and among researchers. Participants were instructed to mark a point along the 10-point Likert scale (0 to 10 cm, indicating no pain to most severe pain). According to a published study, the mean reduction in VAS of 1.0 cm represents the minimal clinical important difference (MCID) of pain alleviation.[27]

Pressure Pain Thresholds (PPTs)

Fischer et al recommended that a specially designed digital pressure algometer could be used to evaluate the pressure pain thresholds (PPTs). PPT is usually defined as the least amount of pressure to provoke pain, and the lower value usually indicates hyperalgesia and peripheral sensitization. Thus, it is recommended that the PPT could be used as an important objective indication of pain.[28] Based on a previously published study, the PPTs of hips were measured at 5cm distally and 2cm anteriorly of the greater trochanter.[29] Before the tests, the patients were instructed to differentiate the pain and sensations of pressure, and they were asked to give a sign as soon as they felt the pain. An experienced assessor performed the assessment with the algometer (Model PTH AF2; Pain Diagnostics and Thermography, Great Neck, NY) by placing the 1 cm^2 rubber tip to the affected hip at a rate of 1 kg/sec. All the measurements were performed by a single assessor blinded to allocation. We performed three repetitive measures at an interval of 60 seconds, and the average values were determined as the final results.

Western Ontario and McMaster Universities Osteoarthritis Index (WOMAC)

The WOMAC was developed in the 1980s and designed as an evaluation tool for knee and hip osteoarthritis. In the past several decades, the WOMAC has been widely used to evaluate clinically patient-relevant changes and therapeutic effects of specific interventions in hip joint disorders. The complete WOMAC scale covers three dimensions: pain, stiffness, and physical function. The total score is 96, and the sub-total scores are 20, 8, and 68 for the above three domains. The Likert version of WOMAC was adopted, with higher scores indicating more severe pain symptoms and disability.[30]

Harris Hip Score (HHS)

The Harris Hip Score (HHS) was originally developed as a standardized assessment following the THA. In recent years, it was also commonly used for hip osteoarthritis and ONFH patients. The HHS consists of four subscales for pain severity, function, absence of deformity, and range of motion. The total score ranges from 0 to 100, with higher scores indicating better outcomes. Generally, the HHS total score of <70 is considered as a poor result; 70–80 is considered fair; 80–90 is good; and 90–100 is excellent.[31]

Magnetic Resonance Imaging (MRI)

MRI examinations were performed at baseline and 12-month follow-up, using T1- and T2-weighted scans, and T2-weighted sequences with fat saturation. One radiologist and one physician who were blinded to allocation evaluated the stages of ONFH and disease progress independently according to the ARCO classification system.

Statistical Analysis

The sample size was calculated using Power Analysis and Sample Size (PASS) software (version 15.0; NCSS) based on the difference of VAS between interventions according to the previous study and our preliminary experiment. Power analysis was performed with $\alpha = 0.05$ (one-sided) and $\beta = 0.20$ (power). The minimum sample size of 60 patients (N=30 for each group) was determined by considering the probable loss to follow-up (20%).

The intention-to-treat principle was applied to all analyses, and the participants' follow-up data were analyzed according to groups they were allocated to originally. Data analysis was performed using R software version 4.0.5.

Descriptive statistics were used to present the patient characteristics. The normally distributed data were presented as means±standard deviations (SDs), and non-normally distributed data as Median (Percentile 25, Percentile 75). Descriptive statistics utilized χ^2 for categorical measures and t-test for continuous measures. The Mann–Whitney U-test was used to evaluate differences between the disease duration since the data were not normally distributed.

To detect the changes of primary outcomes (VAS and PPTs) and secondary outcomes (WOMAC and HHS) over time and the comparisons between groups, we constructed a linear mixed model (LMM) with repeated measures, adjusting for baseline scores of the above outcome variables, and other demographic variables. R package nlme was used to conduct the LMM analysis. Further pairwise comparisons of simple main effects based on the LMMs were performed to explore the differences between the two groups at the 12-month follow-up. Cohen's d was calculated to assess the between-group effect size (the mean difference scores for the ESWT group were subtracted from the mean difference scores for the PRP group and divided by the standard deviation).[32]

We also performed post hoc exploratory analyses to detect the effects of the interventions on the primary outcomes (VAS and PPTs) at 12-month follow-up using tests for interaction, according to the baseline characteristics of the participants. A P-value less than 0.05 was considered statistically significant.

Results
Demographic Characteristics
Among the 68 recruited subjects, 60 eligible participants consented to participate and were randomized to the PRP group (n=30) and ESWT group (n=30). Details of demographic characteristics are presented in Table 1. The PRP group consisted of 13 men and 17 women, while the ESWT group consisted of 9 men and 21 women. In the PRP group, 3 patients were classified as stage I, 11 as stage II, and 16 as stage III, while 3 patients as stage I, 13 as stage II, and 14 as stage III in the ESWT group. There were no significant differences in characteristics between the two groups, including age, sex distribution, disease duration, and body mass index (BMI). Before the end of the 12-month follow-up, two patients at ARCO stage III in the PRP group (2/30) and two in the ESWT group (2/30) decided to receive the THA and were lost to follow-up. The dropout rate was 6.66% for each group. Figure 2 shows the flowchart of the study. Baseline assessments of primary and secondary outcomes for both groups are displayed in Table 2.

Primary Outcomes
Results from LMM analysis with the between-group simple main effects are displayed in Table 2. Trends for the primary outcomes (VAS and PPTs) over time are presented in Figure 3A and B. Our results indicated significant Group × Time interactions between the two groups at 3-month, 6-month, and 12-month follow-up. The VAS scores of the PRP group, when compared to the ESWT group, exhibited significant improvements since 3-month (mean difference = −0.83 points, 95% CI [−1.39, −0.27], P = 0.004) and maintained up to 12-month (mean difference = −0.82 points, 95% CI [−1.39,

Table 1 Demographic Characteristics of the Two Groups

	PRP Group (N=30)	ESWT Group (N=30)	P
Age, mean (SD)	63.4 (11.8)	61.6 (11.8)	0.542
Sex			0.422
Male	13 (43.3%)	9 (30.0%)	
Female	17 (56.7%)	21 (70.0%)	
Disease duration (years), Median (P25, P75)	2.75(1.00, 3.88)	2.00(1.00, 4.75)	0.820
ARCO stages			0.929
I	3 (10.0%)	3(10.0%)	
II	11 (36.7%)	13(43.3%)	
III	16 (53.3%)	14(46.7%)	
BMI, mean (SD)	24.6 (3.78)	24.6 (3.68)	0.969

Abbreviations: PRP, platelet-rich plasma; ESWT, extracorporeal shock wave therapy; P25, 25th percentiles; P75, 75th percentile; ARCO, Association Research Circulation Osseous; BMI, body mass index.

242

Dovepress

Luan et al

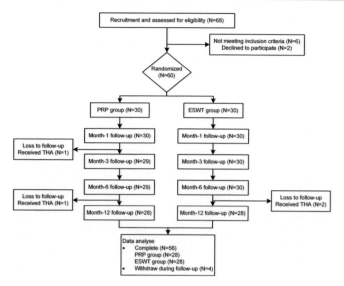

Figure 2 Flow diagram of the study.
Abbreviations: PRP, platelet-rich plasma; ESWT, extracorporeal shock wave therapy; THA, total hip arthroplasty.

−0.25], P=0.005). At 12-month follow-up, the VAS scores of the PRP group (from 6.13 to 3.11) decreased significantly compared to the ESWT group (5.97 to 3.75), with a standard effect size (Cohen d) of 0.73.

Similarly, the LMM showed that the participants in the PRP group had significantly increased PPTs in comparison with the ESWT group, and the between-group differences in the PPTs were statistically significant for six-month post-treatment (3-month: 0.15, 95% CI [0.001 to 0.30], P=0.049, Cohen d=0.51; and 6-month: 0.16, 95% CI [0.01 to 0.30; P=0.041; Cohen d=0.53). However, simple main effects of between-group PPTs comparisons at the 12-month follow-up was not statistically significant (0.11, 95% CI [−0.04, 0.26]; P=0.138; Cohen d=0.38) (Tables 2 and 3).

Secondary Outcomes

For the WOMAC and HHS assessment, there was a trend that the PRP group patients achieved better functional outcomes compared to the ESWT group during follow-up (see Figure 3C and D). Considering the between-group differences, PRP groups showed significantly improved WOMAC and HHS scores compared to the ESWT group since month-3 (WOMAC: P = 0.005, HHS: P = 0.002) and maintained up to the end of follow-up (WOMAC: P = 0.004, HHS: P =0.002). At 12 months, compared to the ESWT group, the estimated mean improvement of PRP group in WOMAC scores was −4.19 (95% CI [−7.00, −1.37], P = 0.004; Cohen d=0.75) and in HHS was 5.28 (95% CI [1.94, 8.62], P = 0.002; Cohen d=0.80), respectively (Tables 2 and 3).

No discrepant MRI evaluations were reported between the radiologist and the physician. At the end of the study, the improvements in radiographic findings of ARCO I–II individuals were observed in two groups (one patient in the PRP group: from ARCO stage II to I, and one in the ESWT group: from ARCO stage I to 0), respectively. And two patients at ARCO stage III (one in the PRP group and one in the ESWT group) progressed to ARCO stage IV. Other participants in both groups remained unchanged on radiographic assessments.

Table 2 Between-Group Comparisons for Primary Outcomes and Secondary Outcomes for the PRP and ESWT Groups at All Follow-Ups

Follow-Up Time	PRP Group (N=30), Mean (SD)	ESWT Group (N=30), Mean (SD)	Treatment Effects (95% CI)[a]	Liner Mixed Model Results, P value[a,c]		
				Group[b]	Time	Group×Time
Primary outcomes						
VAS (0–10)						
Baseline	6.13 (1.28)	5.97 (1.19)	–	0.820	–	–
1-month	3.40 (1.19)	3.10 (1.06)	0.13(−0.42, 0.69)	–	<0.001	0.640
3-month	2.97 (1.30)	3.67 (1.27)	−0.83 (−1.39, −0.27)	–	<0.001	0.004
6-month	3.00 (1.36)	3.83 (1.39)	−0.96 (−1.52, −0.40)	–	<0.001	0.001
12-month	3.11 (1.23)	3.75 (1.11)	−0.82 (−1.39, −0.25)	–	<0.001	0.005
PPTs (kg/cm²/second)						
Baseline	2.11 (0.48)	2.07 (0.45)	–	0.636	–	–
1-month	2.59 (0.37)	2.61 (0.27)	−0.07 (−0.22, 0.08)	–	<0.001	0.341
3-month	2.84 (0.31)	2.63 (0.32)	0.15 (0.001, 0.30)	–	<0.001	0.049
6-month	2.73 (0.31)	2.51 (0.37)	0.16 (0.01, 0.30)	–	<0.001	0.041
12-month	2.68 (0.29)	2.53 (0.27)	0.11 (−0.04, 0.26)	–	<0.001	0.138
Secondary outcomes						
WOMAC (0–96)						
Baseline	41.87 (9.52)	40.67 (8.88)	–	0.727	–	–
1-month	29.00 (7.54)	25.93 (5.76)	1.87 (−0.89, 4.62)	–	<0.001	0.185
3-month	24.45 (6.84)	27.30 (6.45)	−4.05 (−6.82, −1.28)	–	<0.001	0.005
6-month	24.79 (6.75)	28.40 (6.25)	−4.80 (−7.57, −2.04)	–	<0.001	0.001
12-month	25.71 (6.42)	28.36 (5.44)	−4.19 (−7.00, −1.37)	–	<0.001	0.004
HHS (0–100)						
Baseline	51.73 (9.15)	55.64 (9.35)	–	0.227	–	–
1-month	71.25 (9.67)	73.92 (6.16)	1.24 (−2.03, 4.51)	–	<0.001	0.458
3-month	76.07 (8.58)	73.88 (7.79)	5.57 (2.28, 8.86)	–	<0.001	0.002
6-month	75.65 (6.80)	73.07 (7.56)	5.96 (2.67, 9.25)	–	<0.001	<0.001
12-month	74.17 (8.15)	72.37 (5.79)	5.28 (1.94, 8.62)	–	<0.001	0.002

Notes: [a]Between-group difference for mean change from baseline (95% CI); [b]P of Group indicates the baseline comparisons between the two groups; [c]Linear mixed model based on five time points (baseline, 1-month, 3-month, 6-month and 12-month follow-up) and adjusted for baseline of the outcome variables, and other baseline demographic characteristic (age, disease duration, body mass index, sex and ARCO stage).
Abbreviations: PRP, platelet-rich plasma; ESWT, extracorporeal shock wave therapy; VAS, visual analogue scale; PPTs, pressure pain thresholds; WOMAC, Western Ontario and McMaster Universities Osteoarthritis Index; HHS, Harris Hip Score.

Exploratory Subgroup Analysis

Except for ARCO stages, no significant interactions were found in the post hoc exploratory analyses of VAS, including age, gender distribution, disease duration, and BMI. Patients at ARCO stages I and II had statistically greater improvements of VAS than those at ARCO stage III. For the PPTs, significant interactions were found in the age and ARCO stage, which indicated that younger participants with early-stage ONFH were more likely to benefit from PRP injection treatment (see Figure 4).

Discussion

ONFH is a refractory devastating orthopedic disease characterized by pain, stiffness, and joint dysfunction. Up to date, there are still no standardized treatments for these patients. Previous pilot studies proved that both the PRP injection and

244

Dovepress

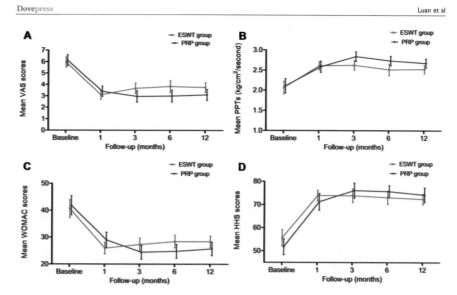

Figure 3 Changes in Visual Analogue Scale (VAS), pressure pain thresholds (PPTs), Western Ontario and McMaster Universities Osteoarthritis Index (WOMAC), and Harris Hip Score (HHS) in the 12-month follow-up period. (**A**) Visual Analogue Scale (VAS); (**B**) pressure pain thresholds; (**C**) Western Ontario and McMaster Universities Osteoarthritis Index; (**D**) Harris Hip Score.
Notes: Data are presented as mean (±95% confidence interval).
Abbreviations: PRP, platelet-rich plasma; ESWT, extracorporeal shock wave therapy.

ESWT might contribute to pain relief and slowing down the progression of ONFH.[16,33] Our current results confirm our hypothesis that there were significant improvements in the PRP group for pain relief and functional recovery compared to the conventional ESWT.

For ONFH patients, the pain symptoms and radiologic findings do not necessarily parallel each other. Among all of its symptoms, pain is one of the most disabling symptoms of ONFH and the unsolved persistent pain is also the main reason for patients to seek THA. In this study, we chose the VAS and PPTs as the primary outcomes, and we confirmed that the pain improvements between the two groups were maintained over time in favor of intra-articular injection (except for PPTs at 12-month). In particular, even though we did not detect the between-group simple main effect of PPTs at 12-month follow-up, we observed the significant Group × Time interactions at 3-month and 6-month for PPTs. In previous studies of musculoskeletal disease, VAS has been widely used for pain assessment, but objective pain assessment tools are still urgently needed. PPTs, as one of the widely used quantitative sensory tests, usually work as an objective supplementary tool. Unfortunately, the measurement protocol of PPTs has not been unified and few prior studies have reported the reference range or the MCID for the PPTs in hip disorders.[34] Our results provided the available evidence-based PPTs in ONFH patients for future reference. Based on our post hoc subgroup analysis of VAS and PPTs, we found that younger early-stage patients (ARCO I and II) achieved better results than those at late stages (ARCO III), similar to the findings in other published studies.[35] Early interventions before the femoral head collapse usually lead to better and long-lasting pain relief.

For hip function assessments, we observed similar patterns of WOMAC and HHS improvements in both groups during the 12-month follow-up. For the radiographic assessments at the end-point of follow-up, the staging progression did not occur in ARCO stages I and II patients in both groups. It is commonly accepted that the natural history of ONFH is of progression, thus our results might be encouraging. Interestingly, the MRI scannings at 12-month showed

https://doi.org/10.2147/JPR.S347961

DovePress

Table 3 Between Group Effect Size Assessed Using Cohen's *d*

Outcomes	Effect Sizes	95% CI
Primary outcomes		
VAS		
1-month	0.12	−0.39 to 0.63
3-month	0.75	0.23 to 1.28
6-month	0.87	0.34 to 1.40
12-month	0.73	0.21 to 1.25
PPTs		
1-month	0.25	−0.26 to 0.75
3-month	0.51	0.001 to 1.03
6-month	0.53	0.02 to 1.05
12-month	0.38	−0.13 to 0.90
Secondary outcomes		
WOMAC		
1-month	0.34	−0.17 to 0.85
3-month	0.74	0.22 to 1.26
6-month	0.88	0.35 to 1.41
12-month	0.75	0.23 to 1.28
HHS		
1-month	0.19	−0.31 to 0.70
3-month	0.86	0.33 to 1.39
6-month	0.92	0.39 to 1.45
12-month	0.80	0.27 to 1.33

Notes: The effect size calculated by the Cohen's d (delta value/SD before and after treatment sessions), interpreted as 0.20–0.40 (small), 0.50–0.70 (moderate), and large (0.80 or higher).
Abbreviations: VAS, visual analogue scale; PPTs, pressure pain thresholds; WOMAC, Western Ontario and McMaster Universities Osteoarthritis Index; HHS, Harris Hip Score.

radiological improvements based on the ARCO stages in two early-stage patients (one patient in the PRP group: from ARCO stage II to I, and one in the ESWT group: from ARCO stage I to 0), accompanied by improved clinical outcomes. It is important to acknowledge that the effectiveness of PRP and ESWT is highly related to the disease stages of ONFH. Generally, THA is inevitable in most cases with femoral head collapse (ARCO stage III, IV) in the long term. We also found that two ARCO stage III patients (one in each group) progressed to ARCO stage IV. It is still unclear how PRP injection and ESWT affect the disease course, and future clinical trials with longer follow-up periods are warranted.

Related evidence about the beneficial effects of ESWT is accumulating in both basic and clinical research. It is commonly recognized that the ESWT promotes many cellular activities, which are critical to neovascularization and bone tissue regeneration.[15] Ludwig et al once reported positive results of ESWT in treating ARCO I–III stage patients.[36] In 2012, Vulpiani et al reported that after four sessions of ESWT treatment at 48–72 h intervals (2400 impulses, 0.50 mJ/mm²), the patients were assessed with VAS scores, HHS, and Roles and Maudsley score at 3, 6, 12, and 24 months. They found patients from ARCO stage I–II groups were more likely to benefit from ESWT than those from the ARCO stage III group.[16] The results of our study are basically in line with those observations obtained in the published studies mentioned above. Results from LMM analysis indicated that both PRP injection and ESWT significantly promoted pain relief and functional recovery in ONFH patients over the 12-month follow-up. Notably, the doses of EFD and pulses varied considerably in the clinical trial protocols, which might explain the potential discrepancies among different studies. Generally, most researchers adopted a total of 2400–6000 impulses (single or multiple points) at 0.16–0.62 mJ/mm in one session. In this study, the ESWT doses were determined as 4000 impulses at 0.50 mJ/mm² for four sessions according to the published evidence and our pilot study experience. Future researches might focus on the intensity and impulses adjustment according to patients' tolerance.

246

Dovepress

Luan et al

Subgroup analyses of VAS

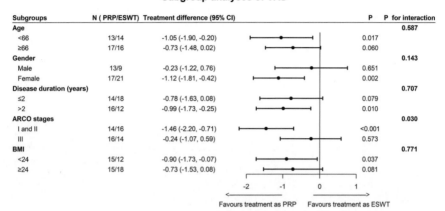

Favours treatment as PRP　　Favours treatment as ESWT

Subgroup analyses of PPTs

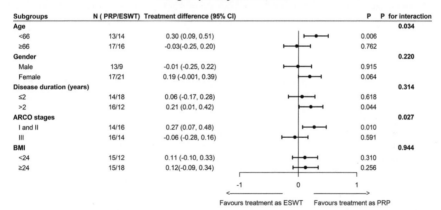

Favours treatment as ESWT　　Favours treatment as PRP

Figure 4 Changes in primary outcomes in two groups by participant characteristics. Subgroup analyses of visual analogue scale and pressure pain thresholds.
Abbreviations: PRP, platelet-rich plasma; ESWT, extracorporeal shock wave therapy; VAS, visual analogue scale; PPTs, pressure pain thresholds; ARCO, Association Research Circulation Osseous; BMI, body mass index.

Promising advances have been made in the surgical treatments for ONFH in the past decades, especially in combination with biological treatments. PRP was originally used in conjunction with the classical core decompression procedure since PRP could augment the therapeutic effects of joint-preserving surgeries for the ONFH. The PRP in association with core decompression has a major regenerative role on necrosis.[17] In intra-articular infiltrations, it could have a pain-reducing role by acting on the synovial membrane, where synovitis is the basis of the joint degenerative process. In a 4.5- to 6-year prospective comparative study, the authors reported that the PRP use after core decompression provided obvious pain relief and functional improvements, which enhanced the survivorship free from THA and retarded ONFH progression.[37] Relatively, the intra-articular injections are less invasive and more

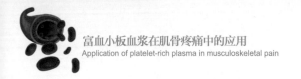

convenient than the surgical procedures, thus the injection therapy might be preferred by the young early-stage patients, especially when the pain symptoms persist. For decades, many studies have explored the possible mechanisms by which PRP promotes repair and tissue regeneration. The PRP treatment has gained widespread attention because of its potential to release a large pool of growth factors, including concentrated levels of vascular endothelial growth factor (VEGF), transforming growth factor-β 1 (TGF-β1), and insulin-like growth factor (IGF).[38] However, few studies have addressed the analgesic effects of PRP. Recently, more and more PRP-related clinical studies focused on its possibility in relieving symptoms and delaying the more invasive surgical treatments in musculoskeletal disease management, especially for osteoarthritis and ONFH. First, some researchers revealed the direct analgesic effects of PRP, which might be achieved by the augmentation of cannabinoid receptors (CB1 and CB2) in pain regulation.[39] Second, recent studies found that a large amount of pain-modulating serotonin (5-hydroxytryptamine, 5-HT) could be discharged from activated PRP, thus the partial analgesic effects could be attributed to the increased 5-HT level. More efforts should be made to further understand the modulatory roles of PRP-derived 5-HT in peripheral nociceptive transmission.[40] Another important possible reason might be the long-lasting effects of PRP in maintaining joint homeostasis.[41] In our study, the intra-articular activation of PRP is finished more physiologically and various biologically active components released from platelets helped promote sequential restoration.

To our knowledge, ultrasound-guided PRP injection for ONFH treatment has rarely been discussed in clinical studies to date, especially in randomized controlled trials. Our current data proved that the intra-articular PRP injection exerted better effects in terms of pain relief and function improvement on ONFH patients when compared to conventional ESWT. A strength of the study was that we conducted the repeated measures analysis using LMMs, and the LMMs are more flexible at handling the dropout and missing data. Another strength of this study was that we reported the relative effect sizes, which indicated the practical significance of the current results for future reference.

The current study still has some limitations. First, the subjects were only followed for up to 12 months, and the follow-up period was relatively short. In this study, we did not perform the MRI at each time point to assess dynamic evolution. Second, we chose the symptomatic ONFH patients as objects of the study. Whether the PRP injection and ESWT influence the disease progression of asymptomatic patients still needs further discussion. Considering the potential PRP preparation and injection regimen variations that existed among different studies, future studies are still required to standardize the PRP treatment protocol.

Abbreviations

PRP, platelet-rich plasma; ESWT, extracorporeal shock wave therapy; THA, total hip arthroplasty; ARCO, Association Research Circulation Osseous; BMI, body mass index; VAS, visual analogue scale; PPTs, pressure pain thresholds; WOMAC, Western Ontario and McMaster Universities Osteoarthritis Index; HHS, Harris Hip Score; LMM, linear mixed model; VEGF, vascular endothelial growth factor; TGF-β1, transforming growth factor-β 1; IGF, insulin-like growth factor.

Data Sharing Statement

The data of this study are available from the first author, Shuo Luan, on request contact luanshuo@mail2.sysu.edu.cn. De-identified data will be made available to qualified researchers by reasonable request.

Ethics Approval and Informed Consent

This study was approved by the Medical Ethics Committee of Sun Yat-sen Memorial Hospital (2019-KY-086). All participants provided written informed consent. The study was conducted according to the guidelines of the Declaration of Helsinki.

Funding

This study was funded by Sun Yat-sen Clinical Research Cultivating Program (SYS-C-202002).

Disclosure

The authors report no conflicts of interest in this work.

248

Dovepress

References

1. Mont MA, Cherian JJ, Sierra RJ, Jones LC, Lieberman JR. Nontraumatic osteonecrosis of the femoral head: where do we stand today? A ten-year update. *J Bone Joint Surg Am*. 2015;97(19):1604–1627. doi:10.2106/JBJS.O.00071

2. Zhao D, Zhang F, Wang B, et al. Guidelines for clinical diagnosis and treatment of osteonecrosis of the femoral head in adults (2019 version). *J Orthop Translat*. 2020;21:100–110. doi:10.1016/j.jot.2019.12.004

3. Cui Q, Jo WL, Koo KH, et al. ARCO consensus on the pathogenesis of non-traumatic osteonecrosis of the femoral head. *J Korean Med Sci*. 2021;36(10):e65. doi:10.3346/jkms.2021.36.e65

4. Di Benedetto P, Niccoli G, Beltrame A, Gisonni R, Cainero V, Causero A. Histopathological aspects and staging systems in non-traumatic femoral head osteonecrosis: an overview of the literature. *Acta Biomed*. 2016;87(Suppl 1):15–24.

5. Yoon BH, Mont MA, Koo KH, et al. The 2019 revised version of association research circulation osseous staging system of osteonecrosis of the femoral head. *J Arthroplasty*. 2020;35(4):933–940. doi:10.1016/j.arth.2019.11.029

6. Bennardo F, Buffone C, Giudice A. New therapeutic opportunities for COVID-19 patients with Tocilizumab: possible correlation of interleukin-6 receptor inhibitors with osteonecrosis of the jaws. *Oral Oncol*. 2020;106:104659. doi:10.1016/j.oraloncology.2020.104659

7. Choi HR, Steinberg ME, Cheng EY. Osteonecrosis of the femoral head: diagnosis and classification systems. *Curr Rev Musculoskelet Med*. 2015;8 (3):210–220. doi:10.1007/s12178-015-9278-7

8. Cao H, Guan H, Lai Y, Qin L, Wang X. Review of various treatment options and potential therapies for osteonecrosis of the femoral head. *J Orthop Translat*. 2016;4:57–70. doi:10.1016/j.jot.2015.09.005

9. Osmani F, Thakkar S, Vigdorchik J. The utility of conservative treatment modalities in the management of osteonecrosis. *Bull NYU Hosp Jt Dis*. 2017;75(3):186–192.

10. Rajpura A, Wright AC, Board TN. Medical management of osteonecrosis of the hip: a review. *Hip Int*. 2011;21(4):385–392. doi:10.5301/HIP.2011.8538

11. Hua KC, Yang XG, Feng JT, et al. The efficacy and safety of core decompression for the treatment of femoral head necrosis: a systematic review and meta-analysis. *J Orthop Surg Res*. 2019;14(1):306. doi:10.1186/s13018-019-1359-7

12. Saito S, Saito M, Nishina T, Ohzono K, Ono K. Long-term results of total hip arthroplasty for osteonecrosis of the femoral head. A comparison with osteoarthritis. *Clin Orthop Relat Res*. 1989;244:198–207.

13. Schreurs BW, Hannink G. Total joint arthroplasty in younger patients: heading for trouble? *Lancet*. 2017;389(10077):1374–1375. doi:10.1016/S0140-6736(17)30190-3

14. Wang CJ, Cheng JH, Huang CC, Yip HK, Russo S. Extracorporeal shockwave therapy for avascular necrosis of femoral head. *Int J Surg*. 2015;24:184–187. doi:10.1016/j.ijsu.2015.06.080

15. Wang CJ, Wang FS, Ko JY, et al. Extracorporeal shockwave therapy shows regeneration in hip necrosis. *Rheumatology*. 2008;47(4):542–546. doi:10.1093/rheumatology/ken020

16. Vulpiani MC, Vetrano M, Trischitta D, et al. Extracorporeal shock wave therapy in early osteonecrosis of the femoral head: prospective clinical study with long-term follow-up. *Arch Orthop Trauma Surg*. 2012;132(4):499–508. doi:10.1007/s00402-011-1444-9

17. Grassi M, Salari P, Massetti D, Papalia GF, Gigante A. Treatment of avascular osteonecrosis of femoral head by core decompression and platelet-rich plasma: a prospective not controlled study. *Int Orthop*. 2020;44(7):1287–1294. doi:10.1007/s00264-020-04628-4

18. Bennell KL, Hunter DJ, Paterson KL. Platelet-rich plasma for the management of hip and knee osteoarthritis. *Curr Rheumatol Rep*. 2017;19(5):24. doi:10.1007/s11926-017-0652-x

19. Lin MT, Wei KC, Wu CH. Effectiveness of platelet-rich plasma injection in rotator cuff tendinopathy: a systematic review and meta-analysis of randomized controlled trials. *Diagnostics*. 2020;10(4). doi:10.3390/diagnostics10040189

20. Fortunato L, Bennardo F, Buffone C, Giudice A. Is the application of platelet concentrates effective in the prevention and treatment of medication-related osteonecrosis of the jaw? A systematic review. *J Craniomaxillofac Surg*. 2020;48(3):268–285. doi:10.1016/j.jcms.2020.01.014

21. Bennardo F, Bennardo L, Del DE, et al. Autologous platelet-rich fibrin injections in the management of facial cutaneous sinus tracts secondary to medication-related osteonecrosis of the jaw. *Dermatol Ther*. 2020;33(3):e13334. doi:10.1111/dth.13334

22. Everts P, Onishi K, Jayaram P, Lana JF, Mautner K. Platelet-rich plasma: new performance understandings and therapeutic considerations in 2020. *Int J Mol Sci*. 2020;21(20):7794. doi:10.3390/ijms21207794

23. Han J, Gao F, Li Y, et al. The use of platelet-rich plasma for the treatment of osteonecrosis of the femoral head: a systematic review. *Biomed Res Int*. 2020;2020:2642439. doi:10.1155/2020/2642439

24. Tao SC, Yuan T, Rui BY, Zhu ZZ, Guo SC, Zhang CQ. Exosomes derived from human platelet-rich plasma prevent apoptosis induced by glucocorticoid-associated endoplasmic reticulum stress in rat osteonecrosis of the femoral head via the Akt/Bad/Bcl-2 signal pathway. *Theranostics*. 2017;7(3):733–750. doi:10.7150/thno.17450

25. Dallari D, Stagni C, Rani N, et al. Ultrasound-guided injection of platelet-rich plasma and hyaluronic acid, separately and in combination, for hip osteoarthritis: a randomized controlled study. *Am J Sports Med*. 2016;44(3):664–671. doi:10.1177/0363546515620383

26. Luan S, Liu C, Lin C, Ma C, Wu S. Platelet-rich plasma for the treatment of adolescent late-stage femoral head necrosis: a case report. *Regen Med*. 2020;15(9):2067–2073. doi:10.2217/rme-2020-0057

27. Ehrich EW, Davies GM, Watson DJ, Bolognese JA, Seidenberg BC, Bellamy N. Minimal perceptible clinical improvement with the Western Ontario and McMaster Universities osteoarthritis index questionnaire and global assessments in patients with osteoarthritis. *J Rheumatol*. 2000;27 (11):2635–2641.

28. Fischer AA. Pressure algometry over normal muscles. Standard values, validity and reproducibility of pressure threshold. *Pain*. 1987;30 (1):115–126. doi:10.1016/0304-3959(87)90089-3

29. Rienstra W, Blikman T, Dijkstra B, et al. Validity of the Dutch modified painDETECT questionnaire for patients with hip or knee osteoarthritis. *Disabil Rehabil*. 2019;41(8):941–947. doi:10.1080/09638288.2017.1413429

30. Bellamy N, Buchanan WW, Goldsmith CH, Campbell J, Stitt LW. Validation study of WOMAC: a health status instrument for measuring clinically important patient relevant outcomes to antirheumatic drug therapy in patients with osteoarthritis of the hip or knee. *J Rheumatol*. 1988;15 (12):1833–1840.

https://doi.org/10.2147/JPR.S347961

DovePress

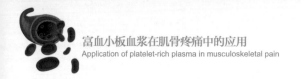

富血小板血浆在肌骨疼痛中的应用
Application of platelet-rich plasma in musculoskeletal pain

31. Harris WH. Traumatic arthritis of the hip after dislocation and acetabular fractures: treatment by mold arthroplasty. An end-result study using a new method of result evaluation. *J Bone Joint Surg Am.* 1969;51(4):737–755. doi:10.2106/00004623-196951040-00012

32. Cohen J. A power primer. *Psychol Bull.* 1992;112(1):155–159. doi:10.1037//0033-2909.112.1.155

33. Xu HH, Li SM, Fang L, et al. Platelet-rich plasma promotes bone formation, restrains adipogenesis and accelerates vascularization to relieve steroids-induced osteonecrosis of the femoral head. *Platelets.* 2020:1–10. doi:10.1080/09537104.2020.1810221

34. Izumi M, Petersen KK, Arendt-Nielsen L, Graven-Nielsen T. Pain referral and regional deep tissue hyperalgesia in experimental human hip pain models. *Pain.* 2014;155(4):792–800. doi:10.1016/j.pain.2014.01.008

35. Mont MA, Jones LC, Hungerford DS. Nontraumatic osteonecrosis of the femoral head: ten years later. *J Bone Joint Surg Am.* 2006;88 (5):1117–1132. doi:10.2106/JBJS.E.01041

36. Ludwig J, Lauber S, Lauber HJ, Dreisilker U, Raedel R, Hotzinger H. High-energy shock wave treatment of femoral head necrosis in adults. *Clin Orthop Relat Res.* 2001;387:119–126. doi:10.1097/00003086-200106000-00016

37. Aggarwal AK, Poornalingam K, Jain A, Prakash M. Combining platelet-rich plasma instillation with core decompression improves functional outcome and delays progression in early-stage avascular necrosis of femoral head: a 4.5- to 6-year prospective randomized comparative study. *J Arthroplasty.* 2021;36(1):54–61. doi:10.1016/j.arth.2020.07.010

38. Giusti I, D'Ascenzo S, Macchiarelli G, Dolo V. In vitro evidence supporting applications of platelet derivatives in regenerative medicine. *Blood Transfus.* 2020;18(2):117–129. doi:10.2450/2019.0164-19

39. Lee HR, Park KM, Joung YK, Park KD, Do SH. Platelet-rich plasma loaded hydrogel scaffold enhances chondrogenic differentiation and maturation with up-regulation of CB1 and CB2. *J Control Release.* 2012;159(3):332–337. doi:10.1016/j.jconrel.2012.02.008

40. Mammadova-Bach E, Mauler M, Braun A, Duerschmied D. Autocrine and paracrine regulatory functions of platelet serotonin. *Platelets.* 2018;29 (6):541–548. doi:10.1080/09537104.2018.1478072

41. Filardo G, Kon E, Roffi A, Di Matteo B, Merli ML, Marcacci M. Platelet-rich plasma: why intra-articular? A systematic review of preclinical studies and clinical evidence on PRP for joint degeneration. *Knee Surg Sports Traumatol Arthrosc.* 2015;23(9):2459–2474. doi:10.1007/s00167-013-2743-1

Journal of Pain Research

Dovepress

Publish your work in this journal

The Journal of Pain Research is an international, peer reviewed, open access, online journal that welcomes laboratory and clinical findings in the fields of pain research and the prevention and management of pain. Original research, reviews, symposium reports, hypothesis formation and commentaries are all considered for publication. The manuscript management system is completely online and includes a very quick and fair peer-review system, which is all easy to use. Visit http://www.dovepress.com/testimonials.php to read real quotes from published authors.

Submit your manuscript here: https://www.dovepress.com/journal-of-pain-research-journal

250

Hindawi
Neural Plasticity
Volume 2021, Article ID 5558138, 11 pages
https://doi.org/10.1155/2021/5558138

Research Article

Ultrasound-Guided Transforaminal Injections of Platelet-Rich Plasma Compared with Steroid in Lumbar Disc Herniation: A Prospective, Randomized, Controlled Study

Zhen Xu [ID], Shaoling Wu [ID], Xiao Li [ID], Cuicui Liu [ID], Shengnuo Fan [ID], and Chao Ma [ID]

Department of Rehabilitation Medicine, Sun Yat-sen Memorial Hospital, Sun Yat-sen University, Guangzhou, Guangdong 510120, China

Correspondence should be addressed to Chao Ma; machao@mail.sysu.edu.cn

Received 3 February 2021; Revised 10 May 2021; Accepted 15 May 2021; Published 27 May 2021

Academic Editor: Xue-Qiang Wang

Copyright © 2021 Zhen Xu et al. This is an open access article distributed under the Creative Commons Attribution License, which permits unrestricted use, distribution, and reproduction in any medium, provided the original work is properly cited.

Transforaminal steroid injection is extensively used as a treatment in cases of herniated disc, but it is associated with complications. In comparison, platelet-rich plasma (PRP) injection has been used in musculoskeletal disorders and could be another option. This study is aimed at comparing the efficacy and safety aspects between ultrasound-guided transforaminal injections of PRP and steroid in patients who suffer from radicular pain due to lumbar disc herniation. In a randomized controlled trial, ultrasound-guided transforaminal injections of either PRP ($n = 61$) or steroid ($n = 63$) were administered to a total of 124 patients who suffer from radicular pain due to lumbar disc herniation. Patients were assessed by the visual analogue scale (VAS), pressure pain thresholds (PPTs), Oswestry disability index (ODI), and the physical function (PF) and bodily pain (BP) domains of the 36-item short form health survey (SF-36) before operation and 1 week, 1 month, 3 months, 6 months, and 12 months after operation. The rate and latency of F-wave were obtained before operation and 12 months postoperation. There was no statistical difference in terms of age and sex between both groups. Statistically significant improvements from the patients' data before operation to data obtained 1-month postoperation were observed in VAS, PPTs, ODI, and PF and BP of SF-36 in both groups and kept for 1 year. F-wave rate and latency were improved significantly at 1-year postoperation in both groups. Intergroup differences during follow-ups over a period of 1 year were not found to be significant in all the above assessment between the PRP and steroid groups. No complications were reported. The results showed similar outcome for both transforaminal injections using PRP and steroid in the treatment of lumbar disc herniation, suggesting the possible application of PRP injection as a safer alternative. The trial was registered in the Chinese Clinical Trial Registry (ChiCTR-INR-17011825).

1. Introduction

Low back pain is one of the most difficult conditions to manage for doctors, patients, and policymakers. Not only does it limit physical activity, life quality is also greatly reduced alongside additional social and economic burden. The point prevalence of low back pain is 12%, with its one-year prevalence being 38% and the lifetime prevalence being approximately 40% [1]. Aging population leads to the rising number of individuals affected by low back pain. Lumbar disc herniation has been identified as the common etiology of low back pain [2]. The treatments for lumbar disc herniation vary from conservative to surgical management, which include analgesics, traction, physical therapy, manipulation, and psychotherapy. However, not all patients are able to be relieved from pain through these treatments.

For over 30 years, epidural steroid injection has been widely used as a treatment for lumbar disc herniation [3, 4], with its effectiveness proven by multiple research [5–7]. It works in anti-inflammation, pain relief, and functional improvement. There are three routes for steroid injection: interlaminar, transforaminal, and caudal routes. The transforaminal route fared better than the other two because it could reach the targeted sites, namely, spinal nerve, anterior epidural space, and the dorsal root ganglion, to counteract the inflammation secondary to compression [8]. However, there are still concerns about the safety of epidural steroid injection. Based on literature, several complications related to epidural steroid injection have been pointed out, including neurotoxicity, pharmacologic effect of steroid (hypercorticism, adrenal suppression, and hyperglycemia), and neurologic injury [8, 9]. Besides, the contraindications of steroid use (allergy, diabetes, severe osteoporosis, pregnancy, severe hypertension, infection, etc.) limit the usage of epidural steroid injection.

Platelet-rich plasma (PRP), a biological product from the centrifugation of autologous blood with a high number of platelets in a small volume of plasma, has a positive effect on pain relief in some musculoskeletal diseases, especially osteoarthritis, tendinosis, and ligament tears [10]. PRP contains high concentration of growth factors (GFs) and cytokines that play important roles in anti-inflammatory, antiapoptotic, and proliferative effects on the neurons and fibroblasts [11]. Although the role of PRP in pain relief looks promising, the effect of transforaminal PRP injection in lumbar disc herniation with radicular pain remains unclear.

Henceforth, this study is aimed at investigating the efficacy and safety of ultrasound-guided platelet-rich plasma injections compared with steroid injections in treating lumbar disc herniation with radicular pain.

2. Materials and Methods

2.1. Study Design and Participant Recruitment. A prospective, randomized, and controlled study was carried out to compare the treatment of lumbar disc herniation with radicular pain with ultrasound-guided transforaminal steroid or PRP injections. This study was approved by the Ethics Committee of Sun Yat-sen Memorial Hospital, and the trial was registered with the Chinese Clinical Trial Registry (registration number: ChiCTR-INR-17011825). This investigation was conducted in accordance with the Declaration of Helsinki. 184 patients were assessed for eligibility based on the inclusion and exclusion criteria listed as follows.

Inclusion criteria are as follows: (1) aged 20-60 years; (2) low back pain with unilateral lower limb radicular pain, duration of more than 3 months; (3) posterolateral lumbar disc herniation of L4/L5 or L5/S1 segment diagnosed by MRI or CT and consistent with the clinical symptoms and signs; (4) degree of pain (VAS) more than 5 and obvious symptoms and clinical signs of nerve root irritation; (5) had received conservative treatment, including physical therapy, manipulation, and nonmorphine treatment; (6) no symptoms of severe nerve damage including motor paralysis, muscle atrophy, and cauda equina syndrome; (7) had no history of spinal surgery.

Exclusion criteria are as follows: (1) infection; (2) had received prior injection treatment in the past 3 months, such as nerve root injection and caudal injection; (3) spinal tumors or tuberculosis; (4) multisegmental lumbar disc herniation, spinal deformity, or spinal stenosis; (5) not suitable for local injection; (6) allergic to the drug used in this study; (7) a history of drug abuse or oral anticoagulation; (8) pregnancy; (9) severe diabetes; (10) clinical diagnosis of heart disease, liver and kidney dysfunction, and hematological diseases; (11) abnormal psychological and cognitive disorders.

52 patients were not enrolled in this study (31 patients either did not meet the inclusion criteria or met the exclusion criteria, while the other 21 patients declined to participate). The randomization sequence was produced by a statistician, who did not contact with patients, using a random number generator. The other 132 patients who were enrolled were simply randomized at a ratio of 1 : 1 to 2 groups: the steroid group (control group, $n = 68$) and the PRP group (experimental group, $n = 64$). The randomization was performed by the nurse, who did not participate in the process of patient assessment, by opening the numbered sealed opaque envelop. A written informed consent was obtained from each patient before enrollment. During follow-ups over 1 year, 4 patients did not receive allocated intervention and 4 others did not follow through. Thus, only 124 patients were included for data analysis (steroid group $n = 63$, PRP group $n = 61$) (Figure 1).

2.2. Study Procedure. The patients who were enrolled to this study underwent physical examination, neurological examination, and laboratory tests. The operation was performed at the operating room in the rehabilitation medicine department of Sun Yat-sen Memorial Hospital.

The procedure of PRP preparation was as follows: 18 ml blood sample was drawn from the anterior elbow vein and mixed with 2 ml of 3.8% (w/v) sodium citrate. The blood sample was then centrifuged at 1600 rpm for 10 minutes at room temperature (RT, 23°C) under aseptic condition to divide the sample into 3 layers. The lower layers composed of red blood cells were subsequently removed. The remaining sample was transferred into a new centrifuge tube and was centrifuged again at 3200 rpm for 10 minutes at RT. 4 ml was collected from the lower part which contains PRP. 1 ml of this PRP was then sent for quantitative analysis of platelet count.

The procedure of operation was as follows. An experienced physician performed the ultrasound-guided transforaminal injection using an ultrasonic device (Konica Minolta Medical & Graphic (Shanghai) Company limited, SONIMAGE HS1 PLUS, Tokyo, Japan) in out-of-plane approach. The patients were prepared in prone position with a pillow under their abdomen. The area of injection was disinfected. The sacral spinous process and the fifth lumbar spinous process transducer were identified when transducer placed longitudinally. The transducer in midline was moved laterally to recognize the lamina, transverse process, and facet joint. Then, the edge of the zygapophyseal joints was obtained when the transducer was moved back. The needle (22 G) was subsequently inserted into the skin using the out-of-plane approach upon determination of injection level to ensure that the needle tip was positioned in the middle of adjacent facet joints. After an inhalation test yielding negative results for cerebrospinal fluid and blood aspiration, the injection was administered (steroid group: 2 ml betamethasone+0.5 ml 0.9% sterile saline+0.5 ml 2% lidocaine; PRP group: 3 ml autologous PRP) (Figure 2). The detail of the ultrasound-guided out-of-plane injection can be found in this reference [12].

In the follow-up, some short-acting analgesics were given to patients when they felt obvious pain. The patients would

Neural Plasticity   3

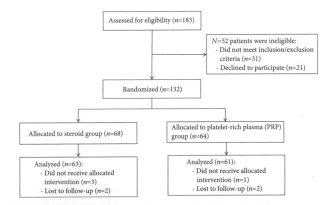

FIGURE 1: Flow diagram of enrolment, randomization, and analysis.

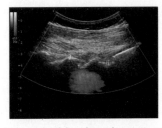

FIGURE 2: Ultrasound-guided transforaminal injection in out-of-plane approach. Ultrasound-guided transforaminal injection was performed, and the needle tip was positioned in the middle of (i) L5/S1 facet joint and (ii) sacral foramina. The red signal represented the spreading of drug in targeted epidural space.

be excluded from this study in follow-up when patients had any one of the following situations: (1) had overloaded pain which affects their life quality; (2) had symptom of motor paralysis, muscle atrophy, or cauda equina syndrome in the follow-up period; (3) transforaminal epidural injection failed to improve pain or function of patients during 3 months postoperation. Treatments including surgery or conservative treatments were given to those excluded patients.

2.3. Assessment and Outcome. The statistics of demographic characteristics, including gender and age, as well as baseline information of patients were collected upon admission of the patients. Baseline information was obtained before operation, which includes visual analogue scale (VAS), pressure pain thresholds (PPTs), the rate and latency of F-wave, Oswestry disability index (ODI), and physical function (PF) and bodily pain (BP) from the 36-item short form health survey (SF-36). Each patient was required to complete the same assessments as the baseline information (except F-wave rate and latency) at 1 week, 1 month, 3 months, 6 months, and

1 year postoperation. F-wave rate and latency were obtained only 1 year postoperation. All assessments were independently performed by two experienced blinded doctors.

The visual analogue scale (VAS) was a method to evaluate the degree of pain. A 10 cm line was used as an indicator whereby one end represents no pain, while the other end represents the most severe pain imagined. The patient was asked to indicate the point on the line which could represent the patient's pain level [13].

The pressure pain thresholds (PPTs) were measured by an algometry device (Pain Diagnostics and Thermography Corporation, Model PTH AF2, Great Neck, NY 11023) according to the procedure recommended by Fischer [14]. A plastic tip was placed at the paraspinal tenderness point in the segment with lumbar disc herniation. Detailed description can be found in our previous article [15].

The rate and latency of F-wave in the affected side were measured by electromyogram. The recording electrode was placed at the muscle belly of abductor halluces of the affected side; the reference electrode was placed at the tendon of abductor halluces; the stimulation electrode was placed at the tibial nerve behind the medial malleolus; the ground wire was placed at the ankle joint between the stimulation electrode and the recording electrode. At stimulation points of the affected side, 20 consecutive stimuli at the frequency of 1 Hz and the width of 0.2 ms were induced, obtaining records of the rate and latency of F-waves at the affected sides.

There were 10 items in the Oswestry disability index (ODI), including pain, individual function, and personal comprehensive function. The minimum score for each item is 0 (good state), whereas the highest score is 5 (poor state). The Oswestry disability index referred to the percentage of the sum of score from all 10 items out of 50.

The 36-item short form health survey (SF-36) consisted of 36 items, which includes one scale on health transition and 8 domains. The score for each domain ranges from 0 (poor health) to 100 (good health). The reliability, validity, and application of the Chinese version SF-36 have been

TABLE 1: Demographic characteristics and baseline information of patients.

	Steroid group ($n = 63$)	PRP group ($n = 61$)	P value
Age (y, median (1st-3rd))	56.0 (50.0-59.0)	56.0 (44.5-60.0)	0.910
Female (N (%))	26 (41.3)	33 (54.1)	0.153
VAS (median (1st-3rd))	6.0 (5.0-7.0)	6.0 (6.0-7.25)	0.106
PPTs (kPa, median (1st-3rd))	598.74 (535.24-607.81)	580.60 (557.92-601.01)	0.703
F-wave rate (%, median (1st-3rd))	82.0 (80-95)	82.0 (80.0-85.0)	0.161
F-wave latency (ms, median (1st-3rd))	48.9 (47.8-50.8)	48.7 (46.9-49.7)	0.217
ODI (%, median (1st-3rd))	27.0 (21.0-43.0)	35.0 (26.35-44.0)	0.193
PF of SF-36 (median (1st-3rd))	65.0 (55.0-80.0)	60.0 (45.0-70.0)	0.091
BP of SF-36 (median (1st-3rd))	41.0 (41.0-52.0)	41.0 (31.0-51.0)	0.428

PRP: platelet-rich plasma; 1st-3rd: 1st-3rd quartiles; PPTs: pressure pain thresholds; VAS: visual analogue scale; ODI: Oswestry disability index; SF-36: the 36-item short form health survey; PF: physical function; BP: bodily pain.

proven [16]. In this study, two domains were recorded, namely, the physical function (PF) and bodily pain (BP) domains.

2.4. Statistical Analysis. With a sample size of 60 patients each group, we calculated that the study would have the power of 80% to detect a 0.9 difference at the significant improvement in VAS between groups from baseline to 6 months with the 2 standard deviation of the change in VAS. The mean and standard deviation were based on data from previous literature and our previous study [17, 18]. Besides, there was an increase of 15% in sample size in each group in case of the loss to follow-up. Two-sided α level was 0.05.

Data were analyzed using the SPSS 23.0 software. The continuous variables were expressed by mean ± standard deviation or medians (1st-3rd quartiles) depending on data distribution, while the discrete variable (such as sex) was described as n (%). The Shapiro-Wilk test was used to test the data distribution of the continuous variables. Continuous data before operation with nonnormal distribution was analyzed using the Mann–Whitney U test, whereas the discrete variable was analyzed by the χ^2/Fisher exact test. To compare the difference between the steroid group and the PRP group over time, the generalized estimating equation was used to estimate the time × treatment interaction. A negative interaction represents the ability of the generalized estimating equation in indicating the difference between the steroid and PRP groups over time. If the interaction existed, the Mann–Whitney U test can be used to compare the difference between both groups at the same time point. The Friedman test was used to evaluate the difference between different time points within one group, while the post hoc test was used to compare the data between preoperation and postoperation in one group. The Wilcoxon signed-rank test was used for paired sample in one group. The difference is considered statistically significant when bilateral $\alpha = 0.05$, $P < 0.05$.

3. Results

3.1. Patient Characteristics. There were 124 patients who completed follow-ups over the period of 1 year with 63 patients in the steroid group and 61 patients in the PRP

group. There was no statistically significant difference in age and gender between both groups ($P > 0.05$) (Table 1). Besides, no statistically significant differences were found in VAS, PPTs, F-wave rates and latency, ODI, and physical function (PF) and bodily pain (BP) domains of SF-36 between the two groups before operation ($P > 0.05$) (Table 1).

3.2. PRP Longitudinal Data. The PRP group consisted of 61 participants who were enrolled and completed the follow-ups over 1 year. There was no significant difference in terms of VAS, PPTs, ODI, and the PF and BP domains of SF-36 in 1 week postoperation compared to corresponding basal values (median (1st-3rd quartiles); 6.0 (6.0-7.3) vs. 5.0 (5.0-6.0), $P = 0.887$; 580.60 kPa (557.92-601.01) vs. 625.96 kPa (571.53-716.68), $P = 0.087$; 35.0% (26.4-44.0) vs. 27.0% (20.0-40.0), $P = 0.125$; 60.0 (45.0-70.0) vs. 75.0 (60.0-90.0), $P = 0.284$; 41.0 (31.0-51.0) vs. 43.0 (41.0-52.0), $P = 0.794$, respectively). Statistically significant improvements were observed in terms of VAS, PPTs, ODI, and the PF and BP domains of SF-36 in 1-month postoperation compared to corresponding basal values (Tables 2 and 3). The median (1st-3rd quartiles) VAS was 6.0 (6.0-7.3), which decreased significantly to 3.0 (3.0-4.0) 1 month after operation ($P < 0.001$). Over the same period of time, PPTs had also significantly improved from 580.60 kPa (557.92-601.01) to 707.60 kPa (612.35-780.18) ($P < 0.001$), and ODI reduced from 35.0% (26.4-44.0) to 22.0% (14.25-42.5) ($P < 0.001$). The PF and BP domains of SF-36 had also significantly improved from baseline (60.0 (45.0-70.0) and 41.0 (31.0-51.0), respectively) to 1 month postoperation (88.0 (76.5-95.0), $P < 0.001$; 52.0 (41.0-62.0), $P < 0.001$, respectively). In the PRP group, statistically significant differences were also observed between baseline VAS, PPTs, ODI, and PF and BP domains of SF-36 and the same set of data from 3 months, 6 months, and 1 year postoperation (Tables 2 and 3). F-wave rate was higher after the administration of transforaminal PRP injection, increasing from 82.0% (80.0%-85.0%) to 95.0% (92.0%-100.0%) 1 year after operation ($P < 0.001$). Significant decrease in F-wave latency was observed in the PRP group, where it decreases from 48.7 ms (46.9-49.7) to 45.2 ms (44.5-46.2) 1 year postoperation ($P < 0.001$) (Table 3).

TABLE 2: Longitudinal outcomes of pain degree and spinal function for the PRP group over time.

Outcome	Time	PRP group ($n = 61$)	P value[#]
	Baseline	6.0 (6.0-7.3)	Ref
	1 week	5.0 (5.0-6.0)	0.887
	1 month	3.0 (3.0-4.0)	<0.001
VAS (median (1st-3rd))	3 months	3.0 (3.0-3.0)	<0.001
	6 months	3.0 (2.0-3.0)	<0.001
	1 year	2.0 (1.0-3.0)	<0.001
	P value over time[†]	<0.001	
	Baseline	580.60 (557.92-601.01)	Ref
	1 week	625.96 (571.53-716.68)	0.087
	1 month	707.60 (612.35-780.18)	<0.001
PPTs (kPa, median (1st-3rd))	3 months	725.75 (698.53-843.68)	<0.001
	6 months	725.75 (694.00-823.27)	<0.001
	1 year	730.28 (694.00-789.25)	<0.001
	P value over time[†]	<0.001	
	Baseline	35.0 (26.4-44.0)	Ref
	1 week	27.0 (20.0-40.0)	0.125
	1 month	22.0 (14.3-42.5)	<0.001
ODI (%, median (1st-3rd))	3 months	20.0 (16.5-29.0)	<0.001
	6 months	20.0 (14.0-29.0)	<0.001
	1 year	19.0 (15.5-30.0)	<0.001
	P value over time[†]	0.001	

PRP: platelet-rich plasma; 1st-3rd: 1st-3rd quartiles; PPTs: pressure pain thresholds; VAS: visual analogue scale; ODI: Oswestry disability index. [#]P value compares difference from baseline using post hoc test or Wilcoxon signed-rank test. [†]P value indicates significance of overall change over time using the Friedman test.

3.3. Steroid Longitudinal Data. The steroid group consisted of 63 patients who completed all the follow-up sessions over 1 year. There was no significant difference in terms of VAS, PPTs, ODI, and the PF and BP domains of SF-36 in 1 week postoperation compared to corresponding basal values (median (1st-3rd quartiles); 6.0 (5.0-7.0) vs. 6.0 (5.0-6.0), $P = 1.000$; 598.74 kPa (535.24-607.81) vs. 598.74 kPa (526.17-694.00), $P = 0.683$; 27.0% (21.0-43.0) vs. 23.0% (20.0-40.0), $P = 0.645$; 65.0 (55.0-80.0) vs. 70.0 (60.0-90.0), $P = 0.152$; 41.0 (41.0-52.0) vs. 47.0 (41.0-61.0), $P = 1.000$, respectively). Significant improvement was observed from baseline VAS, PPTs, ODI, and PF and BP domains of SF-36 to the same set of data from 1 month postoperation (Tables 4 and 5). During this period of time, VAS decreased from 6.0 (5.0-7.0) to 3.0 (3.0-5.0) ($P < 0.001$); PPTs increased from 598.74 kPa (535.24-607.81) to 598.74 kPa (526.17-694.00) ($P < 0.001$); ODI significantly decreased from 27.0% (21.0-43.0) to 18.0% (12.0-29.0) ($P < 0.001$), whereas the PF and BP domains of SF-36 all improved statistically from baseline (65.0 (55.0-80.0) and 41.0 (41.0-52.0), respectively) to 1 month postoperation (88.0 (75.0-95.0), $P < 0.001$; 52.0 (41.0-72.0), $P = 0.004$, respectively). Statistical differences were found between baseline VAS, PPTs, ODI, and PF and BP domains of SF-36 in the steroid group and data obtained from 3 months, 6 months, and 1 year postoperation (Tables 4 and 5). The F-wave rate had significantly increased from 82.0% (80.0-95.0) to 95.0% (90.0-100.0) 1 year postoperation ($P < 0.001$), while the F-wave latency had significantly

decreased from 48.9 ms (47.8-50.8) to 45.2 ms (43.6-46.3) 1 year post operation ($P < 0.001$) (Table 5).

3.4. Intergroup Differences. During the 1-year follow-up period in this study, both the PRP and steroid groups demonstrated obvious improvements in terms of VAS score (Figure 3(a)), PPTs (Figure 3(b)), F-wave rate (Figure 4(a)) and latency (Figure 4(b)), ODI (Figure 3(c)), and the PF (Figure 3(d)) and BP (Figure 3(e)) domains of SF-36. Anyhow, intergroup differences during this 1-year follow-up period were not found to be significant in all tests involved (Figures 3 and 4).

3.5. Safety. No complications or adverse effects were reported after the ultrasound-guided transforaminal injection of PRP or steroid during the 1-year follow-up period.

4. Discussion

This study shows that ultrasound-guided transforaminal injection of both PRP and steroid leads to the significant improvement in the aspects of pain relief, nerve repair, spinal function, and life quality. Furthermore, the outcome after one whole year of follow-up has proven that these improvements stay effective for long term. Besides, no complications or side effects were found during any of the follow-ups.

Results from this study are in accordance with a series of clinical studies which have described the effectiveness of

富血小板血浆在肌骨疼痛中的应用
Application of platelet-rich plasma in musculoskeletal pain

TABLE 3: Longitudinal outcomes of life quality and nerve function for the PRP group over time.

Outcome	Time	PRP group ($n = 61$)	P value[#]
PF of SF-36 (median (1st-3rd))	Baseline	60.0 (45.0-70.0)	Ref
	1 week	75.0 (60.0-90.0)	0.284
	1 month	88.0 (76.5-95.0)	<0.001
	3 months	90.0 (82.5-95.0)	<0.001
	6 months	90.0 (87.5-93.0)	<0.001
	1 year	90.0 (90.0-95.0)	<0.001
	P value over time[†]	<0.001	
BP of SF-36 (median (1st-3rd))	Baseline	41.0 (31.0-51.0)	Ref
	1 week	43.0 (41.0-52.0)	0.794
	1 month	52.0 (41.0-62.0)	0.005
	3 months	82.0 (61.0-94.0)	<0.001
	6 months	74.0 (62.0-85.5)	<0.001
	1 year	74.0 (64.0-87.0)	<0.001
	P value over time[†]	<0.001	
F-wave rate (%, median (1st-3rd))	Baseline	82.0 (80.0-85.0)	Ref
	1 year	95.0 (92.0-100.0)	<0.001
F-wave latency (ms, median (1st-3rd))	Baseline	48.7 (46.9-49.7)	Ref
	1 year	45.2 (44.5-46.2)	<0.001

PRP: platelet-rich plasma; 1st-3rd: 1st-3rd quartiles; SF-36: the 36-item short form health survey; PF: physical function; BP: bodily pain. [#]P value compares difference from baseline using post hoc test or Wilcoxon signed-rank test. [†]P value indicates significance of overall change over time using the Friedman test.

TABLE 4: Longitudinal outcomes of pain degree and spinal function for the steroid group over time.

Outcome	Time	Steroid group ($n = 63$)	P value[#]
VAS (median (1st-3rd))	Baseline	6.0 (5.0-7.0)	Ref
	1 week	6.0 (5.0-6.0)	1.000
	1 month	3.0 (3.0-5.0)	<0.001
	3 months	3.0 (2.0-4.0)	<0.001
	6 months	2.0 (2.0-3.0)	<0.001
	1 year	2.0 (1.0-3.0)	<0.001
	P value over time[†]	<0.001	
PPTs (kPa, median (1st-3rd))	Baseline	598.74 (535.24-607.81)	Ref
	1 week	598.74 (526.17-694.00)	0.683
	1 month	739.36 (607.81-807.39)	<0.001
	3 months	739.36 (698.53-943.47)	<0.001
	6 months	725.75 (694.00-780.18)	<0.001
	1 year	716.68 (694.00-762.04)	<0.001
	P value over time[†]	<0.001	
ODI (%, median (1st-3rd))	Baseline	27.0 (21.0-43.0)	Ref
	1 week	23.0 (20.0-40.0)	0.645
	1 month	18.0 (12.0-29.0)	<0.001
	3 months	20.0 (12.0-29.0)	<0.001
	6 months	20.0 (16.3-29.0)	<0.001
	1 year	20.0 (17.3-40.0)	<0.001
	P value over time[†]	0.001	

1st-3rd: 1st-3rd quartiles; PPTs: pressure pain thresholds; VAS: visual analogue scale; ODI: Oswestry disability index. [#]P value compares difference from baseline using post hoc test or Wilcoxon signed-rank test. [†]P value indicates significance of overall change over time using the Friedman test.

TABLE 5: Longitudinal outcomes of life quality and nerve function for the steroid group over time.

Outcome	Time	Steroid group ($n = 63$)	P value[#]
PF of SF-36 (median (1st-3rd))	Baseline	65.0 (55.0-80.0)	Ref
	1 week	70.0 (60.0-90.0)	0.152
	1 month	88.0 (75.0-95.0)	<0.001
	3 months	90.0 (70.0-95.0)	<0.001
	6 months	90.0 (88.0-95.0)	<0.001
	1 year	90.0 (80.0-95.0)	<0.001
	P value over time[†]	<0.001	
BP of SF-36 (median (1st-3rd))	Baseline	41.0 (41.0-52.0)	Ref
	1 week	47.0 (41.0-61.0)	1.000
	1 month	52.0 (41.0-72.0)	0.004
	3 months	74.0 (51.0-94.0)	<0.001
	6 months	72.0 (62.0-94.0)	<0.001
	1 year	74.0 (62.0-94.0)	<0.001
	P value over time[†]	<0.001	
F-wave rate (%, median (1st-3rd))	Baseline	82.0 (80.0-95.0)	Ref
	1 year	95.0 (90.0-100.0)	<0.001
F-wave latency (ms, median (1st-3rd))	Baseline	48.9 (47.8-50.8)	Ref
	1 year	45.2 (43.6-46.3)	<0.001

1st-3rd: 1st-3rd quartiles; SF-36: the 36-item short form health survey; PF: physical function; BP: bodily pain. [#]P value compares difference from baseline using post hoc test or Wilcoxon signed-rank test. [†]P value indicates significance of overall change over time using the Friedmann test.

epidural PRP injections for treating lumbar disc herniation with radicular pain [19–21]. In a nonrandomized comparative trial performed by Bise et al. on 60 patients with lumbar radicular pain in 2020, the CT-guided epidural PRP injection therapy was shown to cause significant pain reduction and functional improvement, which were measured using the numerical rating scale (NRS) and the Oswestry disability index (ODI). The effects of PRP injection were sustained for 6 weeks with no complications reported [19]. Centeno et al. investigated the efficacy of C-arm fluoroscopy-guided epidural platelet lysate injections in patients with lumbar radicular pain and found significant improvement in pain and function from baseline data to data obtained throughout the 2 years of follow-up period, suggesting the potential of PRP as a promising alternative to epidural steroids [20]. In this study, the PF and BP domains from SF-36 showed significant improvement at 1 month after operation and persisted for at least one year in the PRP group. However, there is no statistically significant difference between the PRP group and the steroid group in terms of the PF and BP domains of SF-36. In a randomized, controlled, and double-blinded study performed on 50 patients with complex chronic degenerative spinal pain, Ruiz-Lopez et al. found similar improvement with SF-36 scores measured at 6 months in the PRP group of fluoroscopically guided caudal epidural injection, whereas the steroid group only showed improvement in the BP of SF-36 [22]. Variation in routes of epidural injection and the type of degenerative spinal pain may attribute to these differences in the results.

F-wave measurement helps to assess conduction of impulse along the peripheral motor nerve, including most of its proximal segment. This investigation revealed the significant decrease in F-wave latencies and increase of F-wave rate in both the PRP and steroid groups, indicating the nerve repair function of PRP and steroid. Steroid has positive effects on the F-wave in peripheral nerve disorder, such as chronic inflammatory demyelinating polyradiculopathy and Guillain-Barré syndrome. One study reported that local steroid injection could help to decrease the F-wave latency in carpal tunnel syndrome [23]. Although no studies were found to support the claim about the impact of epidural PRP injection on F-wave latency and the rate in lumbar radicular pain, several studies have reported the positive role of PRP in nerve healing and reduction of neuropathic pain [24, 25]. Anjayani et al. investigated the efficacy of PRP injection in leprosy peripheral neuropathy, which shows the effect of PRP on nerve regeneration and improvement of peripheral neuropathy sensibility [24].

In recent years, PRP has been widely used in treating musculoskeletal diseases due to its anti-inflammatory properties and ability in promoting the processes of endogenous healing by delivering a high concentration of growth factors and cytokines [23, 26]. These growth factors, such as vascular endothelial growth factor (VEGF), transforming growth factor β-1 (TGFβ-1), platelet-derived growth factor (PDGF), and insulin-like growth factor-1 (IGF-1), are contained within the α-granules of platelets [26–29]. Within 10 minutes after PRP injection, the platelets aggregate and clot at the targeted site with almost 95% of the α-granules load being secreted within 1 hour [21]. Studies have shown that these growth factors are effective in promoting proliferation, angiogenesis, and synthesis of extracellular matrix proteins [26, 30–32].

富血小板血浆在肌骨疼痛中的应用
Application of platelet-rich plasma in musculoskeletal pain

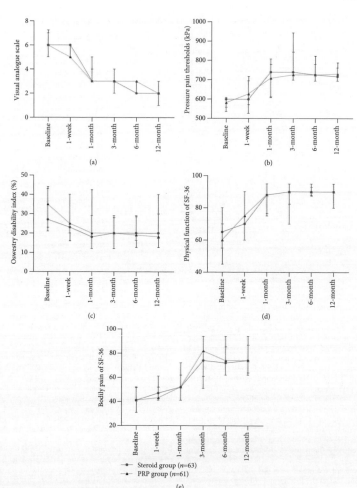

FIGURE 3: Comparison of patient-reported outcomes between the PRP ($n = 61$) and steroid ($n = 63$) groups over time (median, quartile). There was no significant difference in the (a) visual analogue scale, (b) pressure pain thresholds, (c) Oswestry disability index, and (d) physical function and (e) bodily pain domains of the 36-item short form health survey (SF-36) between the PRP group and the steroid group during follow-ups over the course of one year. The error bars represent the 1st quartile and the 3rd quartile.

Therefore, the key rationale behind the application of PRP is to increase the concentration of platelets at the targeted sites so that cytokines and GFs may be released. This will consequently allow the regulation of inflammation and immunological responses of tissue healing [21, 33].

In this investigation, sonography was used to guide transforaminal PRP and steroid injection. The outcomes of nerve root block under the guidance of sonography have proven to be similar to those of injections being guided by either computed tomography scan or X-ray [34–36]. Furthermore, sonography provides the advantages of real-time and dynamic observation with high accuracy, safe, convenient, no radiation, and avoidance of nerve or vessel injury.

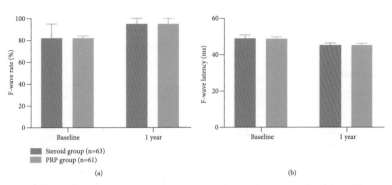

Steroid group (n=63)
PRP group (n=61)

(a)   (b)

FIGURE 4: Comparison of F-wave rate and latency between the PRP ($n = 61$) and steroid ($n = 63$) groups. No significant difference was found in terms of F-wave (a) rate and (b) latency between the PRP group and the steroid group both before and after operation. The error bars represent the 3rd quartile.

No major complications and side effects were reported during the 1-year follow-up period in this study. Only one study reported very rare ischemic complications with lumbar epidural steroid injection by the interlaminar route [37]. Meanwhile, hematomas and infection are known to be the main complications of epidural steroid injection [38, 39]. Henceforth, this makes the autologous PRP a possibly safer alternative with low risks of infection and allergy, since PRP is derived from the patient's own blood and due to the presence of antibacterial proteins in platelets [40]. Furthermore, the systemic side effects of steroid can also be avoided with transforaminal PRP injection [41–43].

Nonetheless, there is currently a lack of standard procedure in PRP production for PRP therapy although a vast variety of formulations and techniques for PRP production is available. Other than that, the cost-effectiveness of PRP treatment remains controversial. On the one hand, the cost of PRP in Europe is reported to be about twice as much as the cost of steroid treatment [44]; on the other hand, a study reported that the cost of PRP therapy for treating orthopedic conditions may actually be less in the long run albeit it appearing to be more expensive than steroid injection in the short term [45].

This study was designed to focus on the long-term treatment effect of transforaminal injection of steroid or platelet-rich plasma (PRP) on lumbar disc herniation. Thus, the evaluation time points were mainly set at 1 month, 3 months, 6 months, and 1 year. The limitation of this study was the lack of short-term evaluation time point, including 2 weeks and 3 weeks. It could be further explored in future clinical trial.

5. Conclusions

This study suggests that ultrasound-guided transforaminal PRP injections yield similar effect as transforaminal steroid injections in treating lumbar disc herniation with radicular pain and that it may be a safer alternative in comparison.

Abbreviations

PRP: Platelet-rich plasma
PPTs: Pressure pain thresholds
VAS: Visual analogue scale
ODI: Oswestry disability index
PF: Physical function
BP: Bodily pain
SF-36:   36-item short form health survey
GFs: Growth factors
NRS: Numerical rating scale
VEGF: Vascular endothelial growth factor
TGFβ-1:   Transforming growth factor β-1
PDGF: Platelet-derived growth factor
IGF-1:   Insulin-like growth factor-1.

Data Availability

Participant original data used to support the findings of this study are available in http://www.medresman.org.cn/pub/cn/proj/search.aspx.

Ethical Approval

This study was approved by the Ethics Committee of Sun Yat-sen Memorial Hospital, and the trial was registered with the Chinese Clinical Trial Registry (registration number: ChiCTR-INR-17011825). This investigation was conducted in accordance with the Declaration of Helsinki.

Disclosure

The sponsors did not participate in the design, participant recruitment, data collections, analysis, and preparation of the paper.

Conflicts of Interest

The authors report no conflicts of interest in this work.

Authors' Contributions

Zhen Xu and Shaoling Wu contributed equally to this work and are the co-first authors.

Acknowledgments

We would like to express our gratitude to all participants for their enthusiastic participation in the trial. This work was supported by grants from the National Natural Science Foundation of China (grant numbers 81771201, 81972152, 81671088, and 81901092) and Sun Yat-sen Clinical Research Cultivating Program (grant numbers SYS-C-201704 and SYS-C-202002).

Supplementary Materials

The supplementary material was the CONSORT 2010 checklist of information to include when reporting a randomized trial. (*Supplementary Materials*)

References

[1] L. Manchikanti, V. Singh, F. Falco, R. Benyamin, and J. Hirsch, "Epidemiology of low back pain in adults," *Neuromodulation*, vol. 17, pp. 3–10, 2014.

[2] C. Lin, A. Verwoerd, C. Maher et al., "How is radiating leg pain defined in randomized controlled trials of conservative treatments in primary care? A systematic review," *European Journal of Pain*, vol. 18, no. 4, pp. 455–464, 2014.

[3] M. D. Ryan and T. K. Taylor, "Management of lumbar nerve-root pain: by intrathecal and epidural injections of depot methylprednisolone acetate," *The Medical Journal of Australia*, vol. 2, no. 10, pp. 532–534, 1981.

[4] A. Kaye, L. Manchikanti, S. Abdi et al., "Efficacy of epidural injections in managing chronic spinal pain: a best evidence synthesis," *Pain Physician*, vol. 18, no. 6, pp. E939–1004, 2015.

[5] G. C. Chang-Chien, N. N. Knezevic, Z. McCormick, S. K. Chu, A. M. Trescot, and K. D. Candido, "Transforaminal versus interlaminar approaches to epidural steroid injections: a systematic review of comparative studies for lumbosacral radicular pain," *Pain Physician*, vol. 17, no. 4, pp. E509–E524, 2014.

[6] N. Quraishi, "Transforaminal injection of corticosteroids for lumbar radiculopathy: systematic review and meta-analysis," *European Spine Journal*, vol. 21, no. 2, article 2008, pp. 214–219, 2012.

[7] R. M. Buenaventura, S. Datta, S. Abdi, and H. S. Smith, "Systematic review of therapeutic lumbar transforaminal epidural steroid injections," *Pain Physician*, vol. 12, no. 1, pp. 233–251, 2009.

[8] S. Cohen, M. Bicket, D. Jamison, I. Wilkinson, and J. Rathmell, "Epidural steroids: a comprehensive, evidence-based review," *Regional Anesthesia and Pain Medicine*, vol. 38, no. 3, pp. 175–200, 2013.

[9] A. Bhatia, D. Flamer, P. Shah, and S. Cohen, "Transforaminal epidural steroid injections for treating lumbosacral radicular pain from herniated intervertebral discs: a systematic review and meta-analysis," *Anesthesia and Analgesia*, vol. 122, no. 3, pp. 857–870, 2016.

[10] S. Mohammed and J. Yu, "Platelet-rich plasma injections: an emerging therapy for chronic discogenic low back pain," *Journal of Spine Surgery*, vol. 4, no. 1, pp. 115–122, 2018.

[11] J. Fang, X. Wang, W. Jiang et al., "Platelet-rich plasma therapy in the treatment of diseases associated with orthopedic injuries," *Tissue Engineering. Part B, Reviews*, vol. 26, no. 6, pp. 571–585, 2020.

[12] Q. Wan, S. Wu, X. Li et al., "Ultrasonography-guided lumbar periradicular injections for unilateral radicular pain," *BioMed Research International*, vol. 2017, Article ID 8784149, 4 pages, 2017.

[13] S. Wu, C. Ma, M. Mai, and G. Li, "Translation and validation study of Chinese versions of the neck disability index and the neck pain and disability scale," *Spine*, vol. 35, no. 16, pp. 1575–1579, 2010.

[14] A. A. Fischer, "Pressure algometry over normal muscles. Standard values, validity and reproducibility of pressure threshold," *Pain*, vol. 30, no. 1, pp. 115–126, 1987.

[15] C. Ma, S. Wu, G. Li, X. Xiao, M. Mai, and T. Yan, "Comparison of miniscalpel-needle release, acupuncture needling, and stretching exercise to trigger point in myofascial pain syndrome," *The Clinical Journal of Pain*, vol. 26, no. 3, pp. 251–257, 2010.

[16] L. Li, H. M. Wang, and Y. Shen, "Chinese SF-36 health survey: translation, cultural adaptation, validation, and normalisation," *Journal of Epidemiology and Community Health*, vol. 57, no. 4, pp. 259–263, 2003.

[17] K. Ökmen and B. M. Ökmen, "The efficacy of interlaminar epidural steroid administration in multilevel intervertebral disc disease with chronic low back pain: a randomized, blinded, prospective study," *The Spine Journal*, vol. 17, no. 2, pp. 168–174, 2017.

[18] K. Akeda, K. Ohishi, K. Masuda et al., "Intradiscal injection of autologous platelet-rich plasma releasate to treat discogenic low back pain: a preliminary clinical trial," *Asian spine journal*, vol. 11, no. 3, pp. 380–389, 2017.

[19] S. Bise, B. Dallaudiere, L. Pesquer et al., "Comparison of interlaminar CT-guided epidural platelet-rich plasma versus steroid injection in patients with lumbar radicular pain," *European Radiology*, vol. 30, no. 6, pp. 3152–3160, 2020.

[20] C. Centeno, J. Markle, E. Dodson et al., "The use of lumbar epidural injection of platelet lysate for treatment of radicular pain," *Journal of experimental orthopaedics*, vol. 4, no. 1, p. 38, 2017.

[21] R. Bhatia and G. Chopra, "Efficacy of platelet rich plasma via lumbar epidural route in chronic prolapsed intervertebral disc patients-a pilot study," *Journal of clinical and diagnostic research: JCDR*, vol. 10, pp. UC05–UC07, 2016.

[22] R. Ruiz-Lopez and Y. Tsai, "A randomized double-blind controlled pilot study comparing leucocyte-rich platelet-rich plasma and corticosteroid in caudal epidural injection for complex chronic degenerative spinal pain," *Pain Practice*, vol. 20, no. 6, pp. 639–646, 2020.

[23] O. Deniz, R. Aygül, D. Kotan et al., "The effect of local corticosteroid injection on F-wave conduction velocity and sympathetic skin response in carpal tunnel syndrome," *Rheumatology International*, vol. 32, no. 5, pp. 1285–1290, 2012.

[24] S. Anjayani, Y. Wirohadidjojo, A. Adam, D. Suwandi, A. Seweng, and M. Amiruddin, "Sensory improvement of leprosy peripheral neuropathy in patients treated with perineural

injection of platelet-rich plasma," *International Journal of Dermatology*, vol. 53, no. 1, pp. 109–113, 2014.

[25] M. Takeuchi, N. Kamei, R. Shinomiya et al., "Human platelet-rich plasma promotes axon growth in brain-spinal cord coculture," *Neuroreport*, vol. 23, no. 12, pp. 712–716, 2012.

[26] P. Wu, R. Diaz, and J. Borg-Stein, "Platelet-rich plasma," *Physical Medicine and Rehabilitation Clinics of North America*, vol. 27, no. 4, pp. 825–853, 2016.

[27] J. Sys, J. Weyler, T. Van Der Zijden, P. Parizel, and J. Michielsen, "Platelet-rich plasma in mono-segmental posterior lumbar interbody fusion," *European Spine Journal*, vol. 20, no. 10, pp. 1650–1657, 2011.

[28] S. Arora, V. Doda, U. Kotwal, and M. Dogra, "Quantification of platelets and platelet derived growth factors from platelet-rich-plasma (PRP) prepared at different centrifugal force (g) and time," *Transfusion and Apheresis Science*, vol. 54, no. 1, pp. 103–110, 2016.

[29] J. Qiao, N. An, and X. Ouyang, "Quantification of growth factors in different platelet concentrates," *Platelets*, vol. 28, no. 8, pp. 774–778, 2017.

[30] E. Anitua, I. Andia, B. Ardanza, P. Nurden, and A. T. Nurden, "Autologous platelets as a source of proteins for healing and tissue regeneration," *Thrombosis and Haemostasis*, vol. 91, no. 1, pp. 4–15, 2004.

[31] N. T. Bennett and G. S. Schultz, "Growth factors and wound healing: part II. Role in normal and chronic wound healing," *American Journal of Surgery*, vol. 166, no. 1, pp. 74–81, 1993.

[32] Y. Kajikawa, T. Morihara, H. Sakamoto et al., "Platelet-rich plasma enhances the initial mobilization of circulation-derived cells for tendon healing," *Journal of Cellular Physiology*, vol. 215, no. 3, pp. 837–845, 2008.

[33] E. Galliera, M. M. Corsi, and G. Banfi, "Platelet rich plasma therapy: inflammatory molecules involved in tissue healing," *Journal of biological regulators and homeostatic agents*, vol. 26, 2 Supplement 1, pp. 35s–42s, 2012.

[34] M. Gofeld, S. J. Bristow, S. C. Chiu, C. K. McQueen, and L. Bollag, "Ultrasound-guided lumbar transforaminal injections," *Spine*, vol. 37, no. 9, pp. 808–812, 2012.

[35] G. Yang, J. Liu, L. Ma et al., "Ultrasound-guided versus fluoroscopy-controlled lumbar transforaminal epidural injections: a prospective randomized clinical trial," *The Clinical Journal of Pain*, vol. 32, no. 2, pp. 103–108, 2016.

[36] Q. Wan, H. Yang, X. Li et al., "Ultrasound-guided versus fluoroscopy-guided deep cervical plexus block for the treatment of cervicogenic headache," *BioMed Research International*, vol. 2017, Article ID 4654803, 6 pages, 2017.

[37] L. Thefenne, C. Dubecq, E. Zing et al., "Un cas rare de paraplegie compliquant une infiltration epidurale lombaire par voie interepineuse," *Annals of Physical and Rehabilitation Medicine*, vol. 53, no. 9, pp. 575–583, 2010.

[38] G. Smith, J. Pace, M. Strohl, A. Kaul, S. Hayek, and J. Miller, "Rare neurosurgical complications of epidural injections: an 8-yr single-institution experience," *Operative Neurosurgery*, vol. 13, no. 2, pp. 271–279, 2017.

[39] J. Lee, E. Lee, G. Lee, Y. Kang, J. Ahn, and H. Kang, "Epidural steroid injection-related events requiring hospitalisation or emergency room visits among 52,935 procedures performed at a single centre," *European Radiology*, vol. 28, no. 1, pp. 418–427, 2018.

[40] Y. Zhu, M. Yuan, H. Meng et al., "Basic science and clinical application of platelet-rich plasma for cartilage defects and osteoarthritis: a review," *Osteoarthritis and Cartilage*, vol. 21, no. 11, pp. 1627–1637, 2013.

[41] M. Younes, F. Neffati, M. Touzi et al., "Systemic effects of epidural and intra-articular glucocorticoid injections in diabetic and non-diabetic patients," *Joint Bone Spine*, vol. 74, no. 5, pp. 472–476, 2007.

[42] R. Mitra, "Adverse effects of corticosteroids on bone metabolism: a review," *PM&R*, vol. 3, no. 5, pp. 466–471, 2011, quiz 471.

[43] S. Kim and B. Hwang, "Relationship between bone mineral density and the frequent administration of epidural steroid injections in postmenopausal women with low back pain," *Pain Research & Management*, vol. 19, no. 1, pp. 30–34, 2014.

[44] T. Gosens, J. Peerbooms, W. van Laar, and B. den Oudsten, "Ongoing positive effect of platelet-rich plasma versus corticosteroid injection in lateral epicondylitis: a double-blind randomized controlled trial with 2-year follow-up," *The American Journal of Sports Medicine*, vol. 39, no. 6, pp. 1200–1208, 2011.

[45] W. Hsu, A. Mishra, S. Rodeo et al., "Platelet-rich plasma in orthopaedic applications: evidence-based recommendations for treatment," *The Journal of the American Academy of Orthopaedic Surgeons*, vol. 21, no. 12, pp. 739–748, 2013.

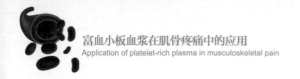

富血小板血浆在肌骨疼痛中的应用
Application of platelet-rich plasma in musculoskeletal pain

·论 著·

超声引导髋关节腔富血小板血浆注射对股骨头坏死的疗效分析

王少玲，栾烁，范胜诺，刘翠翠，栗晓，马超，伍少玲

中山大学孙逸仙纪念医院康复医学科（广州 510120）

【摘要】 目的 探讨分析超声引导下髋关节腔注射富血小板血浆（platelet-rich plasma，PRP）对股骨头缺血性坏死的临床疗效及安全性。方法 回顾分析 2019 年 6 月—2020 年 6 月在中山大学孙逸仙纪念医院康复医学科接受超声引导下髋关节腔 PRP 注射的股骨头坏死患者的临床特征、影像学表现和临床疗效。患者均接受 4 次注射，每次注射间隔 1 周；分别在治疗前和开始治疗后 1、3、6 个月时进行视觉模拟评分（Visual Analogue Scale，VAS）、西安大略和麦克马斯特大学骨关节炎指数（Western Ontario and McMaster Universities Index，WOMAC）、Harris 髋关节功能评分（Harris 评分）等疗效评估和不良事件记录。正态分布资料用均数±标准差表示，行单因素重复测量方差分析；非正态分布资料用中位数（下四分位数，上四分位数）表示，行 Friedman 检验。结果 共纳入患者 29 例，依据国际骨循环研究学会骨坏死分期标准，Ⅰ 期 2 例、Ⅱ 期 11 例、Ⅲ 期 11 例、Ⅳ 期 5 例。治疗前及治疗后 1、3、6 个月的 VAS 评分分别为 7.0（5.5，8.0）、4.0（3.0，5.0）、3.0（2.0，3.0）、3.0（2.0，5.0）分，WOMAC 评分分别为（39.27±11.70）、（28.34±8.08）、（22.82±6.09）、（24.13±7.55）分，Harris 评分分别为 46.0（40.0，64.0）、71.0（57.5，75.0）、78.0（68.0，80.5）、78.0（64.0，80.0）分，各指标治疗前后的差异均有统计学意义（$\chi^2=65.423$，$P<0.001$；$F=46.710$，$P<0.001$；$\chi^2=66.347$，$P<0.001$）。治疗后 1、3、6 个月时与治疗前比较，以及治疗后 3 个月时和治疗后 1 个月时比较，各评分差异均有统计学意义（$P<0.05$）；治疗后 6 个月时与治疗后 3 个月时相比，各评分差异均无统计学意义（$P>0.05$）；治疗后 6 个月时与治疗后 1 个月时相比，WOMAC 评分差异有统计学意义（$P=0.016$），而 VAS 评分和 Harris 评分的差异无统计学意义（$P>0.05$）。随访期间无不良事件报告。结论 超声引导下髋关节腔 PRP 注射能有效缓解股骨头坏死患者的疼痛程度，改善髋关节功能，且效果持续至少 6 个月。但未来需更大样本量的随机对照研究来证实 PRP 对股骨头坏死的长期疗效和安全性。

【关键词】 股骨头坏死；富血小板血浆；超声引导下髋关节腔注射；回顾性研究

Effect of ultrasound-guided intra-articular injection of platelet-rich plasma in the treatment of osteonecrosis of the femoral head: a retrospective study

WANG Shaoling, LUAN Shuo, FAN Shengnuo, LIU Cuicui, LI Xiao, MA Chao, WU Shaoling

Department of Rehabilitation Medicine, Sun Yat-sen Memorial Hospital, Sun Yat-sen University, Guangzhou, Guangdong 510120, P. R. China

Corresponding author: WU Shaoling, Email: wushaolinggz@126.com

【Abstract】 Objective To explore the clinical efficacy and safety of ultrasound-guided intra-articular injection of platelet-rich plasma (PRP) in the treatment of avascular necrosis of the femoral head. Methods We retrospectively collected and analyzed the clinical characteristics, imaging data, and clinical outcomes of patients with femoral head necrosis who received ultrasound-guided intra-articular PRP injection in the Department of Rehabilitation Medicine of Sun Yat-sen Memorial Hospital, Sun Yat-sen University between June 2019 and June 2020. All the patients received 4 injections at one-week intervals. The Visual Analogue Scale (VAS), Western Ontario and McMaster University Osteoarthritis Index (WOMAC), and Harris Hip Joint Function Scale (HHS) were evaluated before treatment and 1 month, 3 months, and 6 months after the first injections. Adverse events were recorded. The normally distributed data were presented as mean±standard deviation, and analyzed by one-way repeated measures analysis of variance; the non-normally distributed data were presented as median (lower quartile, upper quartile), and analyzed by Friedman test.

DOI: 10.7507/1002-0179.202103062
基金项目：中山大学孙逸仙纪念医院临床培育常规项目（SYS-C-202002）
通信作者：伍少玲，Email: wushaolinggz@126.com

West China Medical Journal, May 2021, Vol. 36, No. 5

Results　A total of 29 patients were included. According to the Association Research Circulation Osseous classification standard, 2 patients were classified as stage Ⅰ, 11 as stage Ⅱ, 11 as stage Ⅲ, and 5 as stage Ⅳ. Before treatment and 1 month, 3 months, and 6 months after treatment, the VAS scores were 7.0 (5.5, 8.0), 4.0 (3.0, 5.0), 3.0 (2.0, 3.0), and 3.0 (2.0, 5.0), respectively, the WOMAC scores were 39.27±11.70, 28.34±8.08, 22.82±6.09, and 24.13±7.55, respectively, and the HHS were 46.0 (40.0, 64.0), 71.0 (57.5, 75.0), 78.0 (68.0, 80.5), and 78.0 (64.0, 80.0), respectively. The time effects in VAS (χ^2=65.423, P<0.001), WOMAC (F=46.710, P<0.001), and HHS (χ^2=66.347, P<0.001) were all statistically significant. There were significant differences in each index between the values 1 month, 3 months, and 6 months after treatment and those before treatment respectively, and there was also a significant difference in each index between the value 1 month after treatment and that 3 months after treatment (P<0.05). There was no significant difference in any indicator between the value 6 months after treatment and that 3 months after treatment (P>0.05). Significant difference was shown between the value 6 months after treatment and that 1 month after treatment in WOMAC (P=0.016), but not in VAS or HHS (P>0.05). No obvious adverse event was reported during the follow-up period. **Conclusions**　Ultrasound-guided intra-articular PRP injection can effectively alleviate the pain and improve the hip joint function of patients with femoral head necrosis for at least 6 months. However, randomized controlled studies with a larger sample size and longer-term follow-up are needed in the future to confirm the efficacy and safety of PRP injection in femoral head necrosis.

【Key words】　Osteonecrosis of the femoral head; Platelet-rich plasma; Ultrasound-guided intra-articular injection; Retrospective study

　　股骨头坏死是一种常见的难治性骨关节疾病，流行病学研究显示，我国目前非创伤性股骨头坏死患者已超过 800 万例[1]。股骨头坏死的临床表现为髋关节疼痛、功能障碍，若无及时有效的治疗，70%的患者最终会进展为股骨头塌陷，出现明显疼痛甚至残疾，给患者个人、家庭和社会带来沉重的负担[2]。目前，全髋关节置换术仍是治疗终末期髋关节疾病的常用手段，但该手术创伤大，花费高，且中青年患者一生可能需要接受多次翻修。因此，寻找一种安全有效的治疗方法成为骨关节领域面临的重大挑战[3]。富血小板血浆（platelet-rich plasma，PRP）是自体血经离心后得到的血小板浓缩物，富含多种生长因子，经关节腔内注射后能改善损伤局部微环境，对软骨变性或骨损伤的修复有积极作用[4-5]。因具有制备简单、安全、无免疫反应等优点，PRP 在骨关节炎、骨不连、股骨头坏死等领域中的应用越来越广泛[6-8]。尽管大量基础和临床研究为 PRP 在股骨头坏死中的应用提供了有力证据[9-12]，但以往的临床研究中 PRP 大多作为手术治疗（如髓芯减压术等）的辅助治疗手段，关节腔内直接注射 PRP 的相关临床研究鲜见报道。本研究拟对接受超声引导下关节腔 PRP 注射治疗的股骨头坏死患者的临床疗效及安全性进行回顾性分析，重点探讨 PRP 注射作为保守治疗手段对股骨头坏死疼痛及功能改善的疗效及可能机制。现报告如下。

1　资料与方法

1.1　研究对象

　　选取 2019 年 6 月—2020 年 6 月在中山大学孙逸仙纪念医院康复医学科接受超声引导下髋关节腔 PRP 注射治疗的股骨头坏死患者作为研究对象。纳入标准：① 年龄 25～90 岁；② 股骨头无菌性坏死，病程超过 1 年；③ X 线/CT/MRI 确诊股骨头坏死，并与临床症状、体征相符；④ 疼痛视觉模拟评分（Visual Analogue Scale，VAS）≥4 分；⑤ 根据国际骨循环研究协会（Association Research Circulation Osseous，ARCO）股骨头坏死分期标准[13]，分期为 Ⅰ、Ⅱ、Ⅲ、Ⅳ 期；⑥ 经保守治疗无效，包括非吗啡类药物和物理因子治疗；⑦ 既往无关节手术史。排除标准：① 感染、关节肿瘤或结核；② 贫血、全血血小板计数低于 100×10⁹/L 或凝血功能异常；③ 精神心理异常、认知障碍、其他躯体疾病影响研究结果或不能配合临床随访；④ 注射局部有皮肤感染，不适合局部注射；⑤ 既往 3 个月内曾接受注射治疗；⑥ 孕期及哺乳期。本研究已通过中山大学孙逸仙纪念医院医学伦理委员会审查（审批号：2019-KY-086），临床注册号：ChiCTR1900023601。所有患者均自愿接受治疗并签署知情同意书，随访时间至少 6 个月。所有患者在治疗及随访期间均未接受除 PRP 外的关节腔内注射治疗、物理因子治疗或手术治疗，部分患者因疼痛需服用非甾体类抗炎药物，则将评估推迟至服药 3 d 以后进行。

1.2　研究方法

1.2.1　PRP 制备　本研究制备 PRP 的具体步骤如下：① 制备抗凝管：预先在一次性无菌注射器（上海碧迪医疗器械有限公司，批号：2007118，容量 10 mL）中加入 1 mL 枸橼酸钠抗凝剂。② 采集静脉血：用 18G 针头经肘部浅静脉采血，单侧髋关节注射采血量为 9 mL×2 管，双侧髋关节注射采血量为 9 mL×4 管，采血后缓慢摇晃使抗凝剂和全血充分混匀。③ 离心：采用二次离心法在无菌状态下进行血液离心，第一次离心参数为离心半径 15 cm、转速 1 500 r/min、离心时间 10 min，全血离心后分 3 层，自上而下依次为血浆层、血小板白细胞层、红细胞层，将下层红细胞缓慢排出，剩余部分进行二次离心，离心参数为离心半径 15 cm、转速 2 500 r/min、离心时间 10 min，离心后缓慢排出下层红细胞，留取中间层 2.5 mL 即得 PRP。18 mL 全血（2 管）可得 5 mL PRP。④ 检测：常规对全血样本和 PRP 样本进行细胞成分分析和质量控制，上述方法制备的 PRP 中血小板浓度为全血中血小板浓度的 3~4 倍。所有患者的 PRP 均由同一名医师完成制备。

1.2.2 超声引导下髋关节腔注射 选择彩色超声系统（日本柯尼卡美能达公司，SONIMAGE HS1）和低频凸阵探头（C5-2，3~5 MHz）进行超声引导注射，注射器连接一次性使用无菌注射针头（浙江康德莱医疗器械股份有限公司，0.9×80 TWLB）备用。患者取仰卧位，肢体外展 10~20°，触诊腹股沟区标记股动脉体表位置；常规消毒铺巾，超声探头长轴与股骨颈平行，置于髋关节上方，显示髋臼、股骨头、股骨颈和髋关节腔，确定注射靶点，应用彩色多普勒观察毗邻血管情况，确定进针点和路径；采用"平面外进针"方式，实时调整针尖方向至针尖进入髋关节腔，回抽无积液或血液后注入 PRP 4~5 mL，观察 PRP 的弥散情况（图 1）。拔针后按压进针点 5~10 min，确定无明显出血后再次消毒和覆盖敷料，无痛范围被动活动关节促进 PRP 弥散。告知患者相关注意事项，观察 20 min 无不良反应后方可自行离开。所有股骨头坏死患者治疗方案均为每周注射 1 次，连续治疗 4 周，注射完成后接受居家康复锻炼指导，超声引导注射治疗和康复锻炼均由同一名有多年超声引导下注射经验的康复科医师完成。

1.3 评价指标

记录患者的年龄、性别、体质量指数（body mass index，BMI）、影像学资料等临床资料，根据 ARCO 分期（2019）[13] 标准将患者分为 Ⅰ、Ⅱ、Ⅲ、Ⅳ 共 4 个分期。患者分别于治疗前及首次治疗后 1、3、6 个月进行 VAS、西安大略和麦克马斯特大学骨关节炎指数（Western Ontario and McMaster Universities Index，WOMAC）和 Harris 髋关节功能评分（Harris 评分）的评估[14-15]：① VAS：评估患侧髋关节疼痛程度，分值为 0~10 分；② WOMAC：

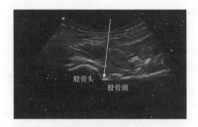

图 1 超声引导髋关节腔注射

白箭示进针方向及注射靶点

共 24 个项目，从疼痛、僵硬和关节功能 3 个方面评估患者髋关节结构和功能状态的改善情况，分值为 0~96 分，分值越低则功能状态越好；③ Harris 评分：包括疼痛、功能、畸形和关节活动度 4 个方面，用于评价各种髋关节疾患，分值为 0~100 分，分值越高则功能状态越好；④ 不良反应：记录患者报告的所有异常情况，如出血或瘀斑、疼痛加剧、关节肿胀、局部皮温升高、局部或全身性感染征象、发热、过敏、腹泻、血象异常等等。

1.4 统计学方法

采用 SPSS 23.0 软件进行统计分析。计量资料若符合正态分布，采用均数±标准差表示；若不符合正态分布，则采用中位数（下四分位数，上四分位数）表示。对于治疗前后不同时间点间的比较，若数据满足正态性、方差齐性，采用单因素重复测量方差分析；若不满足，则采用 Friedman 秩和检验[16]。各个时间点之间的两两比较采用 Bonferroni 法校正 P 值。检验水准 $\alpha=0.05$（双侧）。

2 结果

2.1 临床资料

本研究共纳入患者 29 例（共 41 个患髋），其中男 12 例（41.4%），女 17 例（58.6%）；平均年龄（63.28±17.03）岁；BMI（24.66±3.95）kg/m²。入组基线 ARCO 分期情况为 Ⅰ 期 2 例（6.9%），Ⅱ 期 11 例（37.9%），Ⅲ 期 11 例（37.9%），Ⅳ 期 5 例（17.2%）；注射部位为双侧 12 例（41.4%）、单侧 17 例（58.6%，其中左侧 2 例，右侧 15 例）。

2.2 PRP 注射前后 VAS 评分比较

因治疗前与治疗后各时间点的 VAS 评分数据不满足正态分布，采用 Friedman 检验进行分析；结果显示，不同时间点之间 VAS 评分的差异有统计学意义（$\chi^2=65.423$，$P<0.001$）。两两比较结果显示，治疗后各个时间点的 VAS 评分与治疗前相比，

差异均有统计学意义（P 值均<0.001）；治疗后 3 个月与治疗后 1 个月时的 VAS 评分差异有统计学意义（P=0.036）；而治疗后 6 个月时的 VAS 评分与治疗后 1、3 个月时相比，差异均无统计学意义（P 值均=1.000）。见表 1。

2.3　PRP 注射前后 WOMAC 评分比较

采用单因素重复测量方差分析判断 PRP 注射对股骨头坏死患者 WOMAC 评分的时间效应，经 Mauchly 球形假设检验，因变量的方差协方差矩阵不相等（χ^2=50.700，P<0.001），通过 Greenhouse-Geisser 方法校正 ε=0.490；结果显示，不同时间点之间 WOMAC 评分的差异有统计学意义（校正后 F=46.710，P<0.001）。两两比较结果显示，治疗后各个时间点的 WOMAC 评分与治疗前相比，差异均有统计学意义（P 值均<0.001），其中治疗后 1 个月内 WOMAC 评分平均降低了 10.9 分［95% 置信区间（6.6，15.2）分］；治疗后 1 个月与治疗后 3 个月时的 WOMAC 评分的差异有统计学意义（P<0.001），期间 WOMAC 评分平均降低了 5.5 分［95% 置信区间（2.4，8.5）分］；治疗后 1 个月与治疗后 6 个月时的 WOMAC 评分的差异有统计学意义（P=0.016），期间 WOMAC 评分平均降低了 4.2 分［95% 置信区间（0.5，7.8）分］；而治疗后 6 个月与治疗后 3 个月时的 WOMAC 评分差异无统计学意义（P=0.331）。见表 1。

2.4　PRP 注射前后 Harris 评分比较

因治疗前与治疗后各时间点的 Harris 评分数据不满足正态分布，采用 Friedman 检验进行分析；结果显示，不同时间点之间 Harris 评分的差异有统计学意义（χ^2=66.347，P<0.001）。两两比较结果显示，治疗后各个时间点的 Harris 评分与治疗前相比均有显著改善，差异有统计学意义（P 值均<0.001）；治疗后 3 个月与治疗后 1 个月时的 Harris 评分差异有统计学意义（P=0.007）；但治疗后 6 个月与治疗后 1、3 个月时的 Harris 评分差异均无统计学意义（P 值均=0.622）。见表 1。

2.5　安全性及不良事件发生率

2 例患者报告曾在注射后出现注射部位疼痛加重，但症状持续 2～3 d 后自行消失，6 例患者曾报告短期（1～3 d）服用口服止痛药，所有患者均未报告严重不良反应或并发症。

3　讨论

股骨头坏死是由股骨头静脉淤滞、动脉血供受损或中断使骨细胞及骨髓成分部分死亡引起骨组织坏死，以及随后发生的修复共同导致的股骨头结构改变[17]。研究已初步显示，PRP 主要通过诱导血管生成和成骨促进骨愈合、抑制坏死病变的炎症反应、缓解过量糖皮质激素诱导的细胞凋亡这 3 种机制延缓股骨头坏死进展[18]。本研究初步回顾了超声引导下髋关节腔 PRP 注射对股骨头坏死的临床疗效，结果显示，相比于治疗前，VAS、WOMAC 和 Harris 评分都有不同程度的改善，治疗后 6 个月时，VAS 评分中位数从治疗前的 7 分降低至 3 分（P<0.001），WOMAC 评分从治疗前的（39.27±11.70）分降低至（24.13±7.55）分（P<0.001），Harris 评分中位数由 46 分提高至 78 分（P<0.001），表明 PRP 注射能有效减轻股骨头坏死患者疼痛，改善关节功能。2012 年，Ibrahim 等[19]报道了一例 72 岁的 Ⅲ 期髋关节炎合并股骨头坏死的女性患者接受髋关节腔 PRP 注射治疗，治疗后 1 个月患者 VAS 疼痛评分从 7 分降低至 1 分，髋关节功能及 MRI 股骨头坏死程度均有显著改善。2019 年，一例股骨头坏死晚期的青春期患者在我科接受了 5 次超声引导髋关节腔 PRP 注射，治疗后 9 个月时患者的疼痛程度、关节功能评分及影像学结果均有显著改善[20]。2021 年，Aggarwal 等[21]报道的一项随机对照试验中纳入 40 例股骨头坏死患者（共 53 个髋），随机分为 2 组后行髓芯减压术联合 PRP 注射或行单纯髓芯减压术治疗，平均随访 4.5～6.0 年，末次随访时 PRP 组的 Harris 评分明显改善的患者比例高达 84.0%，显著优于对照组的 67.8%，股骨头坏死进展

表 1　PRP 治疗前后 VAS、WOMAC、Harris 评分的比较（n=29，分）

时间	VAS 评分[$M(Q_L, Q_U)$]	WOMAC 评分（$\bar{x}\pm s$）	Harris 评分[$M(Q_L, Q_U)$]
治疗前	7.0 (5.5, 8.0)	39.27±11.70	46.0 (40.0, 64.0)
治疗后 1 个月	4.0 (3.0, 5.0)*	28.34±8.08*	71.0 (57.5, 75.0)*
治疗后 3 个月	3.0 (2.0, 3.0)*#	22.82±6.09*#	78.0 (68.0, 80.5)*#
治疗后 6 个月	3.0 (2.0, 5.0)*	24.13±7.55*#	78.0 (64.0, 80.0)*
检验统计量	χ^2=65.423	F=46.710	χ^2=66.347
P 值	<0.001	<0.001	<0.001

*与治疗前相比，P<0.05；#与治疗后 1 个月时相比，P<0.05

• 621 •

患者比例为 24%，显著低于对照组的 43%，表明 PRP 可以显著减轻股骨头坏死患者的疼痛程度，改善中期功能预后，延缓股骨头坏死进展。

对 PRP 注射治疗后不同时间点之间的两两比较结果发现，VAS 评分在治疗后 1 个月内改善幅度最大，中位数由治疗前的 7 分降低至 4 分；治疗后 1～3 个月期间，VAS 评分有一定改善，中位数由 4 分降低至 3 分，但改善幅度减小；治疗后 3～6 个月期间 VAS 评分变化不大，提示期间疼痛程度呈稳定状态，无明显恶化。Harris 评分改善趋势与 VAS 评分基本一致，提示 PRP 注射治疗后 VAS 和 Harris 评分改善至少持续 6 个月。WOMAC 评分的两两比较结果提示，治疗后 3 个月内下肢功能有持续性改善，治疗后 1 个月内 WOMAC 评分平均改善了 10.9 分[95% 置信区间 (6.6, 15.2) 分]，治疗后 1～3 个月期间平均改善了 5.5 分[95% 置信区间 (2.4, 8.5) 分]，治疗后 3～6 个月期间下肢功能评分呈维持状态，无明显下降，提示 PRP 注射后下肢功能改善至少持续 6 个月。对于 3 个结局指标出现变化的时间点的不同，我们的考虑与 Han 等[18] 相似，股骨头坏死的症状与骨坏死和滑膜炎症密切相关，而滑膜中的炎症细胞和炎症因子（如白细胞介素-1β、白细胞介素-6、肿瘤坏死因子-α 等）主导了股骨头坏死的疼痛，PRP 注射后在体内发生生理性激活，释放的多种生长因子在关节腔内发挥改善损伤局部微环境和免疫调节作用，总体上抑制了炎症反应，有效减轻了疼痛，因而 VAS 评分和疼痛得分占比较大的 Harris 评分在早期展示了显著的变化，而随着修复和康复锻炼的继续，患者下肢功能、髋关节功能不断改善，并保持了疗效的持续性和稳定性。

近年来，接受全髋关节置换术的股骨头坏死患者比例呈现逐年增长且年轻化的发展趋势[22]，我国人口众多，股骨头坏死发病率高，全髋关节置换术年轻化必将导致翻修率高、手术难度大及并发症概率增加等更多问题。不少学者提出，早期股骨头坏死及年轻患者应优先考虑保髋治疗[3]。髓芯减压术是目前常见的股骨头坏死保髋治疗手段，然而，有研究报道髓芯减压术对于促进坏死区域骨再生无积极作用，其对早期股骨头坏死的治愈率仅为 63.5%[18]，且髓芯减压术同样存在花费大、耗时长、环境要求严、麻醉风险高等问题。超声引导关节腔内注射治疗法具有实时、动态观察、微创、无辐射、准确性高、可在门诊和床旁操作等多种优势，已逐渐成为骨关节炎、骨坏死等疾病的重要治疗手段之一[23]。PRP 因其制备简单、微创、安全、无免疫原性

等优势，近年来在口腔颌面外科、整形外科、骨科等多个领域中广泛应用[24]。值得注意的是，目前 PRP 其对骨坏死的治疗机制尚未完全明确，另外，国内外学者对于 PRP 的标准化制备与保存方法、最佳血小板浓度、细胞成分、是否激活、注射次数及间隔时间等问题尚无统一标准，因而 PRP 用于股骨头坏死规范化治疗方案仍需进一步探讨[25]。

需要特别指出的是，本研究尚存在一定的局限性：首先，本研究为回顾性研究，可能存在一定的选择性偏倚和回忆偏倚；其次，本研究样本量较小，未能对不同 ARCO 分期的患者进行分组，因而无法分析 PRP 对不同分期股骨头坏死的疗效差异；另外，随访时间较短，未能证明关节腔内 PRP 注射对股骨头坏死的长期疗效。

综上所述，本研究结果初步显示了髋关节腔 PRP 注射治疗可有效缓解股骨头坏死疼痛及功能障碍，未来需要更多的高质量随机对照试验进一步证明其长期疗效和安全性。

参考文献

1 Zhao DW, Yu M, Hu K, et al. Prevalence of nontraumatic osteonecrosis of the femoral head and its associated risk factors in the Chinese population: results from a nationally representative survey. Chin Med J (Engl), 2015, 128(21): 2843-2850.

2 Xu HH, Li SM, Fang L, et al. Platelet-rich plasma promotes bone formation, restrains adipogenesis and accelerates vascularization to relieve steroids-induced osteonecrosis of the femoral head. Platelets, 2020: 1-10.

3 赵德伟, 程亮亮. 浅谈全髋关节置换术的年轻化. 中华骨与关节外科杂志, 2019, 12(5): 328-330.

4 Oryan A, Alidadi S, Moshiri A. Platelet-rich plasma for bone healing and regeneration. Expert Opin Biol Ther, 2016, 16(2): 213-232.

5 Akeda K, An HS, Okuma M, et al. Platelet-rich plasma stimulates porcine articular chondrocyte proliferation and matrix biosynthesis. Osteoarthritis Cartilage, 2006, 14(12): 1272-1280.

6 Yancopoulos GD, Davis S, Gale NW, et al. Vascular-specific growth factors and blood vessel formation. Nature, 2000, 407(6801): 242-248.

7 Fiz N, Delgado D, Garate A, et al. Intraosseous infiltrations of platelet-rich plasma for severe hip osteoarthritis: a pilot study. J Clin Orthop Trauma, 2020, 11(Suppl 4): S585-S590.

8 栾烁, 栗晓, 林彩娜, 等. 超声引导下关节腔注射富血小板血浆治疗膝骨性关节炎疗效的回顾性研究. 华西医学, 2020, 35(5): 568-573.

9 Tong S, Yin J, Liu J. Platelet-rich plasma has beneficial effects in mice with osteonecrosis of the femoral head by promoting angiogenesis. Exp Ther Med, 2018, 15(2): 1781-1788.

10 Yokota K, Ishida O, Sunagawa T, et al. Platelet-rich plasma accelerated surgical angio-genesis in vascular-implanted necrotic bone: an experimental study in rabbits. Acta Orthop, 2008, 79(1): 106-110.

• 622 •

West China Medical Journal, May 2021, Vol. 36, No. 5

11 Martin JR, Houdek MT, Sierra RJ. Use of concentrated bone marrow aspirate and platelet rich plasma during minimally invasive decompression of the femoral head in the treatment of osteonecrosis. Croat Med J, 2013, 54(3): 219-224.

12 Pak J, Lee JH, Jeon JH, et al. Complete resolution of avascular necrosis of the human femoral head treated with adipose tissue-derived stem cells and platelet-rich plasma. J Int Med Res, 2014, 42(6): 1353-1362.

13 Yoon BH, Mont MA, Koo KH, et al. The 2019 revised version of Association Research Circulation Osseous staging system of osteonecrosis of the femoral head. J Arthroplasty, 2020, 35(4): 933-940.

14 Dallari D, Stagni C, Rani N, et al. Ultrasound-guided injection of platelet-rich plasma and hyaluronic acid, separately and in combination, for hip osteoarthritis: a randomized controlled study. Am J Sports Med, 2016, 44(3): 664-671.

15 杨富强, 杨晓明, 葛建健. 髓芯减压植骨联合富血小板血浆治疗股骨头缺血性坏死的前瞻随机对照研究. 中华关节外科杂志, 2016, 2: 22-25.

16 D'Ambrosi R, Hantes ME, Mariani I, et al. Successful return to sport in patients with symptomatic borderline dysplasia following hip arthroscopy and T-shaped capsular plication. Knee Surg Sports Traumatol Arthrosc, 2021, 29(5): 1370-1377.

17 中国医师协会骨科医师分会骨循环与骨坏死专业委员会, 中华医学会骨科分会骨显微修复学组, 国际骨循环学会中国区. 中国成人股骨头坏死临床诊疗指南（2020）. 中华骨科杂志, 2020, 40(20): 1365-1376.

18 Han J, Gao F, Li Y, et al. The use of platelet-rich plasma for the treatment of osteonecrosis of the femoral head: a systematic review. Biomed Res Int, 2020, 2020: 2642439.

19 Ibrahim V, Dowling H. Platelet-rich plasma as a nonsurgical treatment option for osteonecrosis. PM R, 2012, 4(12): 1015-1019.

20 Luan S, Liu C, Lin C, et al. Platelet-rich plasma for the treatment of adolescent late-stage femoral head necrosis: a case report. Regen Med, 2020, 15(9): 2067-2073.

21 Aggarwal AK, Poornalingam K, Jain A, et al. Combining platelet-rich plasma instillation with core decompression improves functional outcome and delays progression in early-stage avascular necrosis of femoral head: a 4.5- to 6-year prospective randomized comparative study. J Arthroplasty, 2021, 36(1): 54-61.

22 Kurtz S, Ong K, Lau E, et al. Projections of primary and revision hip and knee arthroplasty in the United States from 2005 to 2030. J Bone Joint Surg Am, 2007, 89(4): 780-785.

23 Byrd JW, Potts EA, Allison RK, et al. Ultrasound-guided hip injections: a comparative study with fluoroscopy-guided injections. Arthroscopy, 2014, 30(1): 42-46.

24 马良彧, 王善正, 郭玉冬, 等. 富血小板血浆治疗骨性关节炎的现状. 中国矫形外科杂志, 2018, 26(15): 1396-1399.

25 Amin I, Gellhorn AC. Platelet-rich plasma use in musculoskeletal disorders: are the factors important in standardization well understood?. Phys Med Rehabil Clin N Am, 2019, 30(2): 439-449.

收稿日期：2021-03-04 修回日期：2021-04-27

本文编辑：孙艳梅

·论 著·

超声引导下关节腔注射富血小板血浆治疗膝骨性关节炎疗效的回顾性研究

栾烁，栗晓，林彩娜，刘翠翠，马超，伍少玲

中山大学孙逸仙纪念医院康复医学科（广州 510120）

【摘要】 目的 探讨分析超声引导下关节腔注射富血小板血浆（platelet-rich plasma，PRP）对不同严重程度膝骨性关节炎的疗效及疗效差异。方法 回顾分析 2018 年 5 月—2019 年 6 月在中山大学孙逸仙纪念医院康复医学科接受超声引导下关节腔 PRP 注射治疗膝骨性关节炎患者的临床特征和 X 线影像学资料，并依据 Kellgren&Lawrence（K&L）分级标准分为 0、Ⅰ、Ⅱ、Ⅲ、Ⅳ级组。各组患者均接受 4 次 PRP 关节腔注射治疗，注射间隔 1 周；并分别于注射治疗前、治疗后 3 个月、治疗后 6 个月完成视觉模拟评分（Visual analogue scale，VAS）、西安大略和麦克马斯特大学（Western Ontario and McMaster Universities Osteoarthritis Index，WOMAC）骨关节炎指数的疗效评估和不良反应评价。结果 共纳入患者 102 例，无 0 级病例纳入；其中，K&L Ⅰ级 20 例、Ⅱ级 37 例、Ⅲ级 31 例、Ⅳ级 14 例；未有不良事件报告。K&L Ⅰ、Ⅱ、Ⅲ级组患者 VAS 评分和 WOMAC 评分均随时间明显改善（$P<0.001$）；各组治疗后 3、6 个月分别与治疗前相比，VAS、WOMAC 评分均改善明显（$P<0.05$）；各组治疗后 3、6 个月 VAS 评分比较，差异均无统计学意义（$P>0.05$）；K&L Ⅰ级组治疗后 3、6 个月 WOMAC 评分比较，差异无统计学意义（$P>0.05$），但 K&L Ⅱ、Ⅲ级组治疗后 3 个月 WOMAC 评分均优于治疗后 6 个月（$P<0.05$）。K&L Ⅳ级组患者随访至 3、6 个月时，VAS 评分和 WOMAC 评分随时间均无明显变化（$P>0.05$）。结论 超声引导下关节腔注射 PRP 操作安全、疗效确切，可有效缓解轻、中度膝骨性关节炎疼痛、改善功能障碍，值得进一步临床推广。

【关键词】 膝骨性关节炎；超声引导注射；富血小板血浆；回顾性研究

A retrospective study of the effect of ultrasound-guided intra-articular injection of platelet-rich plasma in the treatment of knee osteoarthritis

LUAN Shuo, LI Xiao, LIN Caina, LIU Cuicui, MA Chao, WU Shaoling

Department of Rehabilitation Medicine, Sun Yat-Sen Memorial Hospital, Sun Yat-Sen University, Guangzhou 510120, P. R. China
Corresponding author: WU Shaoling, Email: wushaolinggz@126.com

【Abstract】 Objective To explore the clinical efficacy of the ultrasound-guided intra-articular injection of platelet-rich plasma (PRP) in the treatment of patients with different stages of knee osteoarthritis. Methods We retrospectively analyzed the clinical characteristics and X-ray data of patients with knee osteoarthritis who received ultrasound-guided intra-articular injection of PRP in the Department of Rehabilitation Medicine at Sun Yat-Sen Memorial Hospital, Sun Yat-Sen University between May 2018 and June 2019. The patients were grouped according to the Kellgren & Lawrence Classification (K&L 0, Ⅰ, Ⅱ, Ⅲ, and Ⅳ). All the patients received four injections with a one-week interval. The Visual Analogue Scale (VAS) and Western Ontario and McMaster Universities Osteoarthritis Index (WOMAC) were used to evaluate the clinical efficacy before the injection, and 3 and 6 months after the injection. Adverse reactions were recorded. Results A total of 102 patients were included without any grade 0 cases. There were 20 patients in K&L Ⅰ group, 37 in Ⅱ group, 31 in Ⅲ group, and 14 in Ⅳ group. No adverse event was reported. Significant differences of VAS scores and WOMAC index were observed in Ⅰ, Ⅱ and Ⅲ groups at the 3rd and 6th month follow-up (P<0.05). VAS and WOMAC scores of the three groups at the 3rd and 6th month after the treatment were significantly improved compared with those before the treatment (P<0.05). There was no significant difference in VAS score at the

DOI：10.7507/1002-0179.202002248
基金项目：中山大学孙逸仙纪念医院逸仙临床研究培育项目（SYS-C-201704，SYS-C-202002）
通信作者：伍少玲，Email：wushaolinggz@126.com

http://www.wcjm.org

华西医学 2020 年 5 月第 35 卷第 5 期

3rd or 6th month after the treatment three groups ($P>0.05$). For K&L Ⅰ group, there was no statistically significant difference in WOMAC score at the 3rd or 6th month after the treatment ($P>0.05$). However, the WOMAC scores at the 3rd month after the treatment were better than those at the 6th month in K&L Ⅱ and Ⅲ groups ($P<0.05$). There was no significant time-depended changes in VAS score or WOMAC score in K&L Ⅳ group ($P>0.05$). **Conclusion** The ultrasound-guided intra-articular PRP injection is safe and effective for pain relief and function improvement in patients with knee osteoarthritis at the early and middle stage.

【**Key words**】 Knee osteoarthritis; Ultrasound-guided injection; Platelet-rich plasma; Retrospective study

膝骨性关节炎（knee osteoarthritis，KOA）是一种好发于中老年人群的退行性病变。流行病学数据显示，我国症状性 KOA 患病率高达 8.1%[1]，发病情况存在性别差异和地域差异[2]。KOA 患者常见的临床表现包括膝关节疼痛、屈伸活动受限、关节肿胀畸形及肌肉萎缩等，随疾病进展可影响站立及步行功能，给患者自身、家庭和社会造成了沉重的医疗、经济负担[3]。目前，临床常用的 KOA 治疗方法包括健康宣教、物理治疗、药物治疗和手术治疗等[4-5]。随着我国人口老龄化进程加速，阶梯化分级治疗、精准治疗必将成为老年 KOA 患者临床诊疗的必然趋势和要求[6]。关节腔药物注射治疗是 KOA 的经典治疗方法之一，常用注射药物包括糖皮质激素、玻璃酸钠等[7]。近年来，随着国内外基础和临床研究证据不断积累，富血小板血浆（platelet rich plasma，PRP）作为一种新的促进组织修复和镇痛治疗方法，应用越来越广泛。PRP 是指自体全血经离心后得到的血小板浓缩物，治疗浓度通常为生理浓度的 3 倍左右，因 PRP 内富含多种生长因子，且无免疫排斥，有助于促进软骨细胞增殖及组织修复，目前在骨与关节、肌腱疾病、软组织疼痛等领域均有应用[8-10]。既往受医疗技术发展所限，关节腔注射多采用徒手直接注射，常因注射部位不准确直接影响疗效，还有可能加剧病患痛苦、降低治疗依从性等。肌肉骨骼超声作为一种可实时、动态成像方法，具有精准、安全、无辐射、经济等优势，现已成为疼痛注射治疗的常用引导手段[11]。本研究对我科接受超声引导下关节腔 PRP 注射治疗 KOA 患者的系列临床资料进行回顾性分析，比较该方法对不同严重程度 KOA 的疗效及疗效差异。现报告如下。

1　资料与方法

1.1　研究对象

选取 2018 年 5 月–2019 年 6 月在中山大学孙逸仙纪念医院康复医学科接受超声引导下关节腔 PRP 注射治疗 KOA 的患者作为研究对象。纳入标准（同时满足①②）：① 符合美国风湿病学会和欧洲抗风湿联盟制定的标准（满足诊断标准 A，同时满足 B、C、D、E 条中的任意 2 条，可诊断 KOA）：A. 近 1 个月内反复膝关节疼痛；B. X 线片（站立位或负重位）示关节间隙变窄、软骨下骨硬化和（或）囊性变、关节边缘骨赘形成；C. 年龄≥50 岁；D. 晨僵时间≤30 min；E. 活动时有骨摩擦音（感）[12]。② 经保守治疗疗效不佳、注射治疗意愿强烈的患者。排除标准（满足其一）：① 病变关节合并感染（包括局部皮肤感染）、关节肿瘤或结核；② 凝血功能异常；③ 存在严重心肺疾病及严重肝、肾功能不全；④ 合并认知障碍及精神障碍，不能配合治疗及随访；⑤ 膝关节手术治疗史等。本研究已通过中山大学孙逸仙纪念医院医学伦理委员会审查，审批号：2019-KY-097，患者自愿接受治疗并签署知情同意书。

1.2　研究方法

1.2.1　PRP 制备
本研究采用二次离心法制备自体 PRP，具体如下：用预先装有 1 mL 枸橼酸钠抗凝剂的 10 mL 一次性注射器、以 18 G 针头经患者肘前静脉取血 9 mL×4 管（双侧膝关节腔注射取血 9 mL×4 管，单侧取血 9 mL×2 管）；无菌状态下以离心半径 15 cm、转速 1 500 r/min 离心 10 min 后，全血分为 3 层；缓慢排出下层红细胞；将余下部分以离心半径 15 cm、转速 2 000 r/min、离心 10 min；再次离心后，缓慢排出下层红细胞，并留取每管中间层 2.0～2.5 mL 用于注射，即得到 PRP；36 mL 静脉血可获得 8～10 mL PRP。我们对获取的 PRP 制品进行常规质量控制，上述方法制备的 PRP 内血小板浓度为全血血小板浓度的 3～6 倍[13]。

1.2.2　超声引导下膝关节腔注射方案
采用柯尼卡 SONIMAGE HS1 彩色超声系统，高频线阵探头（8～12 MHz）；注射前评估关节腔内滑膜及积液情况，如积液较多，治疗前行积液抽吸。患者仰卧位，患侧膝关节下方垫一薄枕、膝关节屈曲约 15°，常规消毒皮肤，超声引导下采用平面内成像、膝关节外侧入路进针，实时调整针尖方向和深度至髌上囊后，如无积液、回抽无血后，单侧关节腔内注射自体 PRP 4～5 mL，观察其在关节腔内弥散情况。拔针后常规消毒，在可耐受范围内被动活动患者关节 5～8 次，使关节腔内 PRP 充分弥散。观察患者 10 min 无不良反应，并告知注射后注意事项。注射方案采用每周注射 1 次，连续进行 4 周注射治疗。所有患者注射由同一位有资质、经过培训的康复科医师完成。

1.3 评价指标

收集患者年龄、性别、体质量指数（body mass index, BMI）、病程、注射前膝关节 X 线影像学等资料，并根据 KOA 分级诊断标准分为 0、Ⅰ、Ⅱ、Ⅲ、Ⅳ组［基于 X 线片并按照 Kellgren & Lawrence（K&L）分级：0 级无改变（正常）；Ⅰ级，轻微骨赘；Ⅱ级，明显骨赘，但未累及关节间隙；Ⅲ级，关节间隙中度狭窄；Ⅳ级，关节间隙明显变窄，软骨下骨硬化］[14]。

患者分别于注射前，注射后 3、6 个月完成如下评估：① 视觉模拟评分（Visual Analogue Scale, VAS）：评估关节疼痛程度；② 西安大略和麦克马斯特大学（Western Ontario and McMaster Universities Osteoarthritis Index, WOMAC）评估表：采用 WOMAC 骨关节炎指数评分，从疼痛、僵硬和关节功能 3 个方面评估患者症状和功能改善情况，计分范围 0～96 分，分值越高提示关节功能越差；③ 不良反应评价：记录患者报告的所有异常情况，如持续的关节肿胀、疼痛加剧、感染等局部反应，以及过敏、发热、腹泻等其他反应。

1.4 统计学方法

采用 SPSS 20.0 统计软件进行分析。计量资料采用均数±标准差表示，非正态分布的计量资料用中位数（下四分位数，上四分位数）表示。计数资料采用例数、比值或率表示，率的比较采用 χ^2 检验，设定检验水准 $\alpha=0.05$。

采用单因素方差分析比较各组患者年龄、BMI、病程组间差异，各组间两两比较采用 Bonferroni 法（多重比较次数为 6，调整检验水准 $\alpha=0.05/6=0.008$）。各组内 VAS、WOMAC 评分不同时间点比较，如数据满足正态分布、方差齐性，采用重复测量单因素方差分析，各组治疗前及治疗后两两比较采用 Bonferroni 法（调整检验水准 $\alpha=0.05/3=0.017$）；如数据严重不满足正态分布或方差齐性，采用 Friedman 秩和检验，各组内两两比较采用 Bonferroni 法（多重比较次数为 3，调整检验水准 $\alpha=0.05/3=0.017$）。

2 结果

2.1 临床资料

共纳入患者 102 例，其中，男 27 例（26.47%），女 75 例（73.53%）；年龄 36～85 岁，平均（67.28±9.05）岁；BMI（24.70±2.42）kg/m²；病程为 1～15 年，平均（5.91±2.70）年；注射部位为双侧 74 例（72.55%）、右侧 18 例（17.65%）、左侧 10 例（9.80%）。在 K&L 分级中，Ⅰ级 20 例（19.61%），年龄 36～78 岁；Ⅱ级 37 例（36.27%），年龄 54～83 岁；Ⅲ级 31 例（30.39%），年龄 52～85 岁；Ⅳ级 14 例（13.73%），年龄 51～83 岁；无 0 级病例纳入。

4 组间性别、BMI、注射部位的组间比较，差异均无统计学意义（$P>0.05$）；年龄、病程组间比较，差异均有统计学意义（$P=0.018$、0.003）。K&L Ⅰ级组患者年龄小于Ⅱ级（$P=0.006$）、Ⅲ级组（$P=0.003$）；其余各组两两比较，差异均无统计学意义（$P>0.008$）。K&L Ⅳ级组患者病程明显长于 K&L Ⅰ级组（$P=0.006$）和Ⅱ级组（$P=0.0078$）；其余各组两两比较，差异均无统计学意义（$P>0.008$）。患者临床资料，见表 1。

2.2 PRP 注射治疗前后 VAS 评分比较

K&L Ⅰ、Ⅱ、Ⅲ级组患者各时间点 VAS 评分随时间变化（$P<0.001$）；3 组内不同时间点进一步进行两两比较，治疗后 3、6 个月分别与治疗前相比，评分改善均有统计学意义（$P<0.001$）；但各组治疗后 3、6 个月时间点两两比较，差异均无统计学意义（$P=0.021$、0.032、0.018），提示随访期间患者疼痛持续缓解。随访期间各时间点 K&L Ⅳ级组患者 VAS 评分变化比较，差异无统计学（$P>0.05$）。见表 2。

2.3 PRP 注射治疗前后 WOMAC 评分比较

K&L Ⅰ级组 WOMAC 评分随时间变化，提示

表 1 患者临床资料

项目	Ⅰ级 (n=20)	Ⅱ级 (n=37)	Ⅲ级 (n=31)	Ⅳ级 (n=14)	检验统计量	P 值
年龄 ($\bar{x}\pm s$, 岁)	61.65±10.59	68.46±7.28*	69.19±8.72*	68.00±9.41	F=3.524	0.018
性别（男/女，例）	5/15	9/28	10/21	3/11	χ^2=0.819	0.876
BMI ($\bar{x}\pm s$, kg/m²)	23.72±2.31	25.14±2.15	24.68±2.65	25.00±2.62	F=1.598	0.195
注射部位（双侧/右侧/左侧，例）	12/4/4	27/7/3	26/5/0	9/2/3	χ^2=9.018	0.141
病程 ($\bar{x}\pm s$, 年)	4.85±2.30	5.19±1.94	6.81±3.19	7.36±2.76*#	F=4.925	0.003

*与Ⅰ级组比较，$P<0.008$，#与Ⅱ级组比较，$P<0.008$

K&L Ⅰ 级组随访期间患者功能障碍持续改善（$P<0.001$）；组内不同时间点两两比较提示，治疗后 3、6 个月与治疗前分别比较，差异均有统计学意义（$P=0.000、0.002$），治疗后 3 个月和 6 个月比较，差异无统计学意义（$P=0.027$）。K&L Ⅱ、Ⅲ 级组患者 WOMAC 评分随时间变化（$P<0.001$），提示 K&L Ⅱ、Ⅲ 级组膝关节功能改善；组内不同时间点进一步两两比较，治疗后 3、6 个月与治疗前相比，差异均有统计学意义（$P<0.001$）；治疗后 3、6 个月比较，差异亦均有统计学意义（$P<0.001、P=0.015$）。K&L Ⅳ 级组患者，各时间点 WOMAC 评分比较，差异无统计学意义（$P>0.05$）。见表 3。

2.4　安全性及不良事件发生率

所有患者在注射及随访期间，未有不良事件报告。

3　讨论

KOA 是中老年人常见的、慢性退行性疾病，主要病理改变包括膝关节软骨退变、剥脱，骨赘形成及软骨下骨硬化、囊性变，滑膜增厚等[2]。既往研究显示，KOA 的功能预后及疾病进展受较多因素影响，较为明确的危险因素包括高龄、性别（女性）及体重超重（BMI 过高）等。KOA 可导致关节疼痛，活动障碍，影响患者站立、步行和自我照料的能力。有证据显示，严重的 KOA 与心血管事件风险呈正相关，且增加患者全因死亡率[15]。我国患病率随人口老龄化逐年递增，无疑对 KOA 的诊断、治疗和综合健康管理提出了更高要求。

近年来，PRP 因取材制备简便、安全有效、无免疫排斥等优势，在 KOA 临床治疗方面备受国内外学者青睐[16]。PRP 制品在生理状态下激活后，可大量释放血管内皮生长因子、转化生长因子、血小板衍生生长因子、胰岛素生长因子等 10 余种生长因子，通过下调金属蛋白酶、白细胞介素 1β 等促分解代谢基因表达，上调关键细胞外基质如 COL2A1、ACAN、SOX9 等合成代谢，同时有助于调节炎症反应、维持组织内环境稳态，从而有效修复软骨、滑膜、血管等退变结构[17-18]；同时，PRP 注射有助于清除关节腔内炎症因子和坏死组织，有利于抑制炎症反应，为退变组织修复提供了良好的局部微环境。国外研究发现，与传统关节腔内注射药物（如透明质酸、糖皮质激素）相比，PRP 在缓解 KOA 患者疼痛、改善功能障碍方面疗效均等或更显著，其安全性和有效性在大量的基础及临床研究中已得到证实[7]。有学者发表的 meta 分析共纳入 10 项临床随机对照研究，最长随访时间为注射后 12 个月，证实 PRP 关节腔内注射与安慰剂或与透明质酸注射相比，可显著减轻疼痛和促进功能恢复，且随访期间疗效稳定、无不良事件报告[9]。另一项 PRP 与其他注射药物（包括透明质酸、糖皮质激素、安慰剂）及口服非甾体抗炎药物疗效比较的 meta 分析同样指出，PRP 注射可有效改善患者疼痛症状，且缓解期长达 12 个月，因此推荐 PRP 注射作为常规方法以提升临床疗效[19]。有研究报道了 PRP 与透明质酸关节腔内注射的疗效对比研究，结果提示随访至 6 个月，两组患者 WOMAC 评分、国际膝关节委员会评分及 Lequesne 指数均较治疗前基线明显改善（$P<0.05$），且 PRP 组疗效在随访期间持续改善，而透明质酸注射组治疗 6 个月较 3、4 个月时间点评价疗效变差（$P<0.05$），验证了 PRP 关节腔注射疗效

表 2　PRP 注射治疗前后 VAS 评分比较（分）

项目	Ⅰ级（$n=20, \bar{x}\pm s$）	Ⅱ级（$n=37, \bar{x}\pm s$）	Ⅲ级（$n=31, \bar{x}\pm s$）	Ⅳ级[$n=14, M(Q_L, Q_U)$]
治疗前	4.90±1.80	5.62±1.62	6.42±1.59	6.00 (5.00, 7.00)
治疗后 3 个月	2.50±1.67*	3.81±1.52*	4.87±1.75*	5.50 (4.00, 7.00)
治疗后 6 个月	2.75±1.52*	3.97±1.52*	5.13±2.03*	6.00 (4.75, 7.00)
检验统计量	F=27.737	F=39.497	F=22.326	χ^2=2.000
P 值	0.000	0.000	0.000	0.368

*与组内治疗前比较，$P<0.017$

表 3　PRP 注射治疗前后 WOMAC 评分比较（分）

项目	Ⅰ级[$n=20, M(Q_L, Q_U)$]	Ⅱ级[$n=37, M(Q_L, Q_U)$]	Ⅲ级[$n=31, M(Q_L, Q_U)$]	Ⅳ级[$n=14, \bar{x}\pm s$]
治疗前	31.00 (21.25, 35.75)	38.92±11.31	40.10±10.39	47.36±11.46
治疗后 3 个月	14.50 (13.00, 18.00)*	26.65±9.63*	31.65±10.74*	47.21±11.07
治疗后 6 个月	16.50 (15.00, 26.00)*	28.41±9.23*#	32.19±10.40*#	48.36±11.04
检验统计量	χ^2=29.949	F=40.740	F=20.499	F=0.723
P 值	0.000	0.000	0.000	0.443

*与组内治疗前比较，$P<0.017$；#与组内治疗后 3 个月比较，$P<0.017$

的稳定性和持续性[20]。目前，已有多部国内、外临床治疗指南修订了"关节腔药物注射"部分，提出完善对 PRP 关节腔注射疗效评价和深入探究的临床价值[14]。

尽管大量研究证据支持 PRP 关节腔注射治疗 KOA 的临床有效性，然而学术界仍未就 PRP 标准化治疗达成一致，其原因较为复杂：除外既往研究设计存在差异、样本量不足、PRP 制备及注射方法不同等限制因素，未能根据 KOA 患者分级评估疾病进展程度给予梯度治疗和分层疗效观察，也是制约研究结论推广的重要因素。K&L 分级是目前临床 KOA 诊断的最基本和首选方法，具有分级明确、普及程度高等优势。我国专家组于 2019 年发表的《膝骨关节炎阶梯治疗专家共识（2018 年版）》[4] 在《骨关节炎诊疗指南（2018 年版）》[4]基础上，进一步提出了基于临床症状和 K&L 分级划分 KOA 患者初期、早期、中期、晚期，并实施阶梯化分级管理的治疗策略。本研究回顾性分析了超声引导下 PRP 关节腔注射治疗对不同 K&L 分期患者治疗效果及疗效差异，结果发现：随访至治疗后 6 个月，K&L 分级Ⅰ、Ⅱ、Ⅲ 3 组患者注射后 VAS、WOMAC 表现评分均较治疗前明显改善，而 K&LⅣ组患者 PRP 注射治疗改善无统计学意义，提示 PRP 关节腔注射治疗可有效缓解轻、中度 KOA 疼痛和功能障碍，但对于 K&L Ⅳ 患者疗效不明显，上述结果与既往文献结论基本一致。我们认为 VAS 作为主要观察的疗效指标，具有应用广泛、信效度高等优势，可有效评价 PRP 对 KOA 患者疼痛的缓解作用；而治疗后 3 个月 K&LⅡ、Ⅲ组患者 WOMAC 评分优于治疗后 6 个月，可能与入组患者病情特点、WOMAC 评分影响因素较多、回顾样本量偏少及随访时间较短等相关。此外，大部分前瞻性研究基于临床经验，选择性纳入 K&LⅡ、Ⅲ级患者[2,3]，这在一定程度上造成了选择偏倚的风险。鉴于目前样本量较少、不具代表性，PRP 促进 K&LⅣ级疼痛缓解和功能改善的具体机制仍需进一步探讨。

需要指出的是，本研究属于临床回顾性研究，部分组别样本量偏小，可能存在偏倚，且未实现不同 K&L 分级情况患者给予不同次数 PRP 注射的疗效相关性等研究。今后拟进行随访时间更长的前瞻性随机对照研究，并探究 PRP 注射剂量与临床疗效的剂量-反应关系，积累更多循证学依据。

综上所述，本研究结果提示，基于膝关节骨性关节炎 K&L 分级标准，采用超声引导实施精准、可视化关节腔 PRP 注射治疗，可有效改善轻、中度膝骨关节炎患者疼痛、功能障碍及生存质量，是一种精准、安全、有效的治疗手段，值得临床进一步推广。

参考文献

1 Tang X, Wang S, Zhan S, et al. The prevalence of symptomatic knee osteoarthritis in China: results from the China health and retirement longitudinal study. Arthritis Rheumatol, 2016, 68(3): 648-653.

2 中华医学会骨科学分会关节外科学组. 骨关节炎诊疗指南 (2018 年版). 中华骨科杂志, 2018, 38(12): 705-715.

3 中国医师协会急救复苏专业委员会创伤骨科与多发伤学组, 中国医药教育学会骨质疾病专业委员会修复重建学组, 中国老年学和老年医学学会老年病分会骨科专家委员会, 等. 中国老年膝关节骨关节炎诊疗及智能矫形康复专家共识. 临床外科杂志, 2019, 27(12): 1105-1110.

4 周谋望. 骨科康复临床的新进展. 华西医学, 2018, 33(10): 1197-1200.

5 梁翼, 李敏. 骨关节炎非手术治疗进展. 华西医学, 2016, 31(5): 801-802.

6 中华医学会骨科分会关节外科学组, 吴阶平医学基金会骨科学专家委员会. 膝骨关节炎阶梯治疗专家共识 (2018 年版). 中华关节外科杂志(电子版), 2019, 13(1): 124-130.

7 Lin KY, Yang CC, Hsu CJ, et al. Intra-articular injection of platelet-rich plasma is superior to hyaluronic acid or saline solution in the treatment of mild to moderate knee osteoarthritis: a randomized, double-blind, triple-parallel, placebo-controlled clinical trial. Arthroscopy, 2019, 35(1): 106-117.

8 中国医疗保健国际交流促进会骨科分会. 关节腔注射富血小板血浆治疗膝骨关节炎的临床实践指南 (2018 年版). 中华关节外科杂志(电子版), 2018, 12(4): 1-5.

9 Laudy AB, Bakker EW, Rekers M, et al. Efficacy of platelet-rich plasma injections in osteoarthritis of the knee: a systematic review and meta-analysis. Br J Sports Med, 2015, 49(10): 657-672.

10 Alsousou J, Thompson M, Harrison P, et al. Effect of platelet-rich plasma on healing tissues in acute ruptured achilles tendon: a human immunohistochemistry study. Lancet, 2015, 385(Suppl 1): S19.

11 Huang Z, Du S, Qi Y, et al. Effectiveness of ultrasound guidance on intraarticular and periarticular joint injections: systematic review and meta-analysis of randomized trials. Am J Phys Med Rehabil, 2015, 94(10): 775-783.

12 Altman R, Asch E, Bloch D, et al. Development of criteria for the classification and reporting of osteoarthritis. Classification of osteoarthritis of the knee. Diagnostic and therapeutic criteria committee of the American Rheumatism Association. Arthritis Rheum, 1986, 29(8): 1039-1049.

13 Angoorani H, Mazaherinezhad A, Marjomaki O, et al. Treatment of knee osteoarthritis with platelet-rich plasma in comparison with transcutaneous electrical nerve stimulation plus exercise: a randomized clinical trial. Med J Islam Repub Iran, 2015, 29: 223.

14 KELLGREN JH, LAWRENCE JS. Radiological assessment of osteoarthrosis. Ann Rheum Dis, 1957, 16(4): 494-502.

15 Xing D, Xu Y, Liu Q, et al. Osteoarthritis and all-cause mortality in worldwide populations: grading the evidence from a meta-analysis. Sci Rep, 2016, 6: 24393.

16 Le ADK, Enweze L, DeBaun MR, et al. Current clinical

recommendations for use of platelet-rich plasma. Curr Rev Musculoskelet Med, 2018, 11(4): 624-634.

17　Moussa M, Lajeunesse D, Hilal G, *et al*. Platelet rich plasma (PRP) induces chondroprotection via increasing autophagy, anti-inflammatory markers, and decreasing apoptosis in human osteoarthritic cartilage. Exp Cell Res, 2017, 352(1): 146-156.

18　Textor J. Platelet-rich plasma (PRP) as a therapeutic agent: platelet biology, growth factors and a review of the literature. Platelet-Rich Plasma, 2014: 61-94.

19　Campbell KA, Saltzman BM, Mascarenhas R, *et al*. Does intra-articular platelet-rich plasma injection provide clinically superior outcomes compared with other therapies in the treatment of knee osteoarthritis? A systematic review of overlapping meta-analyses. Arthroscopy, 2015, 31(11): 2213-2221.

20　李明, 张长青, 艾自胜, 等. 关节内注射富血小板血浆对膝关节软骨退行性变的治疗作用. 中国修复重建外科杂志, 2011, 25(10): 1192-1196.

21　Pourcho AM, Smith J, Wisniewski SJ, *et al*. Intraarticular platelet-rich plasma injection in the treatment of knee osteoarthritis: review and recommendations. Am J Phys Med Rehabil, 2014, 93(11 Suppl 3): S108-S121.

22　袁林, 郭燕庆, 于洪波, 等. 富血小板血浆治疗Ⅱ-Ⅲ期膝骨关节炎的疗效评价. 中华关节外科杂志(电子版), 2016, 10(4): 386-392.

收稿日期：2020-02-21　修回日期：2020-05-11
本文编辑：凌雪梅